# VIOLENCE AGAINST
# WOMEN

For a catalogue of publications available from ACP-ASIM, contact:

Customer Service Center
American College of Physicians–American Society of Internal Medicine
190 N. Independence Mall West
Philadelphia, PA 19106-1572
215-351-2600
800-523-1546, ext. 2600

Visit our Web site at www.acponline.org

# VIOLENCE AGAINST WOMEN

## A PHYSICIAN'S GUIDE TO IDENTIFICATION AND MANAGEMENT

EDITORS

JANE M. LIEBSCHUTZ, MD, MPH, FACP

SUSAN M. FRAYNE, MD, MPH

GLENN N. SAXE, MD, FRCP(C)

WOMEN'S HEALTH SERIES EDITOR

PAMELA CHARNEY, MD, FACP

AMERICAN COLLEGE OF PHYSICIANS
PHILADELPHIA

*Clinical Consultant:* David R. Goldmann, MD
*Acquisitions Editor:* Mary K. Ruff
*Manager, Book Publishing:* Diane McCabe
*Developmental Editor:* Vicki Hoenigke
*Production Supervisor:* Allan S. Kleinberg
*Production Editor:* Karen C. Nolan
*Editorial Coordinator:* Alicia Dillihay
*Interior and Cover Design:* Patrick Whelan
*Index:* Nelle Garrecht

HV
6626
V56

Manufactured in the United States of America
Composition by UB Communications
Printing/binding by Versa Press

American College of Physicians (ACP) became an imprint of the American College of Physicians—American Society of Internal Medicine in July 1998.

ISBN 1-930-513-11-9

03 04 05 06 07/9 8 7 6 5 4 3 2 1

# Editors

Jane M. Liebschutz, MD, MPH, FACP
Assistant Professor of Medicine
Section of General Internal Medicine
Boston Medical Center
Boston University School of Medicine
Boston, Massachusetts

Susan M. Frayne, MD, MPH
Associate Professor of Medicine
Boston University Schools of Medicine and Public Health
Boston, Massachusetts;
Center for Health Care Evaluation
VA Palo Alto Health Care System
Palo Alto, California

Glenn N. Saxe, MD, FRCP(C)
Associate Professor of Psychiatry
Department of Child Psychiatry
Boston Medical Center
Boston, Massachusetts

# Women's Health Series Editor

Pamela Charney, MD, FACP
Clinical Professor of Medicine
Clinical Associate Professor of Obstetrics & Gynecology and Women's Health
Albert Einstein College of Medicine
Bronx, New York;
Program Director
Internal Medicine Residency
Norwalk Hospital
Norwalk, Connecticut

# Contributors

Arlene D. Bradley, MD
Clinical Director, Women's Health
Roseburg VA Healthcare System
Roseburg Veterans Administration
  Medical Center
Roseburg, Oregon

Marian I. Butterfield, MD, MPH
Assistant Professor
Department of Psychiatry
Duke University Medical Center
Veterans Health Administration
Health Services Research and
  Development
Durham, North Carolina

Jeanne Cawse, AB
Medical Student
University of Massachusetts Medical
  School
Worcester, Massachusetts

Kimberly J. Clermont, MD
Attending Physician and Clinical
  Instructor
Department of Emergency Medicine
North General Hospital
New York, New York;
Clinical Instructor
Department of Internal Medicine
SUNY Downstate Medical Center
Brooklyn, New York

Elizabeth Edwardson, MD
Associate Professor of Emergency
  Medicine
University of Rochester Medical
  Center
Rochester, New York

Mitchell D. Feldman, MD, MPhil
Associate Professor of Medicine
Division of General Internal Medicine
Department of Medicine
University of California, San Francisco
San Francisco, California

Richard Frankel, PhD
Professor of Medicine
Indiana University School of Medicine
Research Scientist
Regenstrief Institute
Indianapolis, Indiana

Susan M. Frayne, MD, MPH
Associate Professor of Medicine
Boston University Schools of Medicine
  and Public Health
Boston, Massachusetts;
Center for Health Care Evaluation
VA Palo Alto Health Care System
Palo Alto, California

Jacqueline M. Golding, PhD
Adjunct Professor
Institute for Health and Aging
University of California, San Francisco
San Francisco, California

Rebecca A. Griffith, MD
University of Medicine and Dentistry of
  New Jersey
Department of Internal Medicine
Morristown Memorial Hospital
Morristown, New Jersey

Sherry L. Hamby, PhD
Research Professor
University of North Carolina, Chapel Hill;
Director, Possible Equalities
Laurinburg, North Carolina

Calvin H. Hirsch, MD
Associate Professor of Medicine,
  Epidemiology, and Preventive
  Medicine
Division of General Medicine
UC Davis Medical Center
Sacramento, California

Julieta Holman, BA
Medical Student
Boston University School of Medicine
Boston, Massachusetts

Melisa M. Holmes, MD
Associate Professor of Obstetrics/
  Gynecology and Pediatrics
Department of Obstetrics/Gynecology
Medical University of South Carolina
Charleston, South Carolina

Carol A. Howland, MPH
Center for Research on Women with
  Disabilities
Department of Physical Medicine and
  Rehabilitation
Baylor College of Medicine
Houston, Texas

Rashna Irani, MD
Resident in Pediatrics
Massachusetts General Hospital
Boston, Massachusetts

Jeffrey R. Jaeger, MD
Assistant Professor of Medicine
University of Pennsylvania Health
  System
Philadelphia, Pennsylvania

Mary P. Koss, PhD
Professor of Public Health, Psychiatry,
  and Psychology
Mel and Enid Zuckerman Arizona
  College of Public Health
University of Arizona
Tucson, Arizona

Jane M. Liebschutz, MD, MPH, FACP
Assistant Professor of Medicine
Section of General Internal Medicine
Boston Medical Center
Boston University School of Medicine
Boston, Massachusetts

Lydia E. Mayer, MD, MPH, FACOG
Fellow, Center for Clinical Bioethics
Assistant Professor of Obstetrics and
  Gynecology
Center for Clinical Bioethics
Georgetown University Medical Center
Washington, DC

Alejandro Moreno, MD, MPH
Adjunct Assistant Professor of Health Law
Health Law Department
Boston University School of Public
  Health
Boston Center for Refugee Health and
  Human Rights
Boston, Massachusetts

Gina A. Moreno-John, MD, MPH
Assistant Clinical Professor
Division of General Internal Medicine
Department of Medicine
University of California, San Francisco
San Francisco, California

Diane S. Morse, MD, MPH
Assistant Professor of Medicine
University of Rochester School of
  Medicine and Dentistry
Rochester General Hospital
Rochester, New York

Maureen Murdoch, MD, MPH
Assistant Professor of Medicine
Center for Chronic Disease Outcomes
  Research
Section of General Internal Medicine
Minneapolis VA Medical Center
Minneapolis, Minnesota

Margaret A. Nosek, PhD
Professor
Department of Physical Medicine and
 Rehabilitation
Center for Research on Women with
 Disabilities
Baylor College of Medicine
Houston, Texas

Anuradha Paranjape, MD, MPH
Assistant Professor of Medicine
Emory School of Medicine
Division of General Internal Medicine
Grady Memorial Hospital
Atlanta, Georgia

Beatrice H. Patsalides, PhD
Psychologist
The Lacanian School of Psychoanalysis
 and the Psychoanalytic Institute of
 Northern California;
Senior Clinical Consultant
Survivors International
San Francisco, California

Nadja G. Peter, MD
Clinical Instructor of Pediatrics
University of Pennsylvania Health System
Children's Hospital of Philadelphia
Philadelphia, Pennsylvania

Mona Polacca, MSW, LICSW
Doctoral Student
Department of Criminology
Arizona State University
 College of Public Health
Tucson, Arizona

Patricia Robinson, MSW, LICSW
Women's Veterans Program Manager
VA Boston Healthcare System
Boston, Massachusetts

Glenn N. Saxe, MD, FRCP(C)
Associate Professor of Psychiatry
Department of Child Psychiatry
Boston Medical Center
Boston, Massachusetts

Eric Sleeper, BA
Medical Student
Boston University School of Medicine
Boston, Massachusetts

Sara L. Swenson, MD
Assistant Clinical Professor
Division of General Internal Medicine
University of California, San Francisco
San Francisco, California

Nancy D. Vogeltanz, PhD
Associate Professor of Neuroscience
Department of Neuroscience
Director of Primary Prevention
Center for Health Promotion and
 Translation Research
University of North Dakota
Grand Forks, North Dakota

Sharon C. Wilsnack, PhD
Chester Fritz Distinguished Professor
Department of Neuroscience
University of North Dakota School of
 Medicine and Health Sciences
Grand Forks, North Dakota

# Acknowledgements

We are greatly indebted to Pamela Charney for her patience and guidance in helping us bring this book from an idea to a reality. An enthusiastic supporter for the entire duration of the project, she gave us a much-needed boost when the tasks at hand seemed most daunting. The book is much improved because of her input.

We must give special thanks to Arlene Bradley, who recruited authors, helped edit Chapters 8 to 12, and wrote Vignettes 2 and 5 (with Maureen Murdoch). Her teaching style and clinical experience influenced the way we think about incorporating violence screening and prevention into routine medical care. We thank her for the mark she has made in this field.

We also want to express sincere gratitude to the staff at ACP-ASIM publishing: Mary Ruff, for advice and knowledge regarding publishing for practicing clinicians; Vicki Hoenigke, for outstanding editorial suggestions; Karen Nolan, for copyediting and supervision of book production; and Alicia Dillihay, for editorial assistance.

We are thankful to all the authors, who contributed from their hearts and taught us so much.

Lastly, this book could not have been written were it not for the many women who survived violence and shared their stories with us. To them, we are grateful.

# Preface

At the turn of the 21st century, patients and the public alike expect that medical doctors will recognize and treat victims of interpersonal trauma. Despite the desire to do so, few clinicians are familiar with how to approach patients about this issue, and even fewer are aware of empiric evidence about what interventions actually work. Part of the dilemma is that clinicians can feel uncomfortable exploring beyond familiar clinical domains into territory with heavy social undercurrents. Furthermore, by definition, someone other than the patient is perpetrating the violence, which shifts the locus of control of the problem away from the patient's behavior or illness. *Violence Against Women: A Physician's Guide to Identification and Management* presents empiric data on treating patients experiencing violence and provides practical clinical approaches.

Two of us (JL and SF) are practicing internists who know exactly the kinds of pressures and demands that are generated by caring for women who have experienced violence. Because of our interest in the field, we were familiar with several texts on violence against women, but we felt there was no single comprehensive and easy-to-use volume specifically oriented towards clinicians practicing in the medical setting.

After the inaugural meeting of the Physicians Against Violence Interest Group at the Society of General Internal Medicine meeting in 1998, Pam Charney approached us to consider writing such a reference for the ACP Women's Health series. We recognized that to meet our objectives we needed strong mental health input because of the complex behavioral and patient-provider interaction issues that arise in caring for patients who have experienced violence. The psychiatrist we recruited as co-editor (GS) was highly qualified for this role because of his expertise in trauma psychiatry and because of his previous experience working alongside internists in an interdisciplinary outpatient treatment team. To widen our perspective, the three of us recruited chapter authors to reflect diversity in discipline, ethnicity, geography, gender, and sexual orientation.

The book is divided into three sections and an Appendix. We have been generous with tables and boxed material because we know that clinicians need to access information quickly and easily. The book can be read from beginning to end but also lends itself to the use of pertinent chapters or sections when clinical questions arise.

The first section, Clinical Issues, comprises Chapters 1 to 6 and provides an overview of the general principles relevant to treating women who have experienced violence. The authors of Chapters 1 to 3 draw on recent studies on epidemiology, screening, and acute violence, paying close attention to data that will be most useful to a clinician. Chapters 4 and 5 break new ground in summarizing principles of referral and managing behaviors that stem from post-traumatic stress disorder. Chapter 6 describes some of the effects that caring for survivors of violence can have upon clinicians themselves. It also gives some important tools and suggestions for clinician self-care.

Chapters 7 to 12 make up the second section, Special Considerations. They focus on particular groups who have an increased vulnerability to experiencing violence and/or decreased ability to seek help. Because clinicians often learn well with case presentations, the last part of the book presents seven Clinical Vignettes. In addition to illustrating the information presented earlier in the book, the Vignettes introduce relevant information not often described in the context of caring for survivors of violence (all Vignettes are fictitious). An Appendix provides useful contact information and resources throughout the United States and Canada.

We have chosen to focus solely on adult patients because the principles, philosophy, and legal issues are very different when caring for children. On the other hand, children grow up to be adults, and therefore the adult sequelae of child abuse is touched upon where appropriate. The book emphasizes domestic violence and sexual trauma, but we touch upon other forms of interpersonal violence as well. As befits the Women's Health series, the focus throughout is on women who have experienced violence, but it is important for clinicians to remember that many men have been the victims of domestic violence and sexual abuse.

Our goal has been to address the important clinical issues that arise in primary care and other medical settings when caring for women who have experienced violence. We aspire to support clinicians in their efforts to provide high-quality medical care to the numerous women in their practices who have survived violence.

*Jane M. Liebschutz, MD, MPH, FACP*
*Susan M. Frayne, MD, MPH*
*Glenn N. Saxe, MD, FRCP(C)*

# Foreword

## From Public Health to Personal Health:
## The Evolution of Clinical Violence Intervention

Ever since barber-surgeons have plied their specialty in the healing of wounds, medicine has responded to trauma. Post-war American medicine is notable for its expansion of emergency medical services, largely through the care of trauma patients. Today, advanced trauma life support, along with basic life support and advanced cardiopulmonary resuscitation, comprise the backbone of the emergency medical system and a well-established regional system of trauma care centers. There has been, however, a subtle shift in emphasis from the word trauma to violence, which in turn reflects a huge shift in our perspective: from the acute physical injury of the trauma victim to the broad ongoing psycho-social harms of the victim of violence. A woman's experience of violence has emerged as a sentinel health event, and clinical violence intervention now includes a spectrum of skills that address the acute and chronic physical, psychological, and social needs of survivors.

The emerging trauma system provided a unique view of the community experience of violence. The keywords of the new specialty of emergency medicine were *fall, accident, trauma,* and *injury;* these were further divided into specific concerns such as *spinal cord injury, head injury, penetrating chest wounds, gunshot injury,* and *motor vehicular accident.* While this vocabulary subsumed numerous injuries that resulted from violence, emergency medicine's technical nature and emphasis on specialized acute management obscured two facets of trauma critical to clinical violence intervention: the social context of deliberate injury and the role of gender in determining social context.

Without a language to mutually explore experiences of violence, physicians treated the mechanism and outcome of each woman's injury in isolation from its social source. The linguistic silence symbolized the absence of a social context that affirmed or protected women who suffered these problems and left survivors feeling isolated or ashamed. Too often, women considered a battering or sexual assault as "just life," attributing their experiences to bad luck or being in the "wrong place at the wrong time." Without putting injury into a social or historical context, there was no way for women or physicians to link the multiple events of trauma in one woman's life, to recognize similarity between women's experiences, to identify problems that arose secondary to violence, or to understand health problems associated with violence. From a research standpoint, there was no way to assess the prevalence, etiology, dynamics, and risk factors of interpersonal violence. Without a language that described women's experience of violence, medicine could not compile an epidemiology of violence against women.

The winds of change in medical perception originated in the advocacy community. In the late 1960s, hundreds of thousands of women formed "rap" or "consciousness raising" groups where they discovered that experiences heretofore believed uniquely private were widely shared. In "speak-outs" women used public venues to tell of sexual assaults they had kept hidden. This new alliance of victims and witnesses generated rape crisis hotlines and other direct support services to rape victims, which were followed by education and training to improve and standardize how police, prosecutors, journalists, and emergency department physicians addressed sexual assault victims. By the early 1970s, community groups had collaborated with nurses, social workers, and other health providers to create hospital-based rape crisis teams that counseled victims, worked closely with police and prosecutors to establish proof of the rapist's identity, and integrated evidence gathering and other forensic skills into the emergency medical response. The words to describe women's experience of sexual assault were incorporated into the language of emergency medicine, and emergency department rape crisis protocols became the first clinical violence intervention in women's health.

Incrementally, the language used in medical records more clearly identified whether injuries were sustained as the result of a deliberate assault. But even recording events as "rape" and "sexual assault" maintained the anonymity of the assailant, and the stereotype of rape remained an acute, isolated event prompting an array of intensive medical, legal, criminal justice, and mental health services for the victim. Lacking a historical context that linked one acute event to another, the woman who returned multiple times to emergency services with injuries remained outside the purview of medical understanding; appearing instead as one whose very identity (i.e., a woman with multiple medical problems and recurrent injury episodes) served to dismiss her from the technological fervor of the emergency department.

Again, a change in our perspective originated in the community. Women's advocates discovered that abusive partners posed a major obstacle to women trying to utilize new opportunities for daycare, employment, legal services, and education. Informal networks of "safe houses" developed, then battered women's support groups, hotlines, and shelters, and finally outreach to justice, health, and social service professionals. Once more, the creation of a support network made it possible for women to name and share their experiences of violence. From this perspective, the stereotypic anonymous rape was now seen as only one small aspect of women's experience of interpersonal violence. Our new vocabulary included *date rape, sexual abuse, marital rape,* and *battered woman.*

The earliest medical responses to woman battering relied on the initiatives of individual health professionals. In 1977, building on hospital-based rape crisis programs, the Ambulatory Nursing Department of the Brigham and Women's Hospital in Boston formed a multidisciplinary committee to develop a therapeutic intervention for victims of domestic violence. The intervention program at Brigham, and a parallel program at Harborview Hospital in Seattle, relied on a multidisciplinary team composed of volunteer social workers and nursing staff. Although efforts to expand hospital-based rape crisis teams to include domestic violence were sporadic and their volunteer base was difficult to sustain, clinician-advocates introduced free-standing domestic violence services at hospitals in Chicago, Hartford, San Francisco, Philadelphia, Minnesota, Wisconsin, and elsewhere. Model protocols for domestic violence intervention were disseminated nationwide. Initially, these efforts concentrated on emergency departments and focused upon acute interventions.

The organization of emergency medicine fostered the development of a clinical database. Trauma remained at the core of the emergency medicine mission, and injury epidemiology was further legitimized by the formation of an Injury Control Center at the Centers for Disease Control in Atlanta. In the mid-1980s, with violence common in national headlines, C. Everett Koop convened a unique—and now historic—Surgeon General's Workshop on Violence and Public Health. A public health surveillance approach to violence was implemented to establish the extent of the problem, identify risk groups and risk factors, and support program development. Patterns of violence among different groups were identified and began to inform intervention efforts. Improved surveillance confirmed the message of advocates that violence against women was epidemic. As we began to address violence as a public health problem, we began to understand the role of gender in constructing an individual's experience of violence.

By 1985, "shoe-leather" epidemiology from the field demonstrated that a disturbing—and growing—proportion of trauma is due to interpersonal violence. From injuries to toddlers, to sexual assault among adolescents, to domestic violence and elder abuse, our understanding of violence began to shift from emphasis on anonymous assault to a problem rooted in the very foundations of social life. The 1990s and beyond have seen an outpouring of research on the prevalence and health effects of episodic and ongoing violence and psychological, physical, and sexual abuse across many women's lifespan.

Researchers introduced simple interview techniques and questionnaires to uncover substantial rates of domestic violence, rape, and child sexual abuse in various medical settings, suggesting that identification is feasible in clinical sites. High rates of patient participation in research on sexual assault and domestic violence confirmed that patients think it appropriate to be asked about their experience of violence. Continuing education and program development as well as the widespread visibility of support for community domestic violence services helped to address health care providers' initial sense of helplessness and belief that identification of violence is a "Pandora's box."

Nevertheless, the predominant strategy remained based on a model of emergency care: to expand the identification of violence against women, assess for trauma-related problems, and implement referrals that place a high priority on immediate safety. Protocols based on this approach use the medical encounter largely for case finding and evidence gathering for subsequent criminal proceedings and typically frame assessment by a physical examination that highlights severe injury.

As we learned to appreciate the ongoing nature of domestic violence, the recurrent risk of sexual assault by abusive partners, and the long-term risk of health and mental health problems among women who experience violence, medical language began to incorporate a longitudinal dimension. The terms *domestic abuse, childhood sexual abuse,* and *elder abuse* communicate the likelihood of previous injuries, a range of psychological harms, and the risk of future injuries.

As the "battered woman's movement" evolved into a nationwide network of domestic violence services, surveys explored the psychological dimensions of violence. Physical abuse is invariably associated with psychological abuse, and it now appears that the threats, isolation, and invidious forms of control associated with the latter carry as poor a prognosis as all but the most severe forms of the former. Women's response to this "domestic terrorism" has been likened to the traumatic stress disorders suffered by soldiers. Although the various survivors of child sexual abuse, rape, domestic violence, and elder abuse have distinct needs, a common thread in their experience is reflected in post-traumatic stress syndromes. In each case, violence is accompanied by a sense of betrayal, vulnerability, and ambivalence about community norms, norms that seem to accept abuse and the abuser. Thus the long-term clinical problems associated with abuse share a common core of hypervigilance, anxiety and phobias, somatic complaints, dissociative disorders, sexual dysfunction, depression, substance abuse, suicide attempts, and risk of revictimization.

Community and hospital-based research suggest that the vast majority of health visits by women who experience violence involve unimpressive injuries, repeated presentations of nonemergency medical problems, and psychosocial and/or behavioral problems elicited by the ongoing experience of trauma, particularly coercive control. Because of this profile, the most appropriate approach is a primary care model of intervention that draws on experience with other issues that overlap with law enforcement and criminal justice concerns, including alcohol and drug use, human immunodeficiency virus (HIV) disease, tuberculosis, and syphilis treatment, birth control, genetic and prenatal testing, and end-of-life care.

Experience suggests that health providers are willing to take on domestic violence as an issue when changes in clinical practice are incremental and consistent with existing values, practices, and skills. The goal of clinical violence intervention is to provide health care in the context of violence, preventing the progression of problems by restoring a woman's sense of control over her material resources, social relationships, and physical environment, a process called *empowerment*. This aim too is best accomplished by considering violence against women as an ongoing concern for primary care. Developing early intervention strategies involves the skills of many medical disciplines, including nursing and social work, and calls upon the expertise of a broad range of clinicians. Meanwhile, because of the emphasis on patient empowerment, clinical violence intervention converges with other intervention strategies (e.g., smoking cessation, medication compliance, cancer screening, HIV prevention, occupational and environmental health, the care of terminally ill patients), where new models of physician/patient relationships are being emphasized. In all of these areas, health care providers already integrate periodic crisis intervention with ongoing monitoring, patient education, patient-centered planning, and liaison with community-based service organizations.

Adapting a primary care model also facilitates the incorporation of clinical violence intervention into routine practice. Mainstreaming and normalization hold the key to the successful institutionalization of clinical violence intervention. Mainstreaming involves making clinical violence intervention part of routine patient care. Normalization implies that work with survivors of violence builds on the skills and patient education techniques clinicians successfully employ in other medical or behavioral health areas. In so doing, both patient and provider are led through what have been identified as the necessary stages of recovery: establishing safety, identifying the trauma, retelling the story, and reconnecting with community.

And so it is that clinical violence serves as a vehicle for health care providers to join a broad spectrum of service providers and community-based groups in a coordinated response to violence against women. In most communities, the objectives of this response are to address three broad areas: new services for victims and perpetrators, coordination and reform of existing services, and prevention of violence against women through strategies to change community norms. This coordinated response allows the community to begin to tackle the crisis of violence against women and is a vehicle for moving from crisis management to prevention.

In this community collaboration, health care is challenged to broaden its traditional perspective, to recognize the strengths of parallel systems while maintaining its core values and commitment to patient care. Public health has a long tradition of working closely with community-based groups in prevention efforts. Clinical medicine brings to the table extensive experience in multidisciplinary cooperation, dogged and continued engagement against seemingly insuperable odds, and a commitment to beneficence and non-malfeasance, patient autonomy, and confidentiality, the last two especially important in the field of women's health.

The challenge of women's health has been not only to introduce a wide-spread change in clinical practice but to enhance and support a model of health care that empowers women. Strategies to meet this goal include

- Improved access to services traditionally underutilized by women (e.g., coronary care units, coronary artery bypass grafting)

- Improved access to women's services (e.g., breast and cervical cancer screening, prenatal care)

- Widespread access to well-organized health care (e.g., many services available during a single appointment)

- Participation in a *new* medicine, a *new* relationship between providers and patients, one that is holistic, nonjudgmental, and gender competent

What is the future of women's health? The answer is "all of the above." But it is in the last—a vision of holistic, nonjudgmental, even empowering care—that women's health shares a connection to the rape crisis and battered women's movements of the 1970s, the precursor of today's community-based violence prevention and intervention services.

Clinical violence intervention is in its infancy but growing rapidly. Domestic violence and public health advocates have long struggled to keep necessary social changes in mind in the midst of burgeoning service demands. Women's health providers now enter the field with the opportunity of insisting that in a gender-competent health care system the quality of care be reflected in the services available to all women.

*Anne Flitcraft, MD*
*Associate Professor of Medicine*
*University of Connecticut School of Medicine*
*Farmington, Connecticut*

# Contents

## CLINICAL ISSUES

## SPECIAL CONSIDERATIONS

# CLINICAL VIGNETTES

# Clinical Issues

# CHAPTER 1

# Violence Against Women: Risk Factors, Consequences, and Prevalence

SHERRY L. HAMBY, PHD

MARY P. KOSS, PHD

## What is Violence Against Women?

Nearly all physicians and health care providers who treat women will see victims of violence. Violence is pervasive in American society, which is one of the most violent societies in the industrialized world. Public attention is largely focused on conventional crime assaults by stranger assailants. Stranger assaults, however, make up a surprisingly small portion of violence. In particular, women are much more frequently victims of violence committed by a husband, boyfriend, former intimate partner, family member, or an acquaintance, rather than a stranger. Furthermore, contrary to many assumptions, assaults committed by intimate partners are usually equally or more severe than assaults committed by strangers (1). The most common type of violence is physical and sexual violence by an intimate partner and thus constitutes the major focus of this book, but clinicians also care for women who have experienced incest, elder abuse, and acquaintance and stranger sexual assault, so these topics are addressed as well.

Violence against women deserves special consideration partly because of the societal and physical vulnerabilities of women. Although recent societal changes have occurred that increase the protection of women, especially in the United States, violence against women still occurs frequently. Persistent societal vulnerabilities include the lower income of women compared to men and positive media portrayals of male violence. Physically, men are on average more than 30 pounds heavier and more than 5 inches taller (2). The average man also has 50% more upper body and 30% more lower body strength than the average woman (3). As a result, most men are generally capable of over-powering and injuring women. Although sexual assaults of men do occur, the majority of all rapes and other sexual assaults are committed against women. These acts are most often perpetrated by men known to the victim.

*Women are more likely to be physically and sexually assaulted by a man known to them than by a stranger.*

In this chapter we define the various kinds of violence that are addressed throughout the rest of the book. We summarize the risk factors for perpetrating and experiencing violence and explain barriers to changing an abusive situation. We then review the physical and psychological consequences of abuse. Finally, we discuss the prevalence of violence against women in the general population and in medical settings.

## Partner Violence

After the birth of their second child, Wendy and Jim's marriage began to fall apart. At first, Jim accused Wendy of squandering their meager income and criticized her for not controlling the children's behavior better. He later took away her bank and credit cards as well as keys to the car as a money-saving measure. He wired the home phone so he could record her phone calls. One day he unexpectedly came home mid-day and found Wendy serving lunch to a former high school boyfriend who was in town for business. After the visitor left, Jim locked the children in their room and began to break Wendy's collection of glass figurines. When she started screaming at him to stop, he beat her into unconsciousness while yelling "whore."

*Partner violence* (also called *domestic violence* and *intimate partner violence*) refers to a wide array of behaviors that are used to coerce, control, and demean women as illustrated in this vignette. According to the American Medical Association, partner violence "is characterized as a pattern of coercive behaviors that may include repeated battering and injury, psychological/emotional abuse, sexual assault, progressive social isolation, deprivation, and intimidation. These behaviors are perpetrated by someone who is or was involved in an intimate relationship with the victim" (4).

The American Medical Association's definition of domestic violence includes psychological abuse, isolation, and other nonphysical forms of abuse. Psychological/emotional abuse is an extremely important form of aggression that is often overlooked by providers. Psychological/emotional abuse includes a wide range of demeaning, threatening, and intimidating words and actions.

Examples of such abuse include insults and threats to take away a woman's children. Other examples of nonphysical abuse include economic control (e.g., taking away bank and credit cards), social isolation (e.g., confiscating keys to the car), and threats to use the legal system against a victim (e.g., by making reports to child welfare or immigration). Many survivors of domestic violence state that the psychological/emotional abuse causes more harm than the physical assault. Psychological/emotional abuse is frequently part of a pattern of power and control that the batterer uses against his victim. It is often the most frequent and pervasive form of abuse in a violent relationship. Despite its importance, psychological/emotional abuse has received comparatively little attention by researchers. Empirical data are largely limited to the impact of physical and sexual assault (1).

When most people think of partner violence, they think of being punched or getting beaten up, but partner violence also includes less injurious forms of physical assault such as pushing and slapping or even malicious destruction of the victim's property, as in the case above. Stalking is increasingly recognized as another important form of partner abuse. Stalking involves repeatedly harassing or threatening someone by doing things such as following a person, making disturbing phone calls, and vandalizing property (5).

Although men are also sometimes assaulted by intimate partners, women are much more likely than men to be injured or killed by a partner and are much more likely to be victims of repeated, severe battering (1). The available data on violence within same-sex couples are addressed in Chapter 12.

## Rape and Sexual Assault

Mona and Rick had met each other at a Halloween costume party and danced together most of the night. Between dances, Rick brought Mona refills on the spiked punch. He offered to escort her home that night because she felt too drunk to drive. When they got to her apartment, she thanked him for the wonderful evening and said that she needed to turn in for the night. He picked her up and carried her inside, while starting to kiss and undress her. She repeated to him that she didn't want to go further, at which point he pinned her down and forcibly raped her.

Sexual assault consists of rape and other acts involving unwanted sexual behavior. Rape refers specifically to the use of force to achieve vaginal, oral, or anal penetration without the victim's consent. The force used can include violence ranging from using a weapon to holding a woman against her will. Force also includes using alcohol or drugs to diminish a woman's capacity to say no, threatening violence, threatening to harm someone else (e.g., her children), and other threatening behavior. Other forms of sexual assault include attempted rape (no penetration), unwanted fondling or kissing, and forcing a woman to have intercourse without using a condom or birth control. Sexual assault can also involve forcing a girl or woman to touch the perpetrator in sexual ways: this form of assault is particularly common with juveniles. Sometimes, sexual aggression occurs without direct physical contact, as in "flashing" or exhibitionism. Although the legal definitions of rape and sexual assault vary by state, from a medical perspective all of these experiences can be traumatic.

## Child Abuse and Neglect

> When Nettie was 11, her 16-year-old brother began touching her back and sitting very close to her while watching TV. One weekend their parents asked him to babysit her while they were out of town. The first night he gave her a long close hug to say good-night. The next night he came into her room and began rubbing his own genitals. He told her to take off her nightgown. She ran out of the room and locked herself in the bathroom. When she tried to tell her mother what happened, her mother told her she was a very naughty girl and that she shouldn't make up stories.

Young girls are at risk for being physically, sexually, and psychologically abused or neglected. The legal definition of these terms does vary from state to state, but physical abuse generally involves any assault that either results in serious harm or has the likely potential of resulting in serious harm or injury. Spanking and other forms of corporal punishment remain legal in every state. Sexual abuse of children does not require any evidence of violence or coercion because any sexual contact with a youth by an adult is illegal. Sexual abuse can also be perpetrated by other juveniles, as in the case above. In most states, sexual contact between juveniles is considered abuse if there is a significant age difference between the youths (for example, a 16-year-old boy fondling a 11-year-old girl). Psychological/emotional abuse in childhood is similar in many ways to psychological/emotional abuse in adult intimate relationships. In addition, children are especially vulnerable to threats of being kicked out of the house or being told they should never have been born.

Neglect is a form of maltreatment that is unique to children and other dependents because of their inability to care for themselves. Neglect is most often a pattern of failing to meet a child's basic needs for food, shelter, supervision, or medical care. The effects of child abuse are often seen well into adulthood.

## Elder Abuse and Abuse of the Disabled

> Ruby, a 74-year-old woman, is morbidly obese and wheelchair bound because of hemiparesis from a stroke. Her caretaker at a private group home has been feeling

overwhelmed with Ruby's care lately because of a large decubitus ulcer. Ruby became agitated during a dressing change and knocked over the sterile gauze and saline before the dressing was complete. The caretaker began swearing at Ruby and forcibly pushed her down on the bed while re-doing the dressing changes.

Elderly women and women with disabilities are sometimes victimized by their family members or caregivers, as in this case. Another very common form of elder abuse is intimate partner violence that persists over the course of a marriage or relationship. In addition, there are other forms of elder abuse, which include neglect, financial exploitation, and psychological abuse. See Chapter 7 for details on elder abuse. Chapter 9 discusses issues on women with physical or mental disabilities.

## Is There a Cycle of Violence?

One of the most well-known findings to emerge from early studies of domestic violence was Lenore Walker's characterization of the "cycle of violence" (6). In the cycle, an act of violence is typically followed by a "honeymoon phase" in which the contrite batterer attempts to reconcile with the victim. The batterer's apologies and promises to be nonviolent in the future help keep the victim in the relationship. This phase is unstable, however, and as the couple settles back into a routine, the tension-building phase begins anew, which is soon followed by more violence.

Although this cycle undoubtedly describes the dynamic of violence in some relationships, abused women and advocates are quick to point out that it by no means describes all violent relationships. Some men never demonstrate a honeymoon phase: they keep the victim close by using death threats, hostage-taking (e.g., locking victim in house, taking victim to isolated cabin), or other violent means. Some survivors of violence report that the violence may follow the pattern of the cycle for a while, but it then escalates into a more constant state of terror (7). At the other end of the spectrum, not all domestic violence inevitably leads to severe battering, and the cycle may end because the couple addresses the problem. The batterer may take steps to stop his violence, or the victim may end the relationship despite the batterer's apologies during any honeymoon phase. Minor violence, in particular, has been shown to stop without formal interventions in some relationships. A 3-year longitudinal study of a nationally representative sample indicated that more than half of the men who were violent in the year before the Year 1 interview ceased or interrupted their violence in subsequent years (8). Although the theory of the cycle of violence was first formulated more than 20 years ago, there is in fact little empirical evidence to support its existence. This is partly because of a dearth of research on the dynamics surrounding individual violence episodes. Most recent research has focused on general correlates of violent relationships or risk markers.

## Risk Factors for Violence Against Women

Risk and vulnerability factors for violence against women are multiple and complex. Although these factors are *associated* with violence against women, current research data cannot point to a definite *cause* of violence. The reason for this is that virtually all research on this topic has been done looking back at violence that has occurred in the past. The possible causes of violence are measured at the same time as the violence, so it is difficult to know which factors caused the violence and which resulted from the violence. Doing research prospectively on the natural history of experiencing violence, that is, following forward in time without any intervention, would be extremely expensive, time-consuming, and ethically challenging. Even in research studies that have examined these questions prospectively, many women will have already experienced considerable violence by the time they enter the study, and teasing out the effects of different risks is complex. This is why the term *risk factors* rather than *causes* is used. The term *risk factors* indicates that these problems are correlated with violence against women but are not necessarily causative.

Risk factors operate at many levels, including individual, interpersonal, and societal/institutional (9). *Individual* risk factors are biological or intrapersonal traits or behaviors of an individual, either perpetrator or victim, that are associated with violence. *Interpersonal* risk factors are traits or behaviors that describe intimate relationships and that may be influenced by societal expectations of gender roles (e.g., male dominance). *Societal* and *institutional* risk factors are systemic influences on the occurrence of violence against women. These factors include the effects of schools, churches, the media, the legal system, and social norms about gender and violence. Societal risk factors include practices and values of a community that allow or encourage gender inequality, objectify women, and glorify violence. In general, although there is wide acknowledgement of the effects of macrolevel risk factors for violence against women (9), they are difficult to document empirically. Therefore, most research has measured interpersonal and individual factors for perpetration and vulnerability to violence.

Some risk factors are associated with the perpetrator of violence, such as history of criminality, and some are associated with vulnerability in a victim. We next review risk factors associated with perpetration of violence, followed by risk factors associated with vulnerability for experiencing violence.

## Risk Factors for Perpetrating Violence Against Women

A body of research has begun to identify some of the characteristics most often associated with violent behavior. These are described briefly and summarized in Box 1-1 (9,10).

It is very important to realize that no single set of characteristics describes all violent men. Most perpetrators will not demonstrate all of the characteristics described here, and even a man with none of these characteristics may behave violently. Conversely, many men who do have these risk factors do not batter. It may be tempting to try to identify which patients are violent and which are not by their physical appearance or other characteristics, but there is no way this can be done reliably. These factors can sometimes be used to identify which perpetrators are *likely* to be the most dangerous or the most

---

**Box 1-1    Risk Factors for Perpetration of Violence**

Individual Risk Factors
- History of violence in the family of origin
- Violent behavior in other settings
- Alcohol abuse
- Other substance abuse
- Unemployment
- Antisocial personality
- Borderline personality
- Insecurity, emotional dependence, low self-esteem
- Poor impulse control
- Belief that use of violence is acceptable in some interpersonal situations
- Head injury
- Neurophysiologic characteristics

Interpersonal Risk Factors
- Attempts to dominate and control partner
- Psychologically/emotionally abusive towards partner
- Relationship conflict or separation
- Poor communication skills
- Jealousy or suspicion

Societal, Population, and Institutional Risk Factors
- The media
- Gender roles and sexual scripts
- Sociocultural policies and practices that disenfranchise women
- Young age (ages 18 to 24, highest risk group)

treatment resistant. Recently, efforts have been made to use profiles of perpetrators to help identify which intervention is likely to be most successful, but such research is still in its infancy.

## Individual Risk Factors

### HISTORY OF VIOLENCE IN THE FAMILY OF ORIGIN

This risk factor refers to the extent to which an individual experienced or witnessed violence in the family-of-origin during his formative childhood years. Childhood exposure to violence is one of the most important correlates of adult violence. Estimates indicate that 42% to 81% of male batterers were exposed to violence as children. It should be noted, however, that exposure to family-of-origin violence is highly correlated with other family-of-origin problems, such as parental alcoholism, so it is likely that many family-of-origin problems contribute to risks for later violence (10,11).

### VIOLENT BEHAVIOR IN OTHER SETTINGS

Many batterers are violent not only towards their wives or girlfriends but also towards other people. Men who use violence in a variety of interpersonal situations are at high risk for using violence in the home. Such men are also generally the most resistant to treatment designed for domestic violence perpetrators (12).

### ATTITUDES TOWARDS VIOLENCE

The extent to which individuals endorse the use of force as acceptable in a variety of interpersonal situations is also associated with violence. This can include specific attitudes excusing violence towards women, such as believing that violence is justifiable after marital infidelity, or more general attitudes towards violence, such as believing that a "real man" does not walk away from a fight (13).

### ALCOHOL ABUSE

Excessive use of alcohol has been consistently associated with domestic violence perpetration. It is important to note that alcohol abuse does not cause violence per se. Not all alcoholics are violent. Estimates range widely, with anywhere from 6% to 85% of violent incidents reported to be related to alcohol, with best estimates closest to 50%. A man's expectations about his behavior when drunk contributes to whether alcohol use leads to violence (10). For example, someone who believes "I only fight when I'm drunk" is more likely to become violent than another person who believes "I drink to relax." Partner alcohol or other drug abuse was the best predictor of acute injury in a sample of domestic violence victims in an emergency department (14,15).

### OTHER SUBSTANCE ABUSE

Other forms of substance abuse have received less attention than alcohol, and the results are less conclusive. After alcohol, cocaine abuse shows the next most reliable association with violence. Illegal drug use is also closely associated with other deviant behaviors, and, again, it can be hard to tease out which factor is most related to violence (10).

### UNEMPLOYMENT

A number of socioeconomic risk factors have also been associated with violence. One of the most reliable associations is with unemployment. Unemployment may reflect several factors that can contribute to violence: a high level of stress, lack of resources, less integration into one's community, and "less to lose" as a consequence of violent behavior. Unemployment is also one of the most consistent risk markers associated with poor treatment outcome. It is important to note, however, that many unemployed men are not violent towards women (10,12).

### ANTISOCIAL PERSONALITY

Antisocial personality refers to a constellation of features such as irresponsibility, general hostility, impulsivity, and poor social relationships characterized by a lack of closeness (16). As many as 25% of batterers have antisocial personality features (although not all batterers meet all diagnostic criteria) and are at particular risk for perpetrating more severe violence (16).

### BORDERLINE PERSONALITY

Borderline personality refers to a constellation of features such as instability, impulsivity, emotional lability, and poor social relationships characterized by intense but erratic attachment (16). Recent efforts to create a profile of batterers suggest that perhaps 25% demonstrate some borderline personality features. Like antisocial batterers, batterers with borderline features generally perpetrate more severe violence than those without significant characterological pathology (17).

### INSECURITY, EMOTIONAL DEPENDENCE, AND LOW SELF-ESTEEM

Other personality traits are even more common among perpetrators of violence. For example, many violent men portray themselves in a negative light, indicating low self-esteem, and many exhibit emotional dependency on their partners and others in their lives, indicating various levels of insecurity (18). Like men with other personality traits and disorders, however, most men with low self-esteem do not perpetrate violence.

### POOR IMPULSE CONTROL

A tendency to act without first reflecting on the consequences of actions is another correlate of partner violence. This can also be accompanied by generally poor mediation of emotional states and aggressive personality styles (10).

PHYSIOLOGY AND NEUROPHYSIOLOGY

Studies have shown that there are correlations between some hormones and neurotransmitters and violence. For example, higher testosterone levels and lower serotonin levels appear to correlate with aggression, but the causal order of such associations is far from clear. In a different approach to identifying biological bases of violence, studies have found that perpetrators of violence have higher rates of head injury than non-perpetrators (9).

## Interpersonal Risk Factors

ATTEMPTS TO DOMINATE AND CONTROL PARTNER

A pattern of dominance indicates relationships that are hierarchical and in which the person with greater advantage uses that advantage to gain status, privileges, or control over his partner. A man's need to have power and control over his partner has been shown to be a major element in domestic violence (19). Common control tactics include not letting victims have contact with family and friends, blocking access to money, and checking up on what the victim does during the day.

PSYCHOLOGICAL/EMOTIONAL ABUSE OF PARTNER

Numerous studies indicate that psychological/emotional abuse and physical violence frequently occur together. Preliminary evidence suggests that men may be more likely than women to simultaneously engage in severe psychological/emotional abuse and physical abuse, which is consistent with clinical data that find that most severe batterers are men. Although health providers sometimes see evidence of physical violence (e.g., bruises), they are unlikely to observe physical violence occurring between partners during an office visit. Therefore, if a health care provider observes any psychological aggression between partners during an office visit, it should be considered a significant warning sign that physical violence may be occurring (20).

RELATIONSHIP CONFLICT OR SEPARATION

Not surprisingly, relationship conflict, separation, and dissatisfaction are linked to domestic violence. When conflict leads to a break up, separation, or divorce, the risks for violence may increase dramatically. In a national survey, 43% of stalking victims indicated that the harassment began after the relationship ended (21). The period around the dissolution of a relationship can be the most dangerous time for many women (10).

> *The period around the dissolution of a relationship can be the most dangerous time for many women.*

### Poor Communication Skills

A limited ability to express oneself verbally to one's partner is also linked to increased violence (22). Communication difficulties can be related to lack of exposure to specific skills during childhood or related to cognitive, psychiatric, or physical limitations.

### Jealousy or Suspicion

An extreme concern about the possible sexual and social exclusiveness of the relationship with one's partner is also correlated with violent behavior. This is sometimes associated with controlling behavior as well (23).

## Societal, Population, and Institutional Risk Factors

### Young Age

Youth is one of the most consistent risk markers for perpetrating violent behavior of all types. Among adults, the age group of 18 to 24 is at the highest risk for perpetrating violence, although risk remains elevated until about age 30. Partner violence rates for youth in dating relationships average around 30% to 35%, which is more than double that for married couples. Even young adolescents assault their dating partners at distressingly high rates (10,24).

### Depiction of Violence in the Media

Pornography and positive portrayals of male violence in the media appear to contribute to high rates of actual violence. Exposure to pornography in laboratory conditions increases men's aggression towards women, and exposure to explicit sexual scenes accompanied by graphic violence decreases empathy toward rape victims (9). Another study found that exposure to violent rock videos increased adversarial sexual beliefs (25).

### Gender Roles and Sexual Scripts

Another aspect of men's power over women expresses itself in traditional and rigid gender roles (19). Traditional gender roles in mainstream United States culture (and in a number of other cultures) dictate that women play subservient roles in relationships with male partners. Sexual scripts cast the man in the role of the pursuer and relegate the woman to the part of gatekeeper. These roles can be used to justify male violence and to limit women's options when they experience violence. Gender roles and sexual scripts are communicated through a variety of social institutions. Even some religious institutions may sometimes promote a subservient role for women. For example, Catholicism does not permit women to be priests, Orthodox Judaism does not permit women to obtain a divorce without the husband's consent, and Conservative Islam insists that women cover themselves from head to toe in front of men or in public.

Cross-cultural studies have found that levels of partner violence vary with other cultural characteristics. Societies that disapprove of partner violence and that provide women with the most economic, political, and social resources are generally the least violent (26,27). In the United States, a state-by-state analysis of wife assault rates found that gender inequality was the factor most highly predictive of variations in rates across states (28). In that study, gender inequality was measured by comparing men's and women's average income, proportion in high-prestige occupations, representation in public office, and legal status (e.g., equal employment opportunity guarantees). A measure of social disorganization was also associated with wife assault.

## Risk Factors for Experiencing Violence

Identifying risk factors for becoming a victim of violence is even more problematic than identifying risks for perpetrating violence. As mentioned earlier, most research on violence against women is collected after the violence has occurred and cannot pinpoint the exact causes of violence. Logically, it seems quite likely that some of the most reliable correlates of victimization, such as depression and anxiety, are consequences rather than causes of victimization. Furthermore, an emphasis on the characteristics of the survivor of violence, exemplified by the focus of much research on why women stay in abusive relationships, perilously approaches victim blaming. Studies of violence against women have found that most survivors of violence do not fit any particular profile (29). Rape and domestic violence cannot be predicted by studying victims. This is because violence against women is primarily a problem originating with the perpetrators, that is, with men behaving violently. Any examination of women's risk for violence must always keep this foremost in mind. In general, risk factors tend to be related to either increased vulnerabilty to becoming a victim of violence or decreased ability to access help once violence has commenced.

### Individual Risk Factors

Women who are survivors of domestic violence are twice as likely to have grown up in violent homes compared to women who have not experienced violence (10). Early victimization increases women's risk for later sexual victimization as well (29). The reasons for this link remain speculative. It is possible that women who grow up surrounded by violence come to see this as a normal part of interpersonal relationships. Past negative experiences with disclosure or attempts to escape may lead them to have low expectations about their ability to cope with violence as adults or may otherwise create a sense of helplessness. Whatever the reason, it is clear that the intergenerational transmission of violence is a contributor to violence against women, for both the perpetrators and the victims.

DRUG AND ALCOHOL USE

Although most data point to alcohol and other drug abuse as a consequence of experiencing violence, some data indicate the use of substances by a woman as increasing vulnerability to experiencing violence (30). This should not be mistaken for blaming the woman for the violence, but it can explain some of the reasons why she may not be able to protect herself from an aggressor or why she may be exposed to violence more often. For example, intoxication from alcohol may impair a woman's physical ability to protect herself, and addiction to cocaine, heroin, and other street drugs may expose a woman to drug-related violence (30-34). See Chapter 10 for detailed information on the relationship between substance abuse and experiencing violence.

### Societal, Population, and Institutional Risk Factors

YOUNG AGE

Younger women are more likely to experience violence. A large-scale survey of women revealed that in 54% of the women who were raped, the rape took place before age 18 (35). The National Crime Victimization Survey by the U.S. Department of Justice found that women ages 19 to 29 were more likely than other adult women to be victims of violence by an intimate. A surveillance study of 2811 women who presented to Philadelphia emergency departments for injuries during a 12-month period found that interpersonal violence was the leading cause of injury in women ages 15 to 44, with the highest rates for women ages 24 to 35 (36).

ECONOMICALLY AND SOCIALLY DISADVANTAGED GROUPS

Old stereotypes about violence suggest that only poor women experience domestic violence. We have known for over 20 years that this is not true: domestic violence is also common among middle and upper class families. Nevertheless, even though women from all backgrounds experience domestic violence, women from economically and socially disadvantaged segments of society experience more violence (37). This includes groups who are marginalized because of their minority status, social class, geographic location (e.g., rural vs. urban), language barriers, political status, and economic status. Although in many cases these groups have different cultural or ethnic backgrounds than the predominant group in their society or country, it is important to be aware that cultural differences can seldom be disentangled from the effects of oppression, discrimination, and lack of resources. Also, racial and ethnic differences are difficult to disentangle from socioeconomic differences, and it appears that at least some of the increased prevalence observed in racial minorities is caused by the lower socioeconomic status of most U.S. minorities (38). Yearly incidence rates among disadvantaged groups range widely, with rates for many groups above the U.S. average (21,39). It should be noted, however, that reliable estimates of violence against women are not available for many disadvantaged groups.

Additionally, domestic violence can force disadvantaged women into worse poverty and hardship because a violent partner may interfere in a variety of ways with a woman's ability to hold steady employment (40)—for example, stalking her at work, destroying work materials such as uniforms, and injuring her in ways that prevent working.

## Physicians and Other Health Care Providers Are Not Immune to Violence

Just as it is true that no class or ethnic group is immune to violence, so it is also important to realize that no occupational group is immune either. A number of studies of health care professionals have begun to document that many providers also have histories of violence (40a–40e,41). Although the focus of this book is on violence against women, some male providers have been victims of child abuse or other forms of violence as well. In short, the data appear to parallel that of the general population.

Perpetration of violence among health providers is a taboo subject, to the point at which there is almost no research examining the topic. One small study found that 15% of health care providers reported that they had perpetrated physical abuse and 3% had perpetrated sexual abuse (41). These rates are lower than for the general population and may indicate that rates of perpetration are lower for providers. It is also likely, however, that providers may be less willing to disclose perpetration than others because of a perceived risk to their professional status.

There are a number of important considerations for providers: personal experiences with violence, emotional reactions to patients with histories of violence, and self-care behaviors to prevent burn-out from caring for such patients. Chapter 6 presents details of studies on experiences of health care providers with childhood abuse, sexual assault, and partner violence.

## The "Why Do Women Stay?" Issue

Health care providers often ask why women stay in violent relationships: "Why don't they just leave?" There are several important points to consider regarding this issue. First, even asking the question in these terms emphasizes the victim's, rather than the perpetrator's, role in the violence. "Why doesn't the perpetrator stop beating her?" would be the more pertinent question.

*Most survivors of violence do actively try to ensure their safety.*

Second, escaping from violence can be an extremely difficult task, with many obstacles hindering a woman's efforts. Third, some assaulted women who show the effects of trauma have been portrayed as passive and unwilling to help themselves, but recent research has shown that most victims try many active ways of addressing the violence (42). It is important not to equate initial lack of success with lack of effort. Four, chronic victimization can lead to depression and other psychological consequences. These conditions may decrease a woman's initiative or self-esteem, thereby impeding her ability to advocate for herself and take action. Five, although it is dangerous to stay, it can be even more dangerous (at least in the immediate term) to leave. A woman may make an informed decision that staying is, for the moment, the safest thing to do.

## Special Focus    Why Do Women Stay in Violent Relationships?

As a health provider, you will come across many people (health care professionals, family members, police, and others) who wonder why a woman does not leave a violent relationship. There are many reasons why it is difficult to leave a violent relationship or in some cases to even seek assistance. Awareness of these issues can be used to fight victim-blaming attitudes.

The main obstacles to leaving can be divided into five categories: Batterer's Behavior, Socioeconomic Obstacles, Institutional Obstacles, Social Network Issues, and Personal Values.

### Batterer's Behavior

- Batterer has threatened to kill victim if she leaves
- Batterer has threatened to kill children if victim leaves
- Batterer has threatened to kill pets if victim leaves
- Batterer has threatened to commit suicide if victim leaves
- Batterer has threatened to fight for custody of victim's children
- Batterer has threatened to kidnap victim's children
- Batterer has escalated the violence or stalked victim when she has tried to leave
- Batterer has promised to change
- Batterer has minimized severity of the violence
- Batterer has blamed victim for the violence
- Batterer has cut off victim's access to outside help and social support

*Continued*

- Batterer has cut up clothes, burned pictures, or destroyed other belongings when victim has prepared to leave
- Batterer has spread rumors that victim is having an affair or has gone crazy
- Batterer has told victim she will never make it without him

## Socioeconomic Obstacles

- Victim has no access to money
- Victim is unemployed
- Victim has limited job experience
- Victim cannot find a job that pays a living wage
- Victim may lose her job if she moves or misses time from work
- Victim does not have a car
- Victim lives in an area with no public transportation
- Victim would lose her health insurance
- Victim would have to leave without her personal belongings
- Victim has trouble calling for help and seeking support

## Institutional Obstacles

- Community services are set up so that the victim is the one expected to leave her home
- Many programs encourage leaving or divorce as the only effective options for the victim
- Local shelters are often full
- Local shelters usually provide services for a limited time
- Local shelters often do not accept women with substance abuse or psychological disorders
- Many programs do not treat members of minority groups equally, offer no bilingual services, and do not adapt programs to different cultural or ethnic groups
- Programs may require that the woman participate in unwanted treatment in order to get the services she wants
- Shelters may not re-admit victims who have previously returned to batterer
- Police may arrest the woman if she has used violence, even in self-defense
- Batterer is unlikely to serve jail time, especially for his first or second conviction
- Courts and batterers' programs support the idea that treatment will change the batterer
- It takes several weeks for AFDC or other public support to be forwarded to a new address
- Welfare reform imposes time limits on eligibility for public assistance
- The victim risks being reported to Child Protective Services for exposing children to violence
- The victim risks losing custody of her children in divorce proceedings
- Health care providers may give the victim a psychiatric diagnosis, which hurts the victim in court
- Victim's religion does not allow divorce

## Social Network Issues

- Family wants couple to stay together
- Family and friends are fearful of getting involved because of danger
- Family is unwilling or unable to provide social or financial support
- Batterer's family uses violence against victim
- Victim and children would lose social support if moved away from friends and family
- Children would have to change schools
- Victim is criticized for having a failed marriage
- Being labeled a "battered woman" may be stigmatizing

## Personal Values

- Victim holds religious beliefs that divorce for any reason is wrong
- Victim believes that a violent father in the home is better than no father at all
- Victim believes that the success of a marriage is the responsibility of the wife
- Victim believes that the man should make the major decisions in a relationship
- Victim's self-esteem is based in large part on perceived success in role of wife or girlfriend
- Victim may feel that relationship problems are her fault
- Victim remembers happier times in the relationship and believes they are possible again
- Victim doubts whether she will be able to have another relationship
- Victim doubts her ability to be self-sufficient
- Victim feels strongly about loyalty, duty, and commitment
- Victim still loves her partner

*Given these obstacles, it is in some ways more amazing that **any** woman is able to leave a violent relationship than that some women remain.*

From Hamby SL. Domestic Violence in Sociocultural Context. Training package. Eastport, ME: Possible Equalities; 1999; with permission.

# Consequences of Violence Against Women

Violence can have devastating consequences for victims. The effects can be loosely divided into psychological and physical categories. Psychological effects include symptoms of trauma-related disorders such as post-traumatic stress disorder (PTSD) and substance abuse (Box 1-2). In addition to the direct effects of abuse, psychological symptoms can be exacerbated by the social isolation that perpetrators often impose on victims. Physical effects include not only injuries but also chronic problems such as headaches, pelvic pain, and irritable bowel syndrome (Box 1-3). Of course, not all women will show all of

---

**Box 1-2    Common Psychological Consequences of Violence for Victims**

- Post-traumatic stress disorder and anxiety symptoms
- Depression
- Suicidal ideation and attempts
- Feelings of helplessness and powerlessness
- Low self-esteem
- Sexual dysfunction
- Self-medication with alcohol or other drugs

---

**Box 1-3    Common Physical Consequences of Violence for Victims**

Direct Effects on Physical Health
- Death
- Traumatic injury
- Unwanted pregnancy
- Adverse effects on pregnancy
- Sexually transmitted diseases

Indirect Effects on Physical Health
- Gynecological symptoms
- Chronic pain
- Gastrointestinal disorders
- Heart disease
- Headaches
- Other medical problems

Increased Medical Utilization
- More frequent physician visits
- More frequent hospitalizations
- More frequent emergency department visits

---

these effects, and some women who have sustained violence may show none of them (7,43,44). These issues are also discussed in Chapters 3 and 5.

## Psychological Consequences

*Post-Traumatic Stress Disorder and Anxiety Symptoms*
Trauma and anxiety symptoms commonly occur after violence and include signs of post-traumatic stress such as intrusive memories or flashbacks, avoidance of settings or stimuli that remind the victim of the violence, and

hypervigilance (7,43). These may persist for many years after the initial violence. Interpersonal violence is one of the most common causes of PTSD and carries the highest risk for PTSD from a variety of traumatic events (45). Early pioneering work in this field described such patterns as Battered Woman Syndrome (46) or Rape Trauma Syndrome (47), but in the current diagnostic system these symptoms are classified as PTSD. PTSD is a useful diagnosis for describing the symptoms of many victims, but it does not fully describe all after-effects of violence and does not take into account the gendered nature of rape and battering. PTSD is discussed in detail in Chapter 5.

## Depression

Depression is a mood disorder characterized by somatic disturbances, anhedonia, difficulty with concentration, and sometimes thoughts of death (16). Depression is one of the consequences of violence that has been most reliably documented by studies of battered women and sexual assault survivors (7,43,44).

## Suicidal Ideation and Attempts

Thoughts of hurting or killing oneself are often the result of feelings of desperation. Suicide attempts are more common among female victims of violence than nonvictims (48). As many as 30% to 55% of rape victims report suicidal ideation after the assault (43).

## Feelings of Helplessness and Powerlessness

Both the batterer's use of control tactics to limit the victim's response to violence and institutional failures to assist victims contribute to the victim's feelings that she has no good options for increasing her safety (7).

## Low Self-Esteem

Batterers often disparage and humiliate their victims. In the context of the social isolation that is also typical of battering, these experiences often lower the victim's sense of self-worth (7).

## Sexual Dysfunction

Victims of sexual assault, including those with a childhood history of sexual trauma, are at particular risk for experiencing later discomfort regarding sexual activity. This can include fear of sex, arousal dysfunction, and decreased sexual interest (43,44).

## Self-Medication with Alcohol or Other Drugs

Another common strategy that victims may use is to turn to the use of alcohol or drugs as an attempt to cope with the overwhelming negative feelings associated with victimization. A recent longitudinal study found that the likelihood of both alcohol and drug use increased after a new assault, even in women with no prior substance use history (30). In that same study, previous illicit drug use, but not alcohol use, increased the chances of becoming victimized. Substance abuse is also common among sexual assault victims (43). See Chapter 10 for a detailed discussion of substance abuse as it relates to victims of violence.

## Physical Consequences

There are numerous physical consequences of being victimized (see Box 1-3). Some of these are direct consequences of the violence and/or sexual assault, such as traumatic injury, unwanted pregnancy, complications of pregnancy, and sexually transmitted diseases. Acute injury is discussed further in Chapter 3. Others, such as gynecological symptoms, chronic pain syndromes, and gastrointestinal problems, are consequences of the effects of traumatic stress, which can influence physical health by various mechanisms. Some of these mechanisms are psychologically based, but emerging literature shows that many of them actually reflect physiologic changes. Such effects are especially common for women who experience long-term or repeated victimization. Many of these effects last for several years after the violence has occurred (48). Although the severity and duration of the violence are important determinants of the extent of the physical consequences, multiple factors contribute to any particular woman's physical response to violence.

Physicians and other health care providers address the many physical sequelae of violence even if they do not identify them as such. Women who have been subjected to violence are, in fact, more likely to seek medical care than to use mental health services, social services, counseling from clergy, victim assistance, or legal aid (49). Because of this increased utilization, health care providers have numerous opportunities to help women who are experiencing the effects of trauma.

> *Physicians from all medical specialties treat female victims of violence.*

### Direct Effects of Violence on Physical Health

#### DEATH

There were 1320 women murdered by intimate partners in the United States in 1998 (the most recent year for which data are available). Intimate partner homicides account for 33% of all murders of women but only 4% of murders of men, reflecting the greater severity of the domestic violence problem for women. Recent trends indicate that this discrepancy is growing because intimate homicide rates have remained fairly steady for women but have declined for men. Gun injuries are the leading cause of death with intimate as well as nonintimate homicides, but knife injuries are more common among intimate than nonintimate homicides (50).

## TRAUMATIC INJURY

Not surprisingly, battered women experience many more traumatic injuries than nonbattered women. Multiple injuries to the face, head, neck, breast, and abdomen are typical, in contrast to accidental injuries, which are more likely to involve the extremities (e.g., arms or legs). Injuries for which there has been a delay in seeking medical care or multiple injuries that are in various stages of healing are commonly seen in victims of intimate violence. Nongenital physical injuries are common among sexual assault victims, and vaginal and perineal trauma are also found in approximately half of rape victims seeking medical care (43,48,51). One study found that one-third of orbital fractures among female ophthalmology patients were caused by sexual or partner assault (52). See Chapter 3 for additional information on acute injuries.

## UNWANTED PREGNANCY

Pregnancy itself is a direct consequence of approximately 5% of all rapes (53). Almost half (47%) of the rapes leading to pregnancy were perpetrated by a husband or boyfriend. Rape-related pregnancy is an understudied source of unwanted pregnancies in the United States.

## ADVERSE EFFECTS ON PREGNANCY

Several studies have found that violence to the mother during pregnancy probably has an adverse effect on the fetus, although the outcomes of pregnancy are so multifactorial that studies have not been consistent about the specific effects of violence. Abused women are more likely than nonabused women to show low maternal weight gain, have more infections, experience pre-term labor, and deliver low-birth-weight infants (54-57). Some studies have found that women who are survivors of abuse are more likely to delay receiving prenatal care until the third trimester (54,58). Abuse during pregnancy has psychosocial effects that are similar to those reported by other victims. Stress levels are elevated, as are risky health behaviors, including increased tobacco, alcohol, and drug use (59,60). See Chapter 8 for more details on the effects of violence on pregnancy.

## SEXUALLY TRANSMITTED DISEASES

Women who have been raped or sexually assaulted are at high risk for contracting sexually transmitted diseases of all types (43). This includes women who are forced to have sex without a condom, a common but often overlooked type of sexual coercion.

## Indirect Effects of Violence on Physical Health

There are effects of violence on physical health that are not directly attributable to acute injury, and there are a number of mechanisms that appear to explain these associations at least in part. One that has received considerable attention is post-traumatic neuroendocrine dysregulation (61-63). Neuroanatomical differences such as lower hippocampal volume have also been found in abuse victims compared to controls, which could represent either an effect of trauma or a risk factor for developing dissociative or other symptoms after trauma (64). Bodily assault and fear may focus attention on internal sensations and contribute to concerns about physical integrity (65). Patients may have somatization disorder: patients with somatization have multiple physical symptoms either without a known physical cause or out of proportion to the patient's known medical conditions (66). The DSM-IV criteria for somatization are presented in Chapter 5. Somatization disorder is seen with increased frequency among patients with a previous trauma history (67-70). This is particularly true for women with childhood trauma who have PTSD. A variety of risky health behaviors are also more common among victims of partner violence than nonvictims. These include excessive alcohol use, cigarette smoking, and street drug use (71-73). Failure to use condoms is a particularly problematic risk behavior for victims of violence. Violent men tend to react violently to requests to use a condom (74). Several studies have shown that women in abusive relationships are less likely to use condoms and to be more likely to be verbally abused when they attempt to discuss condom use (75).

### GYNECOLOGICAL SYMPTOMS

Sexual assault history has been associated with excessive menstrual bleeding, genital burning, painful intercourse, dysmenorrhea (both medically explained and unexplained), and menstrual irregularity (76).

### CHRONIC PAIN

Chronic pain problems of various types are more common among victimized than nonvictimized women. Unfortunately, much of the research in this area includes women with any history of abuse. It is therefore difficult to separate the effects of childhood and adult abuse and to tease out the effects of multiple victimizations (1). Chronic pain syndromes associated with a history of physical and sexual abuse have included pelvic pain, headache, and low back pain.

Chronic pelvic pain is a common problem among women. It accounts for up to 10% of all gynecology visits and is the third most frequent indication for hysterectomy. Research on correlates of chronic pelvic pain indicates that 53% to 64% of patients with this condition have histories of physical and/or sexual abuse (1), which is much higher than any population-based prevalence of abuse.

One small but well-conducted study of patients at a tertiary referral clinic for headache found that chronic headache, especially headache unresponsive to conventional medication, was more common among victimized than nonvictimized women. Furthermore, the presentation of chronic headache appears to differ between abused and nonabused women: 75% of abused women developed headache pain after age 20 compared to 14% of nonabused women after age 20 (77). Fibromyalgia is also seen with higher prevalence among women with a sexual trauma history (78,79).

### GASTROINTESTINAL DISORDERS

Gastrointestinal disorders, especially irritable bowel syndrome, often occur with chronic pelvic pain. Functional gastrointestinal disorders, including irritable bowel syndrome, non-ulcer dyspepsia, and chronic abdominal pain, comprise 35% of gastrointestinal disorder diagnoses and are the most common gastrointestinal conditions seen in primary care (1). Among female gastroenterology patients, 44% to 59% have a history of sexual abuse (1,80,81). Elevated risks for gastrointestinal disorders may also occur among victims of domestic violence (82). However, limited research suggests that a history of victimization and other psychosocial factors cannot distinguish women with functional versus organic gastrointestinal disorders (83,84).

### OTHER MEDICAL PROBLEMS

Victims of domestic violence also seek care for a variety of other health needs, for both chronic and episodic diseases, more than other women (48,65,85,86). Some of these needs are probably directly related to the abuse but may not be identified as a consequence of violence. These include urinary tract infections, vaginitis, neck pain, suicide attempts, and induced abortions (because perpetrators of violence may not cooperate with family planning). Because victimized women are seen for many more medical visits than nonvictimized women, greater attention to the possible contribution of abuse to these other medical problems may improve the overall health of women with victimization histories.

## Increased Medical Utilization

Women with histories of severe sexual and physical assault have many more physician visits per year than nonvictimized women (65). The Cleveland Clinic study of sexual and physical violence against women reported that severely victimized women made physician visits twice as frequently and had medical expenses that were 2.5 times greater than nonvictimized women (65). The largest increase in physician visits occurred not immediately after the assault or even during the first year but 2 years after the assault. Similar findings have been reported elsewhere. Long-term follow-up suggests that victims are not high utilizers before the violence. Research also indicates that victims have higher utilization than nonvictims even after controlling for visits due to injuries sustained in the attack (49). Other services in addition to physician visits are utilized at higher rates as well. A Philadelphia study found that the majority of women who had sought emergency care for injuries more than once in the same year were victims of violence (36). A recent study found that women with current orders of protection because of domestic violence had a 50% relative increase in hospitalization rate for any diagnosis compared with nonabused women (82). A study of HIV-infected women found that a history of victimization conferred a more than 2-fold increase in surgical procedures and a more than 3-fold increase in both emergency department visits and hospitalizations (87).

## Diagnostic Issues

Under-detection of violence histories is a common problem. This is partly because of a continued lack of screening on the part of most providers (88). Screening is extremely important for diagnosis and is addressed in detail in Chapter 2. Proper treatment must include addressing safety issues for patients, discussed in Chapter 2 as well.

It is also important to bear in mind that although survivors of violence have higher rates of many chronic and stress-related illnesses than other groups of women, this by no means indicates that all stress symptoms or other symptoms of unknown etiology are caused by violence. Rare illnesses, hard-to-diagnose illnesses, and atypical symptom patterns are found among victims of violence just as they are in any other group.

Finally, physicians should also be aware that a victimized woman may be prevented or punished by the perpetrator for seeking assistance from legal or social services. A visit to the doctor may be one of the few times she is allowed out of the house on her own. She may also be uncertain about how to approach the topic herself or concerned that her problems will not be taken seriously. For these reasons, it is imperative that physicians become comfortable initiating discussions about physical and/or sexual assault.

## Social Consequences

There are many other consequences of violence against women. Victims of violence sometimes lose their jobs as a result of missed work caused by health problems or stalking by their batterer. Recent research shows that female victims of male physical violence have less steady employment and are more likely to have received welfare (40,89). Rates of homelessness are higher among victimized women (90). Children who witness violence in their homes show many of the same psychological effects as the victims (91) and, as discussed earlier, are at increased risk for subsequent perpetration and victimization. Survivors of violence often become socially isolated and are blocked from seeing family and friends. Few areas of a woman's life are not affected by being a victim of violence.

## Incidence and Prevalence of Violence Against Women

### Physical Violence

Violence against women is common throughout American society. The Department of Justice estimates that at least 2.3% of all women (or 2.7 million) are the victims of violent crime every year (91a). The violent crime rate is higher in the United States than in many other countries. For example, a recent study found that the United States accounted for 70% of murders of women among 25 large, wealthy countries even though it has only 32% of the total female population of those countries (91b). This high rate of femicide appears to be primarily related to the high gun ownership rates in the United States compared with most other industrialized nations.

Intimate violence also occurs with disturbing frequency. Although intimate violence is also a crime, many women do not perceive it as such. Careful assessment shows that it is the most common type of violence women experience. Approximately 10% to 15% of women experience either physical or sexual assault every year: in the United States, this translates into more than 6 million women per year. More than 1.8 million women per year experience assaults serious enough that they could or do produce injury (23). The recent National Violence Against Women Survey indicates that 51% of all women in the United States experience physical assault by any perpetrator at some point in their lifetimes. It also showed that 25% of women have been assaulted by an intimate partner at some point in their lifetimes (35). These same data indicate that most physical assaults of women are by their male intimate partners (in contrast, most physical assaults of men are by other men). Psychological/emotional abuse actually occurs in the majority of all intimate relationships: as many as 75% of all women will be subjected to psychological aggression, particularly in the form of yelling, insults, and swearing, every year (92).

Young women are particularly vulnerable to physical assault. A national study of college students in dating relationships found that 32% have sustained at least some degree of physical assault (93).

# Sexual Assault

Sexual assault is also disturbingly common. More than 300,000 women are raped every year. Almost 18% of women are raped during their lifetimes, which translates into more than 17 million victims in the United States alone (35). As with physical assault, young women in dating relationships report very high rates of sexual assault. A recent national survey found a lifetime prevalence of rape to be 20% and a rate of 15% since age 15 (94). Even high school students are sexually assaulted by acquaintances or boyfriends in surprisingly high numbers, with 20% of female students reporting some form of sexual assault (95). Almost half of these are raped by an intimate partner. A recent study of emergency department patients who had been sexually assaulted indicated that 68% had been assaulted by someone known to them (96). Nearly all rapists are male. The overlap between physical and sexual assault is high: partner rape in the absence of other physical violence is rare (1).

## Special Population Considerations for the Health Care Provider

*Incidence and Prevalence in Emergency Departments*
Emergency departments will see especially high rates of domestic violence. Among women seeking care for injuries, 18% to 30% will have injuries caused by domestic violence (36,72,97,98). Other surveys of emergency department patients have found that 15% to 22% are currently in a violent relationship and that 40% to 60% have lifetime histories of domestic violence (99,100). Domestic violence was the leading cause of injury for women who had two or more injuries in a 1-year period requiring emergency department visits (36).

*Incidence and Prevalence in Primary Care Settings*
A variety of primary care settings also have seen elevated rates of domestic violence. Surveys of primary practice patients have found yearly incidence rates of domestic violence to be 5% to 23% (73,101-103) and 20% for psychological/emotional abuse (103). Rates of psychological/emotional abuse during the span of the current relationship have been reported to be as high as 48% (104). In primary care, prevalence of lifetime adult sexual assault is approximately 30% (103), lifetime partner abuse is 12% to 45% (102,105,106), childhood sexual abuse is 17% to 40%, and childhood physical abuse is 5% to 10% (103,107).

Pregnancy has received considerable attention as a time of particular vulnerability for the occurrence of domestic violence and greater negative outcomes such as miscarriage. Estimates of the incidence of violence during pregnancy suggest that rates are higher than average. Some of this increased risk is because of age differences: pregnant women are on average younger than the general population of adult women (108). One study has found that nearly two-thirds of victimized pregnant women said the abuse worsened during pregnancy (109). Given that pregnancy is a relatively short period of time and also one of increased physical vulnerability, the reported rates are alarmingly high. The post-partum period has also been found to be a period of higher vulnerability (110). See Chapter 8 for a more detailed discussion of the risks and treatment issues associated with pregnancy.

## Special Focus    How Accurate Are Estimates of Violence Against Women?

Determining the exact number of victimized women is complex for a number of reasons. Any review of epidemiological data should be read with the following considerations in mind.

### Strengths of Self-Report Data

Self-report data produce the highest estimates of violence against women for two main reasons (Straus M, Gelles R. Physical violence in American families. New Brunswick, NJ: Transaction Publishers; 1990). First, violence against women almost always occurs in the home or some other private setting, and, usually, only the victim and perpetrator know about it. Second, most assaults do not get reported to the police, and most women do not go to shelters or crisis services. Official statistics can report only what is known to public agencies, and this is a small portion of all violence against women. For example, the Uniform Crime Reports document less than half as many rapes as are identified in self-report surveys (Eigenberg H. The national crime survey and rape: the case of the missing question. Justice Quarterly. 1990;7: 655-71).

The National Family Violence Surveys found that only 7% of physical assaults by husbands were reported to the police (Straus & Gelles). The best self-report surveys ask about the behaviors without labeling them as assault, abuse, or other criminal names and include multiple questions about many forms of violence (Straus & Gelles; Koss M. The measurement of rape victimization in crime surveys. Criminal Justice and Behavior. 1996;23:55-69).

### The Importance of Question Wording

In the past, many studies on violence used terms like "abuse," "domestic violence," "rape," and "assault." It has been shown, however, that questions that describe the actual physical act (e.g., punching, forced sexual contact) reveal many more incidents of violence than those using more emotionally laden terms (Koss M. The measurement of rape victimization in crime surveys. Criminal Justice and Behavior. 1996;23:55-69; Hamby SL, Gray-Little B. Labeling partner violence: when do victims differentiate among acts? Violence Vict. 2000;15:173-86). This is probably because even women willing to disclose may not realize that physical violence includes pushing and slapping and instead think only very severe violence such as assaults with a weapon or those that require emergency medical care should be reported. Similarly,

*Continued*

some women may not realize that sexual assault includes forced kissing, fondling, oral intercourse, and other sexual behaviors in addition to genital intercourse.

Some women may not recognize that forced sexual contact by their husband or other intimate partner is sexual assault. Substantial effort has gone into developing specific questions that describe individual physically and sexually assaultive behaviors to maximize the accuracy of self-report. Unfortunately, many studies of violence against women in health care settings do not use behaviorally based questions; this is an area that needs improvement. The Centers for Disease Control and Prevention has recently released guidelines for uniform definitions for intimate partner violence that should become the standard for future studies (Saltzman L, Fanslow J, McMahon P, Shelley G. National Center for Injury Prevention and Control, Centers for Disease Control and Prevention. Intimate Partner Violence Surveillance: Uniform Definitions and Recommended Data Elements. Version 1.0; 1999).

## Limitations of Self-Report Data

Despite the important advantages of self-report data for uncovering unreported incidents, many believe that most self-report data underestimate the amount of violence against women. Violence is a sensitive subject, and although many women will disclose their trauma histories, especially in a supportive context, the stigma of being labeled a victim can lead to under-reporting (Hamby & Gray-Little). Memory is not perfect, and memory problems can range from simple forgetting of minor incidents that occurred long ago to blocking out painful traumatic experiences as a coping mechanism (Williams LM. Recall of childhood trauma: a prospective study of women's memories of child sexual abuse. J Consult Clin Psychol. 1994;62: 1167-76).

Finally, the vast majority of data on physical violence against women come from the Conflict Tactics Scales (Straus M, Hamby S, Boney-McCoy S, Sugarman D. The Revised Conflict Tactics Scales (CTS2): development and preliminary psychometric data. J Fam Issues. 1996;17:283-316) or similar checklists. Although these checklists can help cue women to think of different types of assaults, they obviously cannot list every possible form of assault. Thus, the more unusual forms of assault are sometimes missed (Hamby S, Poindexter V, Gray-Little B. Four measures of partner violence: construct similarity and classification differences. J Marriage Fam. 1996;58:127-39). Despite these limitations, many studies of reliability and validity indicate that estimates of violence against women are reasonably accurate. Because of underreporting, however, documented rates should be considered lower-bound estimates. This means that the problem may be worse than is currently recognized.

## How Good Are the Data on Violence Rates in Health Care Settings?

In general, the quality of the data about rates of violence in special populations is not as good as it is for the general U.S. population. This is true of data in medical settings as well. Although there have been several studies with large sample sizes, many studies take place in only one, or perhaps a few, clinics or hospitals. A disproportionate number of studies are conducted in medical schools or public clinics that provide easier access to researchers and may not represent patients who seek health care through private practices or hospitals.

The quality of the questions on violence varies also: many studies use only one or two screening questions. Although even a minimal systematic screening will yield five to six times as many domestic violence cases as informal record-keeping (McLeer SV, Anwar R. A study of battered women presenting in an emergency department. Am J Public Health. 1989;79:65-6), few studies of medical populations adopt more comprehensive measures. Research has shown that the number of questions asked has a significant effect on the total incidence rate (Gazmararian A, Lazorick S, Spitz AM, et al. Prevalence of violence against pregnant women. JAMA. 1996;275;1915-20), and it is likely that even more cases would be uncovered with the use of standardized questionnaires.

## Community-Based Studies

The most often-cited data on physical assault come from the National Family Violence Surveys conducted by Straus and Gelles in 1975 and 1985 (Straus & Gelles). Recent data on national rates of sexual assault come from the National Violence Against Women Study (Tjaden P, Thoennes N. Prevalence, Incidence and Consequences of Violence Against Women: Findings from the National Violence Against Women Survey, 1998. National Institute for Justice and Centers for Disease Control and Prevention. November 2000) and the National College Health Risk Behavior Survey (Brenner N, McMahon P, Warren C, Douglas K. Forced sexual intercourse and associated health-risk behaviors among female college students in the United States. J Consult Clin Psychol. 1999;67:252-9).

These surveys are relied upon because they provide data that are not based on samples from high-risk settings such as shelters and police records. Thus, they are used most often as national norms. Most of the violence reported in such surveys is relatively minor (e.g., pushing or other acts that have a low injury potential), and infrequent national surveys do not do a good job of identifying severely battered women. This is in part because such women make up a relatively small portion of all women in the country, and also because batterers may not allow their victims to participate in household-based surveys.

## Statistics from Shelters, Police, and Other High-Risk Settings

Because of the few severely battered women that are identified in community surveys, statistics from shelters and other women's services are also extremely important (Koss M, Goodman L, Browne A, et al. No Safe Haven: Male Violence Against Women at Home, at Work, and in the Community. American Psychological Association; 1994). The descriptions of women who are terrorized by their partners are especially important for health providers because most domestic violence injuries occur in the context of severe battering. These surveys were also among the first to raise community awareness about the domestic violence problem. Knowing the numbers of women served by shelters helps document the severity of the social problem and the need for community resources for victims. Because most victims do not seek help from shelters or other public services, however, they do not give as good an idea about how much violence occurs in our society as a whole.

# Summary

- Violence against women includes physical, sexual, and psychological assaults.

- Every year more than 10% of women experience some form of violence by an intimate partner.

- Over the course of a lifetime, 25% to 50% of women will become a victim of violence.

- Asking women to self-report violence is the best way to identify violence, but even then some women may be hesitant to disclose.

- Women seeking health care report higher rates of recent assault than the general population, so health care providers are in a good position to screen for violence.

- Approximately 25% of non-motor-vehicle injuries seen among female patients of emergency departments are caused by partner violence.

- Health care providers, both male and female, have histories of violence as victims and perpetrators at rates near those of the general population.

- Perpetration of violence is associated with exposure to violence in one's family of origin, other violent behavior, alcohol and substance abuse, emotional instability, attempts to dominate one's partner, societal gender roles, and sociocultural practices.

- Current studies cannot reliably identify whether factors associated with being a victim are causes or consequences of violence. The main reliable risk factor for being a victim is exposure to violence in one's family of origin.

- Psychological effects of violence include depression, anxiety, substance abuse, and suicidal ideation.

- Physical effects of violence include death, injury, chronic pain syndromes, gastrointestinal symptoms, and increased health care utilization. Violence appears to adversely affect pregnancy and existing illness.

## REFERENCES

1. Koss M, Ingram M, Pepper S. Psychotherapists' role in the medical response to male partner violence. Psychother. 1997;34:386-96.
2. National Health and Nutrition Survey Data Tables. National Center for Health Statistics. 1994.
3. Powers S, Howley E. Exercise Physiology: Theory and Application to Fitness and Performance, 3rd ed. Dubuque, IA: Brown & Benchmark; 1997.
4. American Medical Association. Diagnostic and treatment guidelines on domestic violence. Arch Fam Med. 1992;1:39-47.

5. Tjaden P, Thoennes N. Stalking in America: Findings from the National Violence Against Women Survey. U.S. Department of Justice; 1998.

6. Walker LE. The Battered Woman. New York: Harper; 1979.

7. Giles-Sims J. The aftermath of partner violence. In: Jasinski J, Williams L, eds. Partner Violence: A Comprehensive Review of 20 Years of Research. Thousand Oaks, CA: Sage; 1998:44-72.

8. Aldarondo E. Cessation and persistence of wife assault: a longitudinal analysis. Am J Orthopsychiatry. 1996;66:141-51.

9. Crowell N, Burgess A. Understanding Violence Against Women. Washington, DC: National Academy Press; 1996.

10. Kaufman Kantor G, Jasinski J. Dynamics and risk factors in partner violence. In: Jasinski J, Williams L, eds. Partner Violence: A Comprehensive Review of 20 Years of Research. Thousand Oaks, CA: Sage; 1998:1-43.

11. Murphy CM, Meyer SL, O'Leary KD. Family of origin violence and MCMI-II psychopathology among partner assaultive men. Violence Vict. 1993;8:165-76.

12. Hamby S. Partner violence: prevention and intervention. In: Jasinski J, Williams L, eds. Partner Violence: A Comprehensive Review of 20 Years of Research. Thousand Oaks, CA: Sage; 1998:210-58.

13. Haj-Yahia M, Edleson J. Predicting the use of conflict resolution tactics among engaged Arab-Palestinian men in Israel. J Fam Violence. 1994;9:47-62.

14. Kyriacou DN, McCabe F, Anglin D, et al. Emergency department-based study of risk factors for acute injury from domestic violence against women. Ann Emerg Med. 1998;31:502-6.

15. Kyriacou DN, Anglin D, Taliaferro E, et al. Risk factors for injury to women from domestic violence against women [see Comments]. N Engl J Med. 1999;341:1892-8.

16. Diagnostic and Statistical Manual of Mental Disorders (DSM-IV) Washington, DC: American Psychiatric Association; 1994.

17. Holtzworth-Munroe A, Stuart GL. Typologies of male batterers: three subtypes and the differences among them. Psychol Bull. 1994;116:476-97.

18. Murphy CM, Meyer SL, O'Leary KD. Dependency characteristics of partner assaultive men. J Abnorm Psychol. 1994;103:729-35.

19. Koss M, Goodman L, Browne A, et al. No safe haven: male violence against women at home, at work, and in the community. American Psychological Association; 1994.

20. Hamby S, Sugarman D. Acts of psychological aggression against a partner and their relation to physical assault and gender. J Marriage Fam. 1999;61:959-70.

21. Tjaden P, Thoennes N. Extent, nature, and consequences of intimate partner violence: findings from the National Violence Against Women Survey. National Institute of Justice; 2000.

22. Babcock J, Waltz J, Jacobson N, Gottman J. Power and violence: the relationship between communication patterns, power discrepancies, and domestic violence. J Consult Clin Psychol. 1993;61:40-50.

23. Luci P, Foss M, Galloway J. Sexual jealousy in young men and women: aggressive responses to partner and rival. Aggressive Behavior. 1993;19:401-20.

24. Straus M, Gelles R. Physical violence in American families: risk factors and adaptations to violence in 8,145 families. New Brunswick, NJ: Transaction; 1990.

25. Peterson DL, Pfost KS. Influence of rock videos on attitudes of violence against women. Psychol Rep. 1989;64:319-22.

26. Campbell J. Prevention of wife battering: insights from cultural analysis. Response to Victimization of Women and Children. 1991;14:18-24.

27. Levinson D. Family Violence in Cross-Cultural Perspective. Newbury Park, CA: Sage; 1989.

28. Straus M. State-to-state differences in social inequality and social bonds in relation to assaults on wives in the United States. J Comp Fam Stud. 1994;25:7-24.

29. Koss M, Dinero T. Discriminant analysis of risk factors for sexual victimization among a national sample of college women. J Consult Clin Psychol. 1989;57:250-2.

30. Kilpatrick D, Acierno R, Resnick H, Saunders B. A 2-year longitudinal analysis of the relationship between violent assault and substance use in women. J Consult Clin Psychol. 1997;65:834-47.

31. Fagan J. Interactions among drugs, alcohol, and violence. Health Aff (Millwood). 1993;12:65-79.

32. Rivara FP, Mueller BA, Somes G, et al. Alcohol and illicit drug abuse and the risk of violent death in the home. JAMA. 1997;278:569-75.

33. Windle M. Substance use, risky behaviors, and victimization among a US national adolescent sample. Addiction. 1994;89:175-82.

34. Goldstein PJ, Bellucci PA, Spunt BJ, Miller T. Frequency of cocaine use and violence: a comparison between men and women. NIDA Research Monograph Series. 1991;110: 113-38.

35. Tjaden P, Thoennes N. Prevalence, incidence and consequences of violence against women: findings from the National Violence Against Women Survey. National Institute for Justice and Centers for Disease Control and Prevention. 2000;12:1998.

36. Grisso JA, Wishner AR, Schwarz DF, et al. A population-based study of injuries in inner-city women. Am J Epidemiol. 1991;134:59-68.

37. Hamby S. Domestic violence in sociocultural context. Training package. Eastport, ME: Possible Equalities; 1999.

38. Russo NF, Denious JE, Keita GP, Koss MP. Intimate violence and black women's health. Womens Health. 1997;3:315-48.

39. West C. Lifting the 'political gag order': breaking the silence around partner violence in ethnic minority families. In: Jasinski J, Williams L, eds. Partner Violence: A Comprehensive Review of 20 Years of Research. Thousand Oaks, CA: Sage; 1998: 184-209.

40. Browne A, Saloman A, Bassuk S. The impact of recent partner violence on poor women's capacity to maintain work. Violence Against Women. 1999;5:393-426.

40a. Little L, Hamby SL. The impact of a clinician's sexual abuse history, gender and theoretical orientation on treatment issues of childhood sexual abuse. Prof Psychol Res Pract. 1996;27:617-25.

40b. Little L. Risk factors for assaults on nursing staff: childhood abuse and education level. J Nurs Admin. 1999;29:22-9.

40c. Ernst AA, Houry D, Nick TG, Weiss SJ. Domestic violence awareness and prevalence in a first-year medical school class. Acad Emerg Med. 1998;5:64-8.

40d. Cullinane PM, Alpert EJ, Freund KM. First-year medical students' knowledge of, attitudes toward, and personal histories of family violence. Acad Med. 1997;72:48-50.

40e. deLahunta EA, Tulsky AA. Personal exposure of faculty and medical students to family violence. JAMA. 1996;275:1903-6.

41. Karol R, Micka R, Kuskowski M. Physical, emotional, and sexual abuse among pain patients and health care providers: implications for psychologists in multidisciplinary pain treatment centers. Professional Psychology: Research and Practice. 1992;23:480-5.

42. Hamby S, Gray-Little B. Responses to partner violence: moving away from deficit models. J Fam Psychol. 1997;11:339-50.

43. Goodman LA, Koss M, Russo NF. Violence against women: physical and mental health effects. Part I: research findings. Applied and Preventive Psychol. 1993;2:79-89.

44. Mahoney P, Williams L. Sexual assault in marriage: prevalence, consequences, and treatment of wife rape. In: Jasinski J, Williams L, eds. Partner Violence: A Comprehensive Review of 20 Years of Research. Thousand Oaks, CA: Sage; 1998:113-62.

45. Breslau N, Kessler R, Chilcoat H, et al. Trauma and posttraumatic stress disorder in the community: The 1996 Detroit Area Survey of Trauma. Arch Gen Psychiatry. 1998;55: 626-32.

46. Walker L. The Battered Woman Syndrome. New York: Springer Verlag; 1984.

47. Burgess AW, Holmstrom LL. Rape trauma syndrome. Am J Psychiatry. 1974;131: 981-6.

48. Bergman B, Brismar B. A 5-year follow-up study of 117 battered women. Am J Public Health. 1991;81:1486-9.

49. Kimerling R, Calhoun K. Somatic symptoms, social support, and treatment seeking among sexual assault victims. J Consult Clin Psychol. 1994;62:333-40.

50. Rennison C, Welchans S. Intimate partner violence [Statistics]. Bureau of Justice; 2000.

51. Weaver TL, Kilpatrick DG, Resnick HS, et al. An examination of physical assault and childhood victimization within a national probability sample of women. In: Kaufman-Kantor G, Jasinski JL, eds. Out of the Darkness: Contemporary Research Perspectives on Family Violence. Thousand Oaks, CA: Sage; 1997.

52. Hartzell K, Botek A, Goldberg S. Orbital fractures in women due to sexual assault and domestic violence. Ophthalmology. 1996;103:953-7.

53. Holmes MM, Resnick HS, Kilpatrick DG, Best CL. Rape-related pregnancy: estimates and descriptive characteristics from a national sample of women. Am J Obstet Gynecol. 1996;175:320-4; discussion 324-5.

54. Parker B, McFarlane J, Soeken K. Abuse during pregnancy: effects on maternal complications and birth weight in adult and teenage women. Obstet Gynecol. 1994;84:323-8.

55. Schei B, Samuelsen SO, Bakketeig LS. Does spousal physical abuse affect the outcome of pregnancy? Scand J Soc Med. 1991;19:26-31.

56. Berenson AB, Wiemann CM, Wilkinson GS, et al. Perinatal morbidity associated with violence experienced by pregnant women. Am J Obstet Gynecol. 1994;170:1760-9.

57. Shumway J, O'Campo P, Gielen A, et al. Preterm labor, placental abruption, and premature rupture of membranes in relation to maternal violence. J Maternal Fetal Med. 1999;8:76-80.

58. McFarlane J, Parker B, Soeken K, Bullock L. Assessing for abuse during pregnancy. JAMA. 1992;267:3176-8.

59. Amaro H, Fried LE, Cabral H, Zuckerman B. Violence during pregnancy and substance use. Am J Public Health. 1990;80:575-9.

60. Curry MA. The interrelationships between abuse, substance use, and psychosocial stress during pregnancy. J Obstet Gynecol Neonatal Nurs. 1998;27:692-9.

61. Lemieux A, Coe C. Abuse-related post-traumatic stress disorder: evidence for chronic neuroendocrine activation in women. Psychosomatic Med. 1995;57:105-15.

62. Resnick HS, Yehuda R, Pitman RK, Foy DW. Effect of previous trauma on acute plasma cortisol level following rape. Am J Psychiatry. 1995;152:1675-7.

63. Yehuda R. Psychoneuroendocrinology of post-traumatic stress disorder. Psychiatr Clin North Am. 1998;21:359-79.

64. Stein MB, Koverola C, Hanna C, et al. Hippocampal volume in women victimized by childhood sexual abuse. Psychol Med. 1997;27:951-9.

65. Koss MP, Koss PG, Woodruff WJ. Deleterious effects of criminal victimization on women's health and medical utilization. Arch Intern Med. 1991;151:342-7.

66. American Psychiatric Association. Diagnostic and Statistical Manual of Mental Disorders, 4th ed. Washington, DC: American Psychiatric Press; 1994.

67. Springs FE, Friedrich WN. Health risk behaviors and medical sequelae of childhood sexual abuse. Mayo Clin Proc. 1992;67:527-32.

68. McCauley J, Kern DE, Kolodner K, et al. Clinical characteristics of women with a history of childhood abuse: unhealed wounds. JAMA. 1997;277:1362-8.

69. Drossman DA, Leserman J, Nachman G, et al. Sexual and physical abuse in women with functional or organic gastrointestinal disorders. Ann Intern Med. 1990;113:828-33.

70. Walker EA, Katon WJ, Hansom J, et al. Medical and psychiatric symptoms in women with childhood sexual abuse. Psychomatic Med. 1992;54:658-64.

71. Felitti V, Anda R, Nordenberg D, et al. Relationship of childhood abuse and household dysfunction to many of the leading causes of death in adults. The Adverse Childhood Experiences (ACE) Study. Am J Prev Med. 1998;14:245-58.

72. Abbott J, Johnson R, Koziol-McLain J, Lowenstein SR. Domestic violence against women: Incidence and prevalence in an emergency department population. JAMA. 1995;273:1763-7.

73. McCauley J, Kern DE, Kolodner K, et al. The "battering syndrome": prevalence and clinical characteristics of domestic violence in primary care internal medicine practices. Ann Intern Med. 1995;123:737-46.

74. Neighbors C, O'Leary A, Labouvie E. Domestically violent and nonviolent male inmates' responses to their partners' request for condom use: testing a social-information processing model. Health Psychology. 1999;18:427-31.

75. Wingood GM, DiClemente RJ. The effects of an abusive primary partner on the condom use and sexual negotiation practices of African-American women. Am J Public Health. 1997;87:1016-8.

76. Golding J. Sexual assault history and women's reproductive and sexual health. Psychology of Women Quarterly. 1996;20:101-21.

77. Domino JV, Haber JD. Prior physical and sexual abuse in women with chronic headache: clinical correlates. Headache. 1987;27:310-4.

78. Taylor ML, Trotter DR, Csuka M. The prevalence of sexual abuse in women with fibromyalgia. Arthritis Rheum. 1995;38:229-34.

79. Boisset-Pioro M, Esdaile J, Fitzcharles M. Sexual and physical abuse in women with fibromyalgia syndrome. Arthritis Rheum. 1995;38:235-41.

80. Drossman DA, Leserman J, Nachman G, et al. Sexual and physical abuse in women with functional or organic gastrointestinal disorders. Ann Int Med. 1990;113: 828-33.

81. Drossman DA, Talley NJ, Leserman J, et al. Sexual and physical abuse and gastrointestinal illness: review and recommendations. Ann Intern Med. 1995;123:782-94.

82. Kernic MA, Wolf ME, Holt VL. Rates and relative risk of hospital admission among women in violent intimate partner relationships. Am J Public Health. 2000;90: 1416-20.

83. Smith RC, Greenbaum DS, Vancouver JB, et al. Psychosocial factors are associated with health care seeking rather than diagnosis in irritable bowel syndrome. Gastroenterology. 1990;98:293-301.

84. Walker E, Gelfand A, Gelfand M, et al. Medical and psychiatric symptoms in female gastroenterology clinic patients with histories of sexual victimization. Gen Hosp Psychiatry. 1995;17:85-92.

85. Liebschutz JM, Mulvey KP, Samet JH. Victimization among substance-abusing women. Arch Intern Med. 1997;157:1093-7.

86. Muelleman RL, Lenaghan PA, Pakieser RA. Nonbattering presentations to the ED of women in physically abusive relationships. Am J Emerg Med. 1998;16:128-31.

87. Liebschutz J, Feinman G, Sullivan L, et al. Physical and sexual abuse in women infected the human immunodeficiency virus: increased illness and health care utilization. Arch Intern Med. 2000;160:1659-64.

88. Parsons LH, Zaccaro D, Wells B, Stovall TG. Methods of and attitudes toward screening obstetrics and gynecology patients for domestic violence. Am J Obstet Gynecol. 1995;173:381-6; discussion 386-7.

89. Lloyd S, Taluc N. The effects of male violence. Violence Against Women. 1999;5:370-92.

90. Zorza J. Woman battering: a major cause of homelessness. Clearinghouse Review. 1991:25.

91. Wolak J, Finkelhor D. Children exposed to partner violence. In: Jasinski J, Williams L, eds. Partner Violence: A Comprehensive Review of 20 Years of Research. Thousand Oaks, CA: Sage; 1998:113-62.

91a. Rennison CL. Criminal victimization 2001: changes 2000-2001 with trends 1993-2001 [Statistics]. Washington, DC: Department of Justice; 2002.

91b. Hemenway D, Shinoda-Tagawa T, Miller M. Firearm availability and female homicide victimization rates across 25 populous high income countries. J Am Med Womens Assoc. 2002;57:100-4.

92. Straus M, Sweet S. Verbal/symbolic aggression in couples: incidence rates and relationship to personal characteristics. J Marriage Fam. 1992;54:346-57.

93. White J, Koss M. Courtship violence: incidence in a national sample of higher education students. Violence Victims. 1992;6:247-56.

94. Brenner N, McMahon P, Warren C, Douglas K. Forced sexual intercourse and associated health-risk behaviors among female college students in the United States. Journal of Consulting and Clinical Psychology. 1999:67.

95. Davis T, Peck G, Storment J. Acquaintance rape and the high school student. J Adolescent Health. 1993;14:220-4.

96. Ruch L, Gartell J, Amedeo S, Coyne B. The sexual assault symptom scale: measuring self-reported sexual assault trauma in the emergency room. Psychological Assessment. 1991;3:3-8.

97. McLeer SV, Anwar R. A study of battered women presenting in an emergency department. Am J Public Health. 1989;79:65-6.

98. Tilden VP, Shepherd P. Increasing the rate of identification of battered women in an emergency department: use of a nursing protocol. Res Nurs Health. 1987;10:209-15.

99. Ernst AA, Nick TG, Weiss SJ, et al. Domestic violence in an inner-city ED. Ann Emerg Med. 1997;30:190-7.

100. Goldberg WG, Tomlanovich MC. Domestic violence victims in the emergency department: new findings. JAMA. 1984;251:3259-64.

101. Gin NE, Rucker L, Frayne S, et al. Prevalence of domestic violence among patients in three ambulatory care internal medicine clinics. J Gen Intern Med. 1991;6:317-22.

102. Hamburger LK, Sunders DG, Hovey M. Prevalence of domestic violence in community practice and rate of physician inquiry. Fam Med. 1992;24:283-7.

103. Mazza D, Dennerstein L, Ryan V. Physical, sexual and emotional violence against women: a general practice-based prevalence study. Med J Australia. 1996;164:14-17.

104. Rath GD, Jarratt LG, Leonardson G. Rates of domestic violence against adult women by men partners. J Am Board Family Practice. 1989;2:227-33.

105. Elliott BA, Johnson MMP. Domestic violence in a primary care setting. Arch Fam Med. 1995;4:113-9.

106. Freund KM, Bak SM, Blackhall L. Identifying domestic violence in primary care practice. J Gen Intern Med. 1996;11:44-6.

107. Greenwood CL, Tangalos EG, Maruta T. Prevalence of sexual abuse, physical abuse, and concurrent traumatic life events in a general medical population. Mayo Clin Proc. 1990;65:1067-71.

108. Gelles RJ. Violence and pregnancy: are pregnant women at greater risk of abuse? J Marriage Fam. 1988;50:841-7.

109. Stewart DE, Cecutti A. Physical abuse in pregnancy. Can Med Assoc J. 1993;149:1257-63.

110. Gielen AC, O'Campo PJ, Faden RR, et al. Interpersonal conflict and physical violence during the childbearing years. Soc Sci Med. 1994;39:781-7.

# CHAPTER 2

# How Can a Clinician Identify Violence in a Woman's Life?

JANE M. LIEBSCHUTZ, MD, MPH

ANURADHA PARANJAPE, MD, MPH

In light of the high prevalence of violence against women and its potentially severe consequences, an important first step in clinical practice is to identify a history of violence before the patient returns with an acute injury. This chapter presents approaches to routine screening to detect unsuspected violence and focused questions for when violence is suspected. Appropriate responses to the disclosure of ongoing violence, including empathetic statements, a standard safety assessment, and screening for common mental health sequelae of violence, are also described.

## The Importance of Identifying Violence Against Women

Identifying a history of experiencing violence is, in and of itself, a useful intervention because it outwardly recognizes and validates an inherently private experience. Identification can then lead to interventions to increase safety, decrease morbidity, and improve function. Health care providers are in a unique position to identify a history of experiencing violence (i.e., being a victim of violence).

*Identifying a history of violence is itself a useful intervention.*

Providers have the social mandate of confidentiality, trustworthiness, and patient advocacy, as well as distance from the social world of the patient.

Furthermore, knowingly or unknowingly, health care providers have extensive contact with women who have experienced violence: women in abusive relationships will often access the health care system multiple times before the detection of abuse. In one study of help-seeking behaviors of abused women, 86% of the subjects had sought medical assistance during the time they were attempting to leave the relationship (1).

In the early 1990s, the American Medical Association recognized the key role that health care providers can play in intervening on behalf of women experiencing violence and made violence prevention part of its national agenda. It extended the National Campaign Against Family Violence to encompass domestic violence in 1992, urging physicians to screen routinely for domestic violence (2). In 1992, it published diagnostic and treatment guidelines (3). This mandate has translated into JCAHO regulations about protocols for treating victims of domestic violence in hospitals. Although few studies are available to determine the efficacy of universal screening on outcomes such as ongoing violence (4), existing studies suggest that women who have experienced intimate partner violence report that a simple question by a physician or other health care provider was perceived as an essential first step to disclosure and recognition (5). In addition, identification of a history of violence in the medical setting can be a way to access other social support services.

*Inquiry by the physician is an essential first step to the disclosure and recognition of violence.*

For women who use the health care system as an entry to help for abuse, the clinician initiative in asking about abuse is essential. It communicates a willingness to address the issue as part of the overall concern for the patient's health.

Among the first large-scale examples of screening interventions are two recent studies at Health Maintenance Organizations (HMOs), which each implemented a multifaceted approach. In one study, the approach included provider education, support staff training, self-administered patient questionnaires, and visual materials in the waiting area, examination rooms, and bathrooms. These interventions improved a number of measures, including a 4-fold increase in screening rates. Although the improvement in screening was largely due to the self-administered questionnaire, this study highlights the importance of innovative ways to improve detection of violence histories in patients (6). The other study was conducted in two phases: initially, improved infrastructure for referrals, and in the second phase, education for providers and staff members. Preliminary findings showed a significant increase in patient perception that the doctors and the HMO considered domestic violence to be an important health consideration. There was also a 2.5-fold increase in the rates of referrals made to mental health professionals for domestic violence (7). Future research must measure effectiveness of screening on both health and social outcomes.

# Barriers to the Detection of Domestic Violence

Physicians greatly under-detect abuse in their patients. Although documentation in the medical record is only a rough estimate of detection of abuse, in one study domestic violence was listed on the problem list for only 3 (0.8%) of 375 previously victimized women identified through research interviews (8). Another study conducted in an emergency department setting found that medical record identification of domestic violence in female patients presenting for trauma increased from 6% to 30% of women presenting with injury with the introduction of a research nurse, then dropped back to 8% after study personnel were withdrawn (9).

One major cause of under-detection is lack of physician inquiry. In an anonymous survey of physician and patient attitudes, routine physical abuse inquiry was favored by 78% of surveyed patients, yet only 7% recalled being asked about it (10). More recently, a California survey found that a majority of primary care physicians and obstetrician/gynecologists reported routine screening for partner violence in approximately 10% of patients (11). However, those same physicians reported screening for partner violence 79% of the time when patients presented with injuries.

## Physician Barriers

Physician barriers to screening fall into four major categories: lack of knowledge and skills; lack of resources, including time; beliefs; and personal experiences (Table 2-1).

Knowing what to ask and how to ask it can improve violence screening rates. A survey of physicians in Ontario, Canada revealed that fewer than 20% had a standard approach to detecting intimate partner abuse, but that the overwhelming majority felt it would be helpful to have such a standard approach (12). There is some evidence that having attended a talk or workshop on domestic violence in the past 12 months could lead to increased screening, although findings in this area have been inconsistent, perhaps because of the type of educational approach used (11,13). In addition to knowing how to screen for abuse, providers need to know how to react to a disclosure of abuse by a patient. Physicians can feel stymied if they approach abuse in their patients in the same manner as high blood pressure or angina. Recommendations to "just leave" an abusive relationship are rarely followed in the short run, even if leaving is an appropriate long-term solution. Furthermore, such recommendations may have adverse consequences, as discussed below. The question of what to ask and how to counsel such patients is described later in this chapter and in Chapter 4.

Some clinicians attribute difficulty with screening to a lack of resources, including time, to adequately screen for and follow up on abuse histories.

### Table 2-1    Barriers to Screening and Ways to Overcome Them

| Provider Barriers to Screening | Ways to Overcome Barriers |
|---|---|
| Lack of knowledge and skills | Educational programs (didactic and skills-based) |
| Lack of time or resources for referral | Make follow-up appointment to finish discussion Supply office with state and local hotline information and handouts |
| Beliefs | |
|   Fear of offending patient | Recognize that patients believe that it is the clinician's job to ask about abuse |
|   A sense of powerlessness: "There's nothing I can do to help her" | Understand that the clinician's job is to empower the patient, not to solve her problem for her |
|   Patients will volunteer a history of abuse | Screen all patients: few patients volunteer abuse histories without being asked |
|   Only poor women of color experience abuse | Recognize that women of all ages, races, and socioeconomic backgrounds experience abuse |
|   Personal experiences with abuse | Self-care Good support system |

This lack of resources is underscored by findings that HMO-based physicians are least likely to screen new patients (as opposed to follow-up patients) for intimate partner abuse (11). There is also a perception that uncovering an abuse history will be an endless, complicated task, after which it will be impossible to proceed to the next patient, the proverbial "Pandora's Box" or "can of worms" (14). These challenges are even more imposing when clinicians do not have back-up referral resources (social worker, advocate, or mental health professional) for patients who have disclosed an abuse history. With knowledge and skills, however, the task can be efficiently managed. Chapter 4 describes referral mechanisms, and the Appendix gives the phone numbers of statewide hotlines and other domestic violence programs, as well as addresses for Web sites for more information.

Clinician beliefs may also prevent screening for violence. Clinicians are more likely to think about a violence history in a female patient with an acute injury despite the evidence that victimized patients present with other medical issues during times of abuse (11). Some clinicians may believe that screening would offend the patient or may be perceived as prying and consequently not screen the patient, yet patients have reported willingness to be screened and agreement with screening by physicians (10). Some clinicians have the perception that patients will volunteer the information on their own, therefore obviating the need for screening, but survivors report the importance of direct inquiry. Some clinicians believe that violence only occurs among poor women of color and thus may screen middle or upper class white women less often, even though all women are at risk. Physicians also may feel impotent to make changes in their patients if they uncover violence because they may underestimate the effectiveness of intervention. There is no evidence that the physician's gender affects the decision to screen.

A clinician's personal experience with abuse may cause him or her to avoid screening in order to prevent a triggering of strong personal feelings in the clinician. One-sixth of female physicians and medical students may have experienced physical or sexual abuse(15). The ways that a physician's personal experience with violence influences interactions with patients who have experienced abuse, and approaches to overcoming such barriers, are discussed further in Chapter 6.

## Patient Barriers

Although most patients will share an abuse history if the clinician requests it, certain patient factors may deter the patient from disclosing abuse. In ongoing intimate partner abuse, one of the most important factors is fear of retaliation from the partner. The partner may have threatened the patient or her children with injury or even death if she should disclose abuse. She may also fear that sharing information will lead to reporting the violence to police or child protective services, which may anger the perpetrator or may lead to removal of her children from the home (see Chapter 3 for information on mandatory reporting). For immigrant women, the fear of deportation or dependence on the perpetrator for legal residency status may cause such patients to deny abuse.

Another important deterrent to disclosure is feelings of shame. The patient may be very sensitive to judgmental attitudes and feel as if she is to blame. If the abused woman believes that the provider is likely to be judgmental, she may deny the presence of violence even if the provider has initiated a discussion about violence. She may be thinking, "My doctor will think it was my fault for making him [the abuser] mad" or "My doctor will think I'm spineless for not leaving."

*If an abused woman believes that the provider is likely to be judgmental, she may deny the violence.*

Lacking trust in the health care provider or the health care system is an important barrier to disclosing abuse. Women who have experienced intimate partner or childhood abuse may have a particularly hard time trusting others because of the betrayal of trust by the perpetrator. Patients are more likely to disclose abuse in the context of an on-going or established relationship with a provider. In an emergency department setting, in particular, the lack of familiarity with providers, as well as the lack of privacy, may heighten a patient's distrust. Furthermore, an injured patient may be in pain and especially fearful after an episode of violence.

Because abuse may be intermittent or part of a long-standing family relationship, the victim may not recognize her own experience as that of abuse. For example, her father may have told her that his sexual advances on her as a child were part of a normal father–daughter relationship. As described in Chapter 1, actual physical or sexual violence may be a small part in a pattern of emotional dependence and abuse. Asking about emotional abuse may be an important clue to uncovering physical or sexual violence.

## Before Screening for Violence: Establishing a Safe and Receptive Environment

### Office Set-Up

The office environment can indicate to a patient whether violence is an acceptable topic of discussion with the physician. Posters and flyers with information about local rape crisis and domestic violence services visible in the waiting area and in the women's bathroom provide information and create an environment conducive to discussion of violence. Additionally, wallet-sized cards with emergency numbers can be made available in the examining rooms, bathrooms, and the waiting areas. Staff should be trained to recognize signs of active abuse and be familiar with appropriate responses and security measures.

Another way to introduce the topic of abuse is to include a question on the office's written intake form. For example, the following question detected an abuse history in 12% of those screened: "At any time has a partner ever hit you, kicked you, or otherwise physically hurt you?" (16). A written approach might be better in certain situations such as new patient visits because it normalizes the questions, lets the patient know that these are as important as questions about physical illness, and may decrease shame in disclosing abuse. As was mentioned above, the increase in detection of partner abuse in one study was largely because of such intake forms (17).

### Privacy

One of the most important rules is to screen for violence in a private setting. If the patient's partner or family member accompanies her to the appointment, they must be separated from the patient before the clinician asks questions. If the patient does not speak English, then a trained interpreter

*Screening for violence must be done in a private setting.*

should be used rather than a friend or family member. In a shared room, such as an inpatient setting or an emergency department, a curtain that separates patients is not adequate to ensure privacy. Screening in a non-private setting may risk exposing the patient's answers to the perpetrator as well as her own community. She will be less likely to answer truthfully for fear of further abuse or embarrassment. If it is truly impossible to achieve privacy, it is acceptable not to explore violence issues, but this should be documented ("did not question about a history of physical or sexual abuse because of lack of privacy") in the record and a notation made to follow up later.

## Body Language

Shame and self-blame may make the patient sensitive to perceived criticism, so it is important that the clinician's body language and non-verbal cues convey a non-judgmental attitude. For example, squarely facing the patient with a relaxed and open body posture and making direct eye contact demonstrate a willingness to listen. Sitting on the same level (as opposed to standing or sitting on the edge of a high counter) conveys the sense that there is time to hear what is being asked and that the patient is an equal with the clinician. This respectful step, in and of itself, may increase the patient's sense of self-worth. It is also important not to interrupt the patient as she explains herself.

## Routine Screening for Violence

The procedure for identifying abuse differs based on the level of suspicion of ongoing abuse. Routine screening for violence is intended to uncover violence where violence is not suspected based on presenting complaint, physical examination, or other patient characteristics. Strategies for asking about violence when there is some suspicion that it has occurred and issues related to screening for childhood abuse or sexual trauma (rape) are addressed later in this chapter, although the general screening questions may be useful in these situations as well.

Screening for violence involves asking a few targeted questions, which can be incorporated into the medical interview. One of the first dilemmas is where to place the screening questions in the interview. Individual clinician styles vary, so there are a variety of options, including incorporating them into the otherwise routine discussion of sexual activity and contraception, social history, family history, or substance abuse. The American Medical Association recommends that violence screening should occur at every new patient visit and once yearly afterwards. Asking about abuse along with other health prevention measures (guns in the home, seat belt usage, calcium intake, etc.)

---

**Box 2-1    Introducing Screening Questions**

- "One of the things I ask all my patients about is their experiences of violence."
- "Because it is so common, I ask all my patients if they have been hurt by people close to them."
- "I ask all my patients about violence in their lives."

---

will normalize the screening process. The patient will sense that these questions are part of the clinician's routine and that she is not being targeted. A good time for screening is at the yearly physical when there is a general review of the patient's health.

Properly introducing the screening questions (Box 2-1) can be an important factor in the successful identification of individuals at risk. An opening statement such as "One of the things I ask all my patients about is whether violence affects their relationship" is a good way to ease into these questions. Another introduction is "Because it is so common, I ask my patients if they have been hurt by people close to them." By letting the patient know that this is a universal type of inquiry, the patient is less likely to feel singled out or ashamed.

Ideally, screening questions should have a high sensitivity: after screening all women, most women experiencing abuse should be identified. Another feature of a series of good screening questions is that they were developed from a pool of candidate questions. This pool of questions should be comprehensive and contain enough questions to cover all aspects of domestic violence. The questions should be based on behaviors (e.g., "pushed or slapped"), not labels ("abused"). There should be a well-defined gold standard or comparison standard against which candidate questions have been tested for efficacy. The questions should be easy to remember and use. Furthermore, the questions should not induce more shame than the woman may already feel. Questions should not express judgment. Finally, the questions should be validated in a separate study population.

When the available screening questions are scrutinized closely, each has positive features and, unfortunately, drawbacks. Most have not been developed in a scientifically rigorous manner, and some are too unwieldy for a short clinical interaction. We review the best of the available screening measures and describe instruments to screen for domestic violence, adult sexual trauma, child abuse, and elder abuse below.

## Screening for Domestic Violence

The Abuse Assessment Screen (AAS) is a commonly referenced set of screening questions, developed in an antenatal public clinic setting (18). The questions

---

**Box 2-2    Abuse Assessment Screen (AAS)**

---

- "Within the past year, have you been hit, slapped, kicked, or otherwise physically hurt by someone?"
- "Since you have been pregnant, have you been hit, slapped, kicked, or otherwise physically hurt by someone?"
- "Within the past year, has anyone forced you to participate in sexual activities?"

---

Adapted from McFarlane J, Parker B, Soeken K, Bullock L. Assessing for abuse during pregnancy. JAMA. 1992;267:3176-8.

---

in the AAS address the issues of physical violence and violence during sexual contact (Box 2-2). Using these questions, McFarlane et al identified that one in six pregnant women was abused. The standards of comparison were two research questionnaires on violence, but no sensitivity or specificity measures were calculated. The AAS questions focus on violence in the preceding year, thus missing important earlier history. Finally, using this screen may also fail to identify women who are emotionally abused but not physically or sexually abused.

The Partner Violence Screen (PVS) was developed as part of a large study assessing domestic violence prevalence in emergency department settings (Box 2-3) (19). Like the Abuse Assessment Screen, the focus is on experiences in the preceding year. Although both AAS and PVS screen for experiences of physical abuse, the PVS also explores the patient's perceived safety. There are three questions in this screen. Tested against the same two standards as the AAS, the sensitivity of the individual questions ranged from 64% to 71%. Using a prevalence of 24% of partner abuse in the past year, the negative predictive value of the PVS is 89% (20). This means that saying no to the screening questions correctly identifies 89% of these women as not having experienced abuse in the past year. The positive predictive value is much lower, 63%, which indicates that positive responses to the screening questions correctly identify partner abuse 63% of the time. With a lower prevalence in the population being screened, the screen is even less accurate.

Other screens are the HITS and the Woman Abuse Screening Tool (WAST). A written instrument, HITS (Hurts, Insults, Threatens, Screams) was developed to identify current physical or verbal abuse in the family practice setting (21). It comprises four questions, each with a 5-point Likert response scale (Box 2-4). HITS was tested in two study groups: 1) 160 female patients visiting a family practice clinic and 2) 99 women self-identified as victims of violence from domestic violence crisis shelters and emergency departments. A

---

**Box 2-3    Partner Violence Screen (PVS)**

- "Have you been hit, kicked, punched, or otherwise hurt by someone in the past year? If so, by whom?"
- "Do you feel safe in your current relationship?"
- "Is there a partner from a previous relationship who is making you feel unsafe now?"

Adapted from Feldhaus KM, Koziol-McLain J, Amsbury HL, et al. Accuracy of 3 brief screening questions for detecting partner violence in the emergency department. JAMA. 1997;277:1357-61.

---

**Box 2-4    HITS Screening Tool**

How often does your partner:
1. Physically Hurt you?
2. Insult you or talk down to you?
3. Threaten you with harm?
4. Scream or curse at you?

- There is a 5-point frequency format (*Never, Rarely, Sometimes, Fairly Often, Frequently*)
- Possible scores range from 4 to 20
- A HITS score ≥ 10.5 is positive for physical or emotional abuse

Adapted from Sherin KM, Sinacore JM, Li XQ, et al. HITS: a short domestic violence screening tool for use in a family practice setting. Fam Med. 1998;30:508-12.

---

HITS score of greater than 10.5 had a sensitivity of 96% and a specificity of 91% in correctly differentiating the patients in the family practice clinic from the self-identified violence victims. These validity measures should be interpreted with caution because the subjects' study group status (family practice vs. self-identified victim) is used as the reference standard for comparison. Advantages of HITS are that the written format allows for use on self-administered history intake forms and that the acronym is easy to remember. Interpretation of HITS requires calculating a score based on the patient's responses. Although the scoring system is straightforward, it may be cumbersome in a busy clinic setting.

WAST is a seven-question series that asks about abuse in a current relationship (Box 2-5) (22). Emotional aspects of abuse are considered but not sexual abuse. WAST was developed with residents of a battered women's shelter,

---

**Box 2-5    Woman Abuse Screening Tool (WAST)**

---

In general, how would you describe your relationship?
1. A lot of tension
2. Some tension
3. No tension

Do you and your partner work out arguments with
1. Great difficulty
2. Some difficulty
3. No difficulty

Do arguments ever result in your feeling down or bad about yourself?
1. Often
2. Sometimes
3. Never

Do arguments ever result in hitting, kicking, or pushing?
1. Often
2. Sometimes
3. Never

Do you ever feel frightened by what your partner says or does?
1. Often
2. Sometimes
3. Never

Has your partner ever abused you physically?
1. Often
2. Sometimes
3. Never

Has your partner ever abused you emotionally?
1. Often
2. Sometimes
3. Never

---

using the author's personal contacts for comparison. Although the scientific methodology is not ideal, WAST does have the advantage of starting with general questions that lead to more specific questions.

Expert opinion by some authors has suggested the use of a simple, open-ended question. Examples include "What happens when you and your partner [or boyfriend/ husband/ lover] get into a fight?" or "How does your partner treat you?"

---

**Box 2-6    Screen for a Lifetime of Intimate Partner Violence (STaT)**

- "Have you ever been in a relationship in which your partner has pushed or Slapped you?"
- "Have you ever been in a relationship in which your partner Threatened you with violence?"
- "Have you ever been in a relationship in which your partner has thrown, broken, or punched Things?"

---

Adapted from Paranjape A, Liebschutz J. STaT: a three question screen for intimate partner violence. J Womens Health. 2003; in press.

---

We recently developed a screen for lifetime intimate partner violence (including the domains of physical, sexual, and emotional violence) among emergency department patients (Box 2-6) (23). A positive response to any one of the three items on our screen, which is called STaT, has a sensitivity of 97%. A negative response to all three questions on STaT has a specificity of 75%. Assuming a prevalence of 35% lifetime history of intimate partner violence in the population being screened, the positive predictive value of STaT is 67%, and the negative predictive value is 97.4%. This means that 67% of women who answer yes to one or more of the questions have actually experienced intimate partner violence. In contrast, among women who answer no to all three questions only 2.6% have experienced intimate partner violence. Thus, a positive answer to one question makes a violence history quite likely, whereas a negative answer to all three questions essentially rules it out. Although the screen's questions do not directly address sexual trauma, these questions were actually found to be more sensitive for identifying sexual trauma than questions specifically addressing sexual assault. This is probably because sexual assault within the context of a relationship is almost always accompanied by physical abuse. This screen is awaiting validation in a larger sample.

## Screening for Adult Sexual Trauma

Sexual trauma may or may not occur within the context of an intimate relationship. Sexual trauma includes a spectrum of experiences, from sexual harassment to rape. Most standard questions on sexual assault incorporate three elements that define sexual assault: indications that sexual contact occurred, that there was coercion (force or threat of force), and that there was a lack of consent (or an inability to consent because of cognitive limitations, altered state of consciousness, or being a minor). A sexual assault that includes vaginal, anal, or oral penetration is often referred to as rape. Examples of screening

---

**Box 2-7    Suggested Screening Questions for Sexual Assault**

- "Have you had any sexual encounters that you did not want because you were forced, threatened with force, or because you felt you had to?"
- "Has anyone forced you to have sexual relations against your will?"
- "Has anyone made you have sex by using force or by threatening to harm you or someone close to you?"

---

questions for sexual trauma include "Have you had any sexual encounters you did not want because you were forced, threatened with force, or felt you had to?" or "Has anyone ever used force or the threat of force to make you have sexual relations against your will?" (Box 2-7). The CDC and National Institute for Justice jointly sponsored the National Violence Against Women Survey, which used separate questions for vaginal, oral, or anal penetration, and attempted rape (24). The questions all follow the same basic template used for vaginal intercourse: "Has a man or boy ever made you have sex (have oral sex, have anal sex, attempted to have sex) by using force or threatening to harm you or someone close to you?" In order to determine the accuracy of the answers to each question, the survey qualified each question with a statement such as "Just so there is no mistake, by 'sex' we mean putting a penis in the vagina." Narrowly focused questions are not likely to be useful to clinicians for primary screening purposes and do not address other potentially traumatic types of nonconsensual sexual contact (e.g., genital fondling or sexual assault perpetrated by another woman). We recommend using more general questions. There are no published data for sensitivity and specificity of sexual assault questions.

## Screening for Childhood Physical and Sexual Abuse, Including Incest

Unlike screening for intimate partner violence, screening for childhood abuse should occur at a first patient visit but does not need to be repeated every year. Questions about childhood abuse may be particularly useful to ask when there is suspicion of childhood abuse due to a diagnosis of somatization disorder or a chronic pain syndrome.

Questions on childhood sexual abuse differ from the general sexual assault questions in that they do not include coercion (because by definition a minor cannot give consent) but do have a broader definition of the sexual act and age at the time of the victim's abuse. The CDC-sponsored Behavioral Risk Factor Survey System used the following question for childhood sexual abuse: "Before you were 18, did anyone ever touch you in a sexual place or make you touch them when you did not want them to?" (25). Questions on childhood physical abuse specify the elements of age (less than 18), a perpetrator such as a parent or guardian or another trusted adult, and acts of violence. For example, the same survey asked, "Before you were 18, was there any time when you were punched, kicked, choked, or received a more serious physical punishment from a parent or other guardian?"

## Screening for Elder Abuse

Screening for intimate partner violence should not stop when a patient becomes elderly: the screening questions described above also apply to this population. Routine screening for elder abuse by someone other than an intimate partner is covered in Chapter 7. First, the clinician should establish who the patient's caregiver is, if any: "Who helps you with the things that you have trouble doing yourself?" This is particularly important if the clinician determines that the patient's cognitive capacity is limited (see Table 7-2 in Chapter 7). Next, the clinician should introduce a general question, such as "Do you feel safe where you live?" This should be followed by questions that probe for evidence of physical or sexual abuse, neglect, psychological abuse, and financial exploitation (see Box 7-4 in Chapter 7).

# Questions to Ask in Cases of Increased Suspicion

## Recognizing Signs of Abuse

In addition to screening all patients for a history of exposure to violence, it is important to ask about violence when elements of the clinical presentation increase the clinician's index of suspicion. Accordingly, clinicians should be familiar with the signs that suggest ongoing abuse. For example, the presence of multiple injuries or chronic somatic symptoms in the patient or hearing the patient describe controlling behaviors by her partner should increase the clinician's suspicion that the patient may be in a violent relationship.

Although many abusive relationships do not result in injury requiring medical attention, the possibility is high enough that a provider should suspect intentional violence whenever a patient presents with injuries of any type. Scenarios with an increased likelihood of intentional violence include inconsistencies between the patient's history and physical examination or a delay in seeking medical care for a significant injury. Common types of injury seen in battered women include injuries to the central parts of

*Screen for intentional violence when patients present with injuries of any type.*

the body (breasts, abdomen, or chest wall), multiple sites of injuries or those in different stages of healing, and repeated or chronic injuries (3). Chapter 3 discusses the clinical presentation of acute violence.

Numerous health care concerns other than acute injuries bring women experiencing domestic violence to their doctors' offices. These symptoms often take the form of chronic pain syndromes. Studies have shown that victims of abuse are more likely to present with chronic pelvic pain, irritable bowel syndrome, and frequent headaches (26,27). Such somatic symptoms should raise the index of suspicion for current or previous abuse. Depression and post-traumatic stress disorder (PTSD) also frequently occur in abused women. Sexual dysfunction, dyspareunia, and chronic pelvic pain should raise a suspicion for previous sexual trauma or current intimate partner violence.

Certain partner behaviors are characteristic in abusive relationships. An abusive and controlling partner may insist on being present for the physical examination, may hover near the examination room door, or may answer questions for his partner. Such behaviors should trigger questioning about abuse after ensuring privacy with the patient. Privacy can be obtained by insisting that the physical examination is always completed without observation by friends or family members.

## How to Frame the Questions

If the clinical presentation raises the possibility of abuse, the clinician needs to ask about it specifically because women usually do not volunteer information about abuse spontaneously. Some of the most potent emotions of an abused patient include intense shame and a perception of herself as abnormal (28). Furthermore, she may think that if no one says anything, then the abuse must not be bad enough to be noticed. To overcome these barriers, it is important to universalize the experience. For example, if a clinician says that he or she sees these problems in other patients, abuse can be seen as more of a "normal" problem seen in a health care encounter. One such approach might be, "Often when I see a woman with this kind of problem, it is because someone has hurt her. Has that happened to you?" This also lets the patient know that the clinician recognizes that there may be such a problem, thus breaking the feeling of invisibility. This approach is particularly helpful in the case of acute injuries.

In the case of chronic, unexplained physical symptoms (e.g., pain), the clinician must be cautious about using cause-and-effect language in order to avoid suggesting to the patient that the symptoms are "all in her head." For example, the clinician might say, "We know that there are a number of triggers that can lead to imbalances in the chemicals in our bodies that control pain. Experiencing violence is a common trigger, even if the violence happened long ago. Therefore, I ask all my patients who suffer from pain whether

---

**Box 2-8    Examples of Questions When There Is Suspicion of Abuse**

- "Often when I see a woman with this kind of problem, it is because someone has hurt her. Has that happened to you?"

- "We know that there are a number of triggers that can lead to imbalances in the chemicals in our bodies that control pain. Experiencing violence is a common trigger, even if the violence happened long ago. Therefore, I ask all my patients who suffer from pain whether they have experienced physical violence or have been forced to have sexual contact against their will. Has anything like that ever happened to you?"

- "Being in a relationship is often very difficult and can cause us lots of pain and suffering. Many women who have physical problems like yours have suffered from violence in their homes. Could this have happened to you?"

- "When I see problems like these in other patients, often they were hurt as children, either through harsh physical punishment or by being forced to be sexual with a grown-up or family member. Could this have happened to you?"

---

they have experienced physical violence or have been forced to have sexual contact against their will. Has anything like that ever happened to you?"

Other questions have been suggested and may be more appropriate for particular scenarios. These questions assign no blame and are more likely to draw out a history of abuse (Box 2-8).

## When the Physician Suspects But the Patient Does Not Disclose

There are many reasons why a patient might choose not to disclose abuse, even in response to direct inquiry. It is important to respect your patient's decisions about the timing of disclosure. Simultaneously, it may be useful to educate the patient and offer resources for help, even if she does not take advantage of them at that moment (see the Appendix).

> *Even if a patient does not disclose violence, providing education and referral information is useful.*

In qualitative interviews with abused women, the women recalled the advice they received from physicians as extremely useful, even if they did not take advantage of the advice at that time (28). Furthermore, education may pave the way for disclosure at a later visit.

Another important step is to refer the patient back to a clinician who knows her. Patients often have stronger, more trusting relationships with

clinicians they have seen on an on-going basis. A clinician treating a pat.
for a single time (e.g., an acute or episodic care visit) should ask the patient.
permission to inform her primary care physician of her condition and then
contact the primary care physician about the suspicion for abuse. If the patient says no, however, it is important to respect that decision. If it is a patient
with whom there will be follow-up visits, the clinician should periodically ask
about abuse at subsequent visits because it may take years before a patient is
comfortable enough to disclose abuse.

## Initial Response When the Patient Discloses a History of Abuse

### Empathetic Statements

One of the biggest questions for many clinicians is what to do once abuse is uncovered. There are a couple of general rules (much like the rules of asking about
abuse): maintain a non-judgmental
stance and show empathy and sincerity. Because a common characteristic of any violence is isolation
of the victim, a clinician's empathy
and sincerity can lessen the victim's
feeling of isolation and begin the healing process. At the same time, it is important not to re-create a powerless state in the patient by trying to "rescue"
her or "fix" the situation.

*Do not re-create a powerless state in the patient by trying to "rescue" her or "fix" her situation.*

Empathy can be expressed in a number of ways. Empathetic statements
should include an acknowledgement of pain or violation without judgement.
For patients who have experienced any sort of violence, useful statements include: "I can see how upset this makes you feel," "What you have gone through
seems very painful," "It must have been [lonely/scary/frightening/painful/ter-
rifying/upsetting] for you." Some clinicians disagree about using statements
such as "I'm sorry that this has happened to you" because this may provoke a
response such as "It's not your fault" from the patient. Other clinicians find it
to be a sincere expression of empathy.

### Neutralizing Shame and Guilt

A powerful role for the clinician is to help neutralize the patient's shame and
guilt. Survivors of trauma often feel responsible for the violence, particularly
if they have not yet recovered fully from the experience. Clinicians can neutralize this shame by letting the patient know that this is a common experience and by reminding the patient that violence is not an acceptable behavior
toward anyone. It is important not to dismiss provocative, angry, or inappropriate behaviors the survivor reports she exhibited before the abuse. She may
be convinced that her actions brought on the violence and will think that the

ally know" what happened. Rather, it is important to com-

nce is never an acceptable response to any behavior, no

priate the patient's behavior may have been.

; are listed in Box 2-9. A powerful statement that doesn't

e is the simple statement, "You don't deserve to be hurt,

no matter what." Examples of specific statements include "Although you were walking alone at night, you didn't deserve to be hurt," "Although you allowed your ex-husband to come into the house, you didn't deserve to be beaten up," and "I know you were drinking that night, but you didn't deserve to be raped."

### Avoiding Judgmental Questions

Questions such as "What did you do to provoke him?," "Why don't you just leave?," or "Why didn't you defend yourself?" should be avoided. They will be heard by a victim of abuse as judgmental. Instead, an open-ended inquiry about the circumstances of her abuse and the triggering factors of abuse ("Can you tell me what happened?") will convey an interest in the victim as a person; it may also help her verbalize feelings that she has not been able to articulate before.

## "Why Doesn't She Just Leave?"

Leaving an abusive relationship does not necessarily improve the outcome for victims of abuse. It may be that, in the long run, women who leave abusive relationships are safer. However, in the short term, the act of leaving or even contemplating leaving can precipitate dangerous levels of violence. The majority of deaths related to domestic violence occur around times of leaving. Therefore, clinicians should not be cavalier about advising women to leave an abusive relationship.

---

**Box 2-9    Empathetic Responses to Disclosure of Abuse**

- "No one deserves to be hurt by [someone they love/know/trust]."
- "You don't deserve to be hurt, no matter what."
- "I can see how upset this makes you feel."
- "What you have gone through seems very painful."
- "It must have been [lonely/scary/frightening/painful/terrifying/upsetting] for you."
- "Shame and guilt are common reactions to this [kind of violence/experience]."
- "I'm sorry that this has happened to you."

---

Numerous obstacles may prevent a woman from leaving an abusive relationship. These may include threatening behavior of the perpetrator (e.g., threats against her, her children, or her family), socioeconomic obstacles (e.g., the family wants the couple to stay together, the children would have to change schools), and obstacles relating to the woman's personal values (e.g., religious beliefs regarding divorce, issues of self-esteem, feelings of love and loyalty for her partner). These and other significant obstacles that prevent a woman from leaving an abusive relationship are discussed in greater detail in Chapter 1.

> *Leaving an abusive relationship may end the abuse but also ends the relationship's positive aspects.*

For women who do want to leave an abusive relationship, it is important to identify each of the barriers to leaving and to develop strategies to overcome them. Input from an expert (e.g., mental health professional) may be useful at this stage. Chapter 4 discusses strategies for mobilizing various support systems to help the patient decide when and how to leave the abusive situation as safely as possible.

## Safety Assessment

Once the patient has disclosed abuse, it is important to assess her risk of immediate danger. A number of studies have looked at the risks associated with homicide and serious injury from interpersonal violence. These retrospective studies provide only general associations and not specific causes. There are no prospective studies examining interventions to reduce serious injury or homicide because, although violent relationships are common, serious injury is a low-frequency event. The factors commonly associated with homicide or serious injury include a pattern of increasing frequency/severity of battering, the presence of firearms, substance abuse by either the patient or the perpetrator, a history of other violence (i.e., against people outside the home) by the perpetrator, and intense jealousy in the perpetrator. Table 2-2 presents questions that can be included in a standard safety assessment, including an assessment of the patient's risk of suicide.

### Increased Frequency and Severity of Battering

A pattern of escalating violence may predict subsequent injury or homicide. The escalating violence may occur in the form of more frequent abuse (once a week instead of once a month or once a year) or in the form of more serious injuries (ranging from bruises or cuts to contusions, burns, fractures, head

**Table 2-2    Questions to Ask in a Standard Safety Assessment**

| Risk Factor for Serious Injury | Questions |
|---|---|
| Overall safety | "Do you feel safe going home today?" |
| Increased frequency and severity of abuse | "When was the most recent time that you were hurt by your partner?"<br>"How about the time before that?"<br>"Has the violence gotten worse or more frequent?" |
| Presence of firearm | "Is there a gun in your home?"<br>"Has your partner ever threatened you with a knife or gun?" |
| Substance abuse | "Do you think your partner uses drugs or alcohol?"<br>"Is he intoxicated regularly?"<br>"What happens when he uses drugs or alcohol?"<br>CAGE-D questions (Box 2-10) |
| Other violent behaviors by partner or a criminal record | "Has your partner ever been arrested for any crime? Any violent crime?"<br>"Has your partner ever been violent outside the home?"<br>"Has he hurt pets or destroyed property?"<br>"Has anyone ever taken a restraining order out on your partner?" |
| Intense jealousy | "Does your partner try to control all aspects of your life?"<br>"Is your partner violently jealous?" |
| Suicide risk | "Do you think of suicide as a way out of the relationship?"<br>"Have you ever considered, threatened, or attempted suicide?"<br>"Do you have a plan for doing so?" |
| Homicide risk | "Do you ever think of killing or hurting someone as a way out of the relationship?"<br>"Have you considered killing or hurting someone or have you planned to kill or hurt someone?" |

injuries, and internal injuries). The murder or mutilation of pets can also increase the subsequent risk for serious human violence.

## Firearms

There is an association between the risk of serious injury or death and the use of firearms in interpersonal violence. A study of injuries from domestic assaults (intimate partner or other family member) showed that use of firearms increased the risk of death 12 times compared to other forms of violence (29). Just having firearms in the home confers an increased risk of homicide associated with domestic violence. A case control study in three counties in Tennessee, Ohio, and Washington examined the risk factors for violent death

---

**Box 2-10    CAGE-D Questions for Alcohol and Drug Abuse**

- "Have you ever felt you ought to Cut down on your drinking or drug use?"
- "Have people Annoyed you by criticizing your drinking or drug use?"
- "Have you ever felt bad or Guilty about your drinking or drug use?"
- "Have you had a drink or used drugs the first thing in the morning to steady your nerves or to get rid of a hangover?" (Eyeopener)

Adapted from Midanik L, Zahnd E, Klein D. Alcohol and drug CAGE screeners for pregnant, low-income women: the California perinatal needs assessment. Alcohol Clin Exp Res. 1998;22:121-5; and Bradley KA, Boyd-Wickizer J, Powell SH, Burman ML. Alcohol screening questionnaires in women: a critical review [see Comments]. JAMA. 1998;280:166-71.

---

of women in the home (30). If the perpetrator was an intimate acquaintance or a relative, a gun in the home was independently associated with a 7-fold increased likelihood of homicide.

## Substance Abuse

Substance abuse in either the victim or the perpetrator is associated with increased risk of death or serious injury by an intimate partner or family member. In the previously cited study on violent death of women in the home, use of illicit drugs in the home conferred a 28-fold increase in risk of death when the perpetrator was an intimate, relative, or close acquaintance (30). Alcohol abuse was shown to be associated with increased risk of death but was not an independent factor beyond a history of domestic violence (30). Multiple other studies of serious injury and death caused by interpersonal violence show an association with drugs and alcohol in both the victim and the perpetrator.

A well-validated screening tool, CAGE questions can be used to screen for alcohol abuse. Adding the phrase "and drugs" to the CAGE questions can also detect drug abuse (Box 2-10). Answering yes to one or more questions indicates risk of substance use disorder (31,32). For further discussion on the association between substance abuse and violence, see Chapter 10.

## Perpetrator Has History of Other Violent Behaviors

In studies of women who have incurred severe injuries from their partners, the perpetrators often had histories of violence outside the home as well. Male perpetrators of family violence who have criminal records for a wide variety of crimes, including property destruction, violence, and drug or alcohol-related crime, are more likely to fit a sociopathic batterer description. These men are more likely to use guns or other weapons and to commit more serious violent acts (33). Another indication of the potential of general violent behavior is the presence of an active or previous restraining order. A study of 18,369 men in Massachusetts evaluated the profile of men against whom a restraining order was issued for domestic violence. Seventy-five percent had previous criminal records, of whom two-thirds had convictions for violent offenses (34).

## Perpetrator Has a History of Intense Jealousy

In descriptions of perpetrators of family violence, controlling behaviors and intense jealousy appear to be associated with a risk of more severe injury. This has been noted in qualitative studies of battered women, as well as in case studies of homicides of women by their male partners. Examples of behaviors indicating a high level of jealousy include accusing the woman of having affairs, showing up unexpectedly at her work or home to make sure she is there, making her account for every minute of her day, and wiretapping her telephone.

## Suicide Risk

The patient's safety may be threatened not only by the perpetrator but also by herself: she may commit suicide. There is clearly an association between suicide attempts and a history of trauma, as described in Chapter 5. That may be because of severe depression or a sense that suicide is the only escape from the abuse. Although suicidal ideation by the patient has not been shown to be a risk factor for homicide by the partner, it does indicate a situation that is potentially lethal. Suicide screening therefore needs to be part of the safety assessment. Table 2-2 indicates some questions that can be useful when screening for suicide risk.

Occasionally, a woman may feel that killing the perpetrator is the only way to stop the continuing abuse or may become so enraged that she feels she must commit homicide. Examples of questions to ask regarding homicidal ideation are given in Table 2-2.

## What to Do After Risk for Serious Injury Has Been Assessed

If the patient reveals one or more risk factors for serious injury, the clinician may say to her, "I am concerned for your safety because you have some of the risks for serious injury or even death because of this relationship. Would you be willing to speak with someone about ways to keep you [and your children] safe?" When there is risk of suicide or homicide and the clinician has any doubt about the patient's ability to remain safe, the clinician will need to obtain a psychiatric evaluation with possible involuntary admission to a psychiatric facility (clinicians have to be familiar with local regulations regarding involuntary commitment). When there is evidence of child abuse, the clinician may need to file a report with the state department of protective services, depending on the laws in that region regarding mandatory child abuse reporting. Depending on the state, there may also be laws mandating reporting of partner violence, elder abuse, or abuse of people with disabilities (see Chapters 3, 7, and 9). Outside of these specific conditions, the level of action by the patient depends on her readiness to act and the resources available for her to draw upon. The patient should be encouraged to develop a safety plan. The clinician can help her with this by consulting with domestic violence advocates who have specific training in safety plan development. Such advocates can be consulted in person or through local or national hotlines. Local police forces that have domestic violence offices may also be used as a resource for safety planning (see Chapter 3).

A clinician can communicate to the patient that the condition of the relationship as she, the patient, describes it poses a risk of serious injury or death. Because the vast majority of abusive relationships do not result in serious injury or death, a clinician can be somewhat reassured if none of the above risk factors are present. Follow-up and referral after uncovering abuse is extensively outlined in subsequent chapters.

## Screening for Depression and Post-Traumatic Stress Disorder

### Depression

Because depression is a common mental illness associated with experiencing violence, it is important to evaluate victims of violence for undiagnosed depression. The DSM-IV criteria for diagnosing a major depressive episode are listed in Box 2-11. Major depressive disorder is defined by one or more major depressive episodes without mania and not caused by medical illness or substance use effects. SIGECAPS is a useful mnemonic for remembering some of the symptoms of depression:

- Sadness
- Insomnia or hypersomnia
- Guilt
- Energy loss
- Concentration difficulties
- Appetite change or weight loss
- Psychomotor retardation or agitation
- Suicidal ideation

---

**x 2-11   DSM-IV Criteria for Major Depressive Episode**

---

A. Five or more symptoms that have been present during the same 2-week period and represent a change from previous functioning. At least one of the symptoms is either depressed mood *or* loss of interest or pleasure.

1. Depressed mood most of the day, nearly every day, as indicated by subjective report or observation made by others
2. Markedly diminished interest or pleasure in all, or almost all, activities most of the day, nearly every day
3. Significant weight loss when not dieting or weight gain *or* decrease or increase in appetite nearly every day
4. Insomnia or hypersomnia nearly every day
5. Psychomotor retardation or agitation nearly every day (observable by others, not just subjective feelings)
6. Fatigue or loss of energy nearly every day
7. Feelings of worthlessness or excessive or inappropriate guilt nearly every day
8. Dimished ability to think or concentrate, or indecisiveness, nearly every day
9. Recurrent thoughts of death (not just fear of dying), recurrent suicidal ideation without a specific plan, or a suicide attempt or a specific plan for committing suicide

B. Symptoms cause significant distress or impairment in social, occupational, or other important areas of functioning.

C. Symptoms are not caused by direct physiological effects of a substance (medication/drug of abuse) or a general medical condition.

D. Symptoms are not caused by bereavement after the loss of a loved one. If such symptoms persist more than 2 months after the loss or are characterized by marked functional impairment, morbid preoccupation with worthlessness, suicidal ideation, psychotic symptoms, or psychomotor retardation.

E. No evidence of mania.

---

Adapted from Diagnostic and Statistical Manual of Mental Disorders. Washington, DC: American Psychiatric Association; 1994.

## Post-Traumatic Stress Disorder (PTSD)

PTSD does not occur in all cases of trauma but does occur in enough cases that a clinician should evaluate for undiagnosed PTSD when a history of domestic violence, sexual trauma, or childhood abuse is revealed. The DSM-IV criteria for PTSD are listed in Box 2-12. There are few short case-identification instruments for diagnosing PTSD and none that have been evaluated and published for

## Box 2-12  DSM-IV Criteria for Post-Traumatic Stress Disorder (PTSD)

A. Exposure to traumatic event in which:
1. The person experienced/witnessed or was confronted with events that involved actual or threatened death or serious injury, or a threat to the physical integrity of self or others;
AND
2. The person's response involved intense fear, helplessness, or horror

B. Re-experiencing the traumatic event through one or more of the following:
1. Recurrent and intrusive distressing recollections of the event, including images, thoughts, or perceptions
2. Recurrent distressing dreams of the event
3. Acting or feeling as if the event were recurring (including a sense of reliving the experience, illusions, hallucinations, dissociative flashback episodes)
4. Intense psychological distress at exposure to internal or external cues that symbolize or resemble an aspect of the traumatic event
5. Physiological reactivity on exposure to internal or external cues that symbolize or resemble an aspect of the traumatic event

C. Persistent avoidance of stimuli associated with the trauma and numbing of general responsiveness as demonstrated by three or more of the following:
1. Efforts to avoid thoughts, feelings, or conversations associated with the trauma
2. Efforts to avoid activities, places, or people that arouse recollections of the trauma
3. Inability to recall an important aspect of the trauma
4. Markedly diminished interest or participation in significant activities
5. Feeling of detachment or estrangement from others
6. Restricted range of affect
7. Sense of foreshortened future

D. Persistent symptoms of *increased arousal* as shown by two or more of the following:
1. Difficulty falling or staying asleep
2. Irritability or outbursts of anger
3. Difficulty concentrating
4. Hypervigilance
5. Exaggerated startle response

E. Duration of symptoms for >1 month

F. Symptoms cause significant distress or impairment in functioning in social, occupational or other important areas of functioning

Modifiers
*Acute*: duration of symptoms less than 3 months
*Chronic*: duration of symptoms 3 months or more
*Delayed onset*: onset of symptoms is at least 6 months after traumatic event

Adapted from Diagnostic and Statistical Manual of Mental Disorders. Washington, DC: American Psychiatric Association; 1994.

---

**Box 2-13    Short Screening Scale for DSM-IV Post-Traumatic Stress Disorder (PTSD)**

To be asked after disclosure of traumatic event(s).

*Yes to any three of the following five questions:*
1. "Do you avoid being reminded of this experience by staying away from certain places, people, or activities?"
2. "Have you lost interest in activities that were once important or enjoyable?"
3. "Do you feel more isolated or distant from other people?"
4. "Do you find it hard to have love or affection for other people?"
5. "Do you feel that there is no point in planning for the future?"

*Yes to both of these questions:*
6. "Since this experience, have you had more trouble than usual falling asleep or staying asleep?"
7. "Do you become jumpy or get easily startled by ordinary noises or movements?"

If the patient screens positive, refer to mental health professional for full diagnostic evaluation.

---

Adapted from Breslau N, Davis GC, Andreski P, Peterson E. Traumatic events and post-traumatic stress disorder in an urban population of young adults. Arch Gen Psychiatry. 1991;48:216-22.

---

non-psychiatric settings. One available instrument, a seven-symptom scale for lifetime PTSD, is given in Box 2-13 (35). Its questions feature symptoms of numbing, avoidance, and hyper-arousal because these tend to be more sensitive and specific for PTSD than symptoms of re-experiencing the event. If a patient appears to screen positive for the disorder, it is important to refer the patient to a mental health professional for full diagnostic evaluation (see Chapters 4 and 5).

# Patient Education

Although general knowledge of domestic violence dramatically increased in the 1990s, many women do not know what constitutes abuse or that there are resources to get help. Qualitative studies have shown that abused women found education about abuse and information about resources useful at a later time, even if they did not disclose abuse or discuss it with the clinician at the time (28). Thus, patient education can be an important intervention.

Patient education about domestic violence can be divided into two parts. The first part can include a simple explanation of behaviors that constitute an

---

**Box 2-14    Educating the Patient**

---

What Constitutes Abuse

- "When one partner controls the other person through things like financial control or isolation from family and friends, this may be a sign that the relationship is abusive."
- "Any relationship that involves threats of force or use of physical force may be abusive."
- "When a woman is forced to have sex without her consent, that is considered a sexual assault, even if she has been with that partner for a long time."

Resources for Help

- "There are people to talk to who can help women in abusive relationships."
- "There are places a woman [you] can go if she [you] want(s) to leave an abusive relationship."
- "I am here to help if you ever have a problem like this."

General Outreach

- "There are resources to help if you, a friend, or a family member ever experiences such a problem."

---

abusive relationship (Box 2-14). For example: "When one partner controls the other person through financial control or isolation from family and friends, this may be a sign that the relationship is abusive," "Any relationship that involves threats of force or use of physical force may be abusive," and "When a woman is forced to have sex without her consent, that is considered a sexual assault, even if she has been with that partner for a long time." It is particularly useful to have written material to give the patient. Many state domestic violence coalitions can supply medical practices with such materials at little or no cost (see the Appendix for phone numbers).

The second part of this focused education should provide the patient with resources for someone who experiences abuse. For example, a clinician may state, "There are people to talk to and places a woman can go if she wants to leave an abusive relationship." A very potent statement is "I am here to help if you should ever have a problem like this." This conveys caring on the part of the clinician, which is an important part of building trust in the provider–patient relationship. If there is low suspicion and the patient says no to all the screening questions, the clinician can end the discussion with "There are resources to help if you, a friend, or a family member should ever experience such a problem." This conveys the clinician's willingness to address such issues and acknowledges the widespread existence of abuse in our society.

# Summary

Identification of a history of interpersonal violence requires an environment of safety, trust, and adequate privacy. Disclosure of abuse may itself be an important therapeutic intervention for some women. A safety assessment including evaluation for depression and suicidality and other co-morbid conditions can help to assess the short-term risk of serious injury or death. These screens can appropriately focus subsequent interventions.

---

**Summary Box    Sample Screening Questions for Various Forms of Violence**

---

Introducing the Line of Questioning
- "One of the things I ask all my patients about is their experience of violence."

Screening for Lifetime Domestic Violence
- "Have you been in a relationship in which your partner has pushed or slapped you?"
- "Have you ever been in a relationship in which your partner threatened you with violence?"
- "Have you ever been in a relationship in which your partner has thrown, broken, or punched things?"

Screening for Current Domestic Violence
- "Do you feel safe in your current relationship?"
- "Is there a partner from a previous relationship who is making you feel unsafe now?"

Screening for Domestic Violence When There Is Suspicion of Abuse
- "Often when I see a woman with this kind of problem, it is because someone has hurt her. Has that happened to you?"

Screening for Sexual Assault
- "Have you had any sexual encounters when you did not want to because you were forced or threatened with force or felt you had to?"

Screening for Childhood Physical Trauma
- "Before you were 18, was there any time when you were punched, kicked, choked, or received a more serious physical punishment from a parent or other guardian?"

Screening for Childhood Sexual Trauma
- "Before you were 18, did anyone ever touch you in a sexual place or make you touch them when you did not want them to?"

Elder Abuse
- "Who helps you with the things that you have trouble doing yourself?"
- "Do you feel safe where you live?"

---

**Summary Box    Tasks for the Medical Practitioner**

---

Establish an Environment Conducive to Disclosure of Trauma
- Privacy
- Confidentiality
- Written materials in office area

All Patients
- Screen at new patient visits for all types of trauma
- Screen yearly for partner violence and elder abuse (if applicable)
- Educate about violence

Patients with Injuries, Chronic Somatic Symptoms, or Suspicious Partner Behavior
- Ask about violence
- Educate, even if she does not disclose trauma

Patients Who Disclose Violence
- Show empathy
- Perform safety assessment
- Screen for comorbid depression with suicidality and PTSD
- Refer to other social services (see Chapter 4)

---

# REFERENCES

1. Curnow SA. The open window phase: helpseeking and reality behaviors by battered women. Appl Nurs Res. 1997;10:128-35.
2. Council on Scientific Affairs, AMA. Violence against women: relevance for medical practitioners. JAMA. 1992;267:3184-9.
3. American Medical Association Diagnostic and Treatment Guidelines on Domestic Violence. Arch Fam Med. 1992;1:39-47 (published erratum appears in Arch Fam Med 1992;1:287).
4. US Preventive Services Task Force. Guide to Clinical Preventive Services. 3rd ed. Bethesda, MD; 2000-2002.
5. Rodriguez MA, Quiroga SS, Bauer HM. Breaking the silence: battered women's perspectives on medical care. Arch Fam Med. 1996;5:153-8.
6. Thompson RS, Rivara FP, Thompson DC, et al. Identification and management of domestic violence: a randomized trial. Am J Prev Med. 2000;19:253-63.
7. McCaw B, Berman WH, Syme SL, Hunkeler EF. Beyond screening for domestic violence: a systems model approach in a managed care setting. Am J Prev Med. 2001;21:170-6.
8. Saunders DG, Hamberger LK, Hovey M. Indicators of woman abuse based on a chart review at a family practice center. Arch Fam Med. 1993;2:537-43.
9. McLeer SV, Anwar RA, Herman S, Maquiling K. Education is not enough: a systems failure in protecting battered women. Ann Emerg Med. 1989;18:651-3.
10. Friedman LS, Samet JH, Roberts MS, et al. Inquiry about victimization experiences. Arch Intern Med. 1992;152:1186-90.

11. Rodriguez MA, Bauer HM, McLoughlin E, Grumbach K. Screening and intervention for intimate partner abuse: practices and attitudes of primary care physicians. JAMA. 1999;282:468-74.

12. Ferris LE, Tudiver F. Family physicians' approach to wife abuse: a study of Ontario, Canada practices. Fam Med. 1992;24:276-82.

13. Elliott L, Nerney M, Jones T, Friedmann P. Barriers to universal screening for domestic violence. J Gen Intern Med.1998;13(Suppl 1):121.

14. Sugg NK, Inui T. Primary care physicians' response to domestic violence. JAMA. 1992; 267:3157-60.

15. deLahunta EA, Tulsky AA. Personal exposure of faculty and medical students to family violence. JAMA. 1996;275:1903-6.

16. Freund KM, Bak SM, Blackhall L. Identifying domestic violence in primary care practice. J Gen Intern Med. 1996;11:44-6.

17. Thompson RS, Rivara FP, Thompson DC, et al. Identification and management of domestic violence: a randomized trial. Am J Prev Med. 2000;19:253-63.

18. McFarlane J, Parker B, Soeken K, Bullock L. Assessing for abuse during pregnancy. JAMA. 1992;267:3176-8.

19. Feldhaus KM, Koziol-McLain J, Amsbury HL, et al. Accuracy of 3 brief screening questions for detecting partner violence in the emergency department. JAMA. 1997;277: 1357-61.

20. DeHovitz JA, Kelly P, Feldman J, et al. Sexually transmitted diseases, sexual behavior, and cocaine use in inner-city women [see Comments]. Am J Epidemiol. 1994;140:1125-34.

21. Sherin KM, Sinacore JM, Li XQ, et al. HITS: a short domestic violence screening tool for use in a family practice setting. Fam Med. 1998;30:508-12.

22. Brown J, Lent B, Brett P, et al. Development of the woman abuse screening tool for use in family practice. Fam Med. 1996;28:422-6.

23. Paranjape A, Liebschutz J. STaT: a three question screen for intimate partner violence. J Womens Health. 2003; in press.

24. Tjaden P, Thoennes N. (National Institute for Justice and Centers for Disease Control and Prevention). Prevalence, incidence and consequences of violence against women. Findings from the National Violence Against Women Survey, 1998. November 2000.

25. Bensley LS, Eenwyk JV, Simmons KW. Self-reported childhood sexual and physical abuse and adult HIV-risk behaviors and heavy drinking. Am J Prev Med. 2000;18:151-8.

26. Alpert EJ. Violence in intimate relationships and the practicing internist: new "disease" or new agenda? Ann Intern Med. 1995;123:774-81.

27. Drossman DA, Talley NJ, Leserman J, et al. Sexual and physical abuse and gastrointestinal illness: review and recommendations. Ann Intern Med. 1995;123:782-94.

28. Liebschutz J, Rich J. Shame, mistrust and loss of control: a qualitative analysis of barriers between battered women and physicians [Abstract]. J Gen Intern Med. 1998; 13(Suppl):8.

29. Saltzman L, Mercy J, O'Carroll P, et al. Weapon involvement and injury outcomes in family and intimate assaults. JAMA. 1992;267:3043-7.

30. Bailey JE, Kellermann AL, Somes GW, et al. Risk factors for violent death of women in the home. Arch Intern Med. 1997;157:777-82.

31. Midanik L, Zahnd E, Klein D. Alcohol and drug CAGE screeners for pregnant, low-income women: the California perinatal needs assessment. Alcohol Clin Exp Res. 1998;22:121-5.

32. Bradley KA, Boyd-Wickizer J, Powell SH, Burman ML. Alcohol screening question-naires in women: a critical review [see comments]. JAMA. 1998;280:166-71.

33. Gondolf EW. Who are those guys? Toward a behavioral typology of batterers. Violence Vict. 1988;3:187-203.

34. Isaac NE, Cochran D, Brown M, Adams SL. Men who batter: profile from a restraining order database. Arch Fam Med. 1994;3:50-4.

35. Breslau N, Davis GC, Andreski P, Peterson E. Traumatic events and posttraumatic stress disorder in an urban population of young adults. Arch Gen Psychiatry. 1991;48:216-22.

# CHAPTER 3

# Patient Management After Acute Intimate Partner Violence or Sexual Assault

MITCHELL D. FELDMAN, MD, MPHIL

SARA L. SWENSON, MD

GINA A. MORENO-JOHN, MD, MPH

A cute, intentional, interpersonal violence can occur in many different contexts (Box 3-1). It may present as a single event or as recurrent episodes: each has different implications for diagnosis and management. This chapter addresses the management of patients who present for medical care after an incident of physical or sexual assault. Patients who present because of injuries or infections caused by the assault are the main focus, but patients for whom recent exposure to violence is discovered incidentally during the medical encounter are also discussed. Although the focus here is upon acute violence episodes, it is important to emphasize that intimate partner violence is generally a chronic issue that is best addressed through a treatment and intervention model akin to those for smoking cessation or chronic illness (1).

The patient who presents after an acute violence episode offers a unique opportunity for detailed assessment and intervention. Ideally, the treatment of an acute violence episode should set in motion referral, ongoing support, and efforts that can facilitate the patient's long-term ability to deal with the physical and emotional consequences of abuse. There are four general guidelines for transforming the medical treatment of an acute violence event into a successful violence intervention (Box 3-2).

> *An acute violence episode offers a unique opportunity for intervention.*

---

**Box 3-1    Contexts of Acute, Intentional, Interpersonal Violence**

- Domestic violence
- Nondomestic partner violence
- Acquaintance violence
- Anonymous assault
- Date rape
- Child abuse/incest
- Elder abuse
- Hate crimes

---

**Box 3-2    General Guidelines for Managing Acute Intimate Partner Violence/Sexual Assault**

- Incorporate evaluation/treatment into overall medical care.
- Remain attentive to power dynamics within the medical encounter.
- Adopt an interdisciplinary approach.
- Involve the primary care provider.

---

First, the clinician should incorporate evaluation and treatment of intimate partner violence and sexual assault into the medical treatment process. This can be accomplished by screening for acute violence, validating and supporting the patient's experience, obtaining a more detailed violence history, assessing for complicating factors such as substance abuse and mental illness, and devising a safety plan (see Chapter 2).

Second, the clinician must remain attentive to the dynamics of control and power within the medical encounter. Given the unequal power between medical providers and patients, the clinician unwittingly may cause the woman to re-experience the traumatic event. This may undermine her sense of control over her medical care. Thus, to the greatest extent possible, the clinician should give the patient a sense of control over her evaluation and treatment. This includes the clinician

*Give the patient a sense of control over her evaluation and treatment.*

explaining how he or she is going to touch the patient during the evaluation (before and during the physical examination, diagnostic procedures, and treatments) and requesting the patient's permission to perform an examination and provide treatment. The clinician should pay particular attention to communication and control issues during those portions of the examination outside of the patient's view, such as during the examination of the head, posterior torso, and pelvis. The clinician should encourage the patient to verbally communicate about or stop the evaluation if it is physically or emotionally uncomfortable.

Third, the clinician must adopt an interdisciplinary approach. The complex needs of domestic violence/sexual assault victims range from injury assessment and treatment, reproductive counseling, substance abuse, and other mental health treatment to housing and financial assistance, safety planning, and the placement of a restraining order. Even the most dedicated professional lacks the time and expertise to manage these issues alone. The clinician should, with the patient's consent, enlist the expertise of nurses, social workers, mental health professionals, law enforcement, and community domestic violence workers to formulate an ongoing treatment plan and ensure adequate follow-up (see Chapters 4 and 5).

Fourth, if the acute evaluation is performed by a clinician other than the primary care provider, the examining clinician should make every attempt to reconnect the patient with her continuity care provider. The treating clinician should obtain consent from the patient to contact and provide the primary care provider with clinical information.

## Acute Intimate Partner Violence

### Evaluation

*Clinical Presentation*
Detection of intimate partner violence requires a high index of suspicion. Most women do not spontaneously volunteer their history and rarely present with dramatic injuries. Instead, the clinician should look for clues in the history and physical examination that suggest intimate partner violence. For example, patients with nonspecific somatic symptoms (especially pain), psychological distress (including depression, suicidal ideation, and anxiety), and an illogical explanation for their injury or an explanation that is inconsistent with the presentation of the injury should be specifically screened for intimate partner violence. Similarly, clues in the physical examination such as soft tissue injuries, injuries at different stages of healing, and injuries to the central parts of the body (breasts, abdomen, and chest wall) all point to the possibility of intimate partner violence. Because intimate partner violence can present without any such clinical "red flags," screening for domestic violence should be a routine part of the care for patients seen in the acute setting (see Chapter 2).

*Initial Assessment*
When a woman presents for care in the aftermath of an acute violence episode, medical staff should take measures to ensure her safety and emotional well being during the evaluation and treatment. Before the full medical interview, the clinician should first evaluate the patient for injuries that require immediate attention. This should include the assessment and initial treatment of life-threatening injuries, pain, extreme anxiety, and/or emotional dissociation.

Interpreters, if required for patients who do not speak English, should be professional, hospital-affiliated translators rather than friends or family members (see Chapter 11 for more details on use of interpreters). All friends and family should be asked to leave the room during the medical interview and physical examination. Violence may occur in same-sex relationships, and it may also be perpetrated by female relatives and personal care attendants of vulnerable or elderly persons. Thus, clinicians should not assume that a patient's female friend, care provider, or family member can safely be present. Moreover, fear of future retaliation leads some women to request that the perpetrator remain in the examination room: a patient who makes such a request should be re-questioned in private regarding her preferences. If a woman continues to feel unsafe or fearful in the medical setting, staff can post security officers outside the examination room. If the patient is admitted, similar precautions may be necessary to ensure her safety. However, it is important to recognize that security officers may escalate the perpetrator's anger and vindictiveness. Clinical judgement should be used in deciding how to optimize the safety of the patient and health care staff. Clinicians should check with the hospital security department to be sure there is a plan in place for violent visitors and should familiarize themselves with the protocol.

### The Medical Interview

#### ASSESSING FOR A HISTORY OF VIOLENCE

Taking a history from a patient in the aftermath of an acute violence episode can be difficult even for an experienced clinician. When abuse is suspected, the medical interview must be handled carefully to help the patient feel comfortable in disclosing the history of violence. First, the clinician should prepare for the interview by assessing the physical environment. Is the room private and quiet? Will the room enhance the patient's sense of safety and comfort? Do seating arrangements allow enough personal space for the patient? Does she have access to an exit should she feel overly threatened during the interview? Next, the clinician must prepare himself or herself with the aims of minimizing internal and external distractions and enhancing focus on the patient. The clinician should also attempt to eliminate outside intrusion by asking co-workers to take phone calls, hold beepers, and prevent other interruptions.

Patients generally favor a direct approach, even when being asked about the details of an acute violence episode. Leading with open-ended questions helps to create a safe, comfortable environment while providing an opportunity to assess the patient's emotional state. Having accomplished this, the clinician should use direct, non-judgmental questions. He or she should

*Ask the patient direct, non-judgmental questions.*

also phrase the questions in a way that suggests that such injuries are not usual, so that the patient does not feel that she is abnormal. For example, the clinician can ask, "Many people come in with injuries like yours, and often they are the result of a family member or partner hurting them. Is this what happened to you?" (Other questions to ask and ways to frame them are discussed in greater detail in Chapter 2.) Even women with obvious injuries may not consider themselves to be victims of battering, assault, abuse, or intimate partner violence; thus, these terms are best avoided. The clinician should also refrain from attempts to coerce the patient into revealing a past or present history of violence.

The clinician should strive to conduct the interview itself in a nonjudgmental, empathetic manner. Empathy is an underutilized therapeutic skill that can help the patient feel safe and promote a sense of support and trust. In the context of an acute violence episode, helpful techniques for communicating empathy include (2):

- *Reflect:* "You seem frightened."
- *Legitimize:* "I can understand why you would feel upset."
- *Partner:* "We can work together to help you feel better."

Early in the interview, the clinician should attempt to diminish any feelings of shame that the patient may have by clearly stating that others have suffered from intimate partner violence, that such violence is unacceptable, and that the patient is not responsible for what happened. The clinician should avoid questions that imply that the patient is responsible for the violence, for example, questions such as "Why don't you leave him?" or "What did you do to make him mad?"

### AFTER A HISTORY OF VIOLENCE HAS BEEN DISCLOSED

If the patient admits to a violence-related injury or illness, the clinician should then attempt to establish a chronology of the violence by asking about the first episode, most recent episode, and most serious episode (3). Assessing the patient's safety is essential. The clinician should ask about the presence of risk factors for serious injury or homicide. These risk factors are discussed more fully in Chapter 2.

*Assessing patient safety is essential.*

The patient should be encouraged to develop an emergency escape and/or a safety plan. The clinician can help her directly by brainstorming about strategies, but consultation with a trained domestic violence advocate is also recommended, either in person or by using a local or national hotline. Hotline staff receive extensive training in safety-plan development. Local police forces sometimes have specific domestic violence offices that also help with such

---

**Box 3-3    Risk Factors for Serious Injury or Homicide**

- Increasing frequency and severity of violence
- Presence of firearms in the home or in the possession of the perpetrator
- Substance abuse by either the patient or perpetrator
- History of other violence (i.e., against others outside the home)
- Intense violence in the perpetrator

---

*Intimate partner violence often escalates when the woman attempts to leave the abuser.*

planning. It is imperative to educate the patient that partner violence often escalates as the woman leaves, or attempts to leave, the relationship with the abuser. Thus, a woman who plans not to return home should inform co-workers and the person(s) with whom she will stay about the potential for ongoing violence attempts against herself or those close to her.

Finally, if the patient has children the clinician should ask whether they have witnessed or experienced the violence. Clinicians should be aware of resources for abused children in their region and of laws regarding mandatory child abuse reporting (see Appendix).

The clinician should also evaluate the patient's emotional state during the initial medical encounter and assess for depression, acute stress disorder, suicide risk, and other psychological distress. Many abused women meet the diagnostic criteria for post-traumatic stress disorder (PTSD). Consequently, clinicians working with domestic violence and sexual assault victims should learn how to screen for PTSD and acute stress disorder. Depression is also common in intimate partner violence victims. An estimated 25% of abused women will attempt suicide, and of those half will try more than once. Moreover, up to one-third of such suicide attempts take place on the day of a medical encounter for violence-related injuries. Thus, clinicians should screen for depression, and particularly for suicidal and homicidal ideation. Screening for PTSD, depression, and suicide risk are explained in detail in Chapter 2.

The patient should also be assessed for other mental and behavioral disorders often seen in women with a violence history, including eating disorders, panic or other anxiety disorders, sexual difficulties, and substance use. Of note, the clinician may detect an apparent discordance between the patient's emotional state and the history of recent trauma. For example, even though the patient has just been assaulted she may appear unusually calm or hypersexual. She may also be confused and have a fragmented memory of the assault.

Patients with PTSD or severe depression should generally be offered prompt psychiatric evaluation. Emergency intervention may be necessary for patients with suicidal or homicidal ideation. Clinicians need to be familiar with local regulations regarding involuntary commitment. Most states have similar regulations for involuntary commitments for individuals at risk for harming themselves or others or not being able to care for themselves because of a psychiatric illness. It can be traumatic to involuntarily commit the patient, so mental health experts need to work closely with the patient.

*Physical Examination*

MINIMIZING PATIENT DISCOMFORT

The physical examination often represents a particularly threatening or uncomfortable part of the medical encounter for a recently traumatized woman. To support the patient through this portion of the evaluation, the clinician should pay special attention to the issues of power and control, as well as the need for a team approach as outlined above. Before the patient disrobes, the clinician should explain what the examination will entail and request the patient's permission to conduct the examination. The clinician should remind the patient that she can stop the examination at any time.

> *Remind the patient that she can stop the examination at any time.*

OVERALL SURVEY

Even when the complaint is localized, every patient should be asked to undress for a complete physical examination. This allows the clinician to evaluate and treat unseen injuries and to assess for signs of previous injury or abuse. The examination should be performed with the patient's consent and only after its rationale has been explained. A chaperone should be present if indicated. Regardless of whether or not she has disclosed or admitted to abuse, the clinician should explain that he or she routinely checks all patients who have an injury in one area of the body for injuries in other areas, even if the patient is not aware of any other injuries.

The physical examination should begin with vital signs, including temperature to assess for infections such as pelvic inflammatory disease; weight and an evaluation of overall nutritional status; and general appearance as indicators of possible neglect or forced isolation. The skin should be examined for signs of recent or old trauma such as scars, abrasions, ecchymoses, and fractures; thermal injuries or other burns; and rashes indicative of sexually transmitted diseases. To avoid detection, intimate partners typically injure central parts of the body concealed by clothing. Thus, examination should include visual inspection of the breasts, careful abdominal examination for signs of internal trauma and tenderness suggestive of pelvic inflammatory disease or urinary tract infection, and chest and back evaluation for rib fractures or costo-vertebral angle tenderness indicating possible renal contusion or pyelonephritis. Ear-nose-throat evaluation should include visualization of the oropharynx for gonorrhea or other sexually transmitted disease, missing teeth, and tongue or mucosal lacerations. More detailed examinations should be tailored to the individual injuries encountered, such as ophthalmologic and ear-nose-throat evaluation for facial injuries and focused musculoskeletal examination for possible sprains or fractures.

Forced sex, unprotected intercourse, and unplanned pregnancy are common manifestations of intimate partner abuse, particularly in adolescents. Moreover, many sexual assault victims do not initially report this history on presentation to the emergency department or urgent care setting. Consequently, clinicians should consider performing a pelvic examination and pregnancy test in the context of any acute violence episode, not only after disclosed sexual abuse. The evaluation and management of pelvic injuries, rape, and sexual abuse are covered in the section, Acute Sexual Assault Episode.

DETECTION OF TRAUMATIC INJURIES

Physical abuse causes a variety of injuries, including contusions, hematomas, abrasions, lacerations, burns, sprains, and fractures (Box 3-4). When

---

**Box 3-4    Common Injuries Resulting from Intimate Partner Violence**

Central Injuries
- Breasts, abdomen, chest, back, or genitals

Repetitive Injuries
- Injuries in different stages of healing
- Frequent visits for trauma or "accidents"
- Radiographic evidence of multiple old fractures

Injury Types
- Pattern injuries
- Thermal injuries (cigarette or appliance burns)
- Water immersion injuries
- Human bite marks
- Fingertip contusions, especially on nonexposed areas
- Nasal/orbital fractures
- Spiral wrist fractures
- Injuries not explained by patient history

a woman presents for treatment of trauma-related injuries, three features should heighten suspicion of intimate partner abuse: a pattern of central body injuries, evidence of frequent or repetitive injuries, and specific types of injuries.

Accidents or other unintentional trauma generally produce peripheral injuries, such as contusions, lacerations, or wrist/ankle fractures. As mentioned earlier, women who have been hurt by their partners are more likely to suffer injuries to central areas of the body such as their breasts, abdomen, or chest than non-battered trauma patients and are much more likely to sustain injuries to the head, neck, or face.

The strongest predictor of intimate partner violence is the frequency, rather than severity, of injuries. Providers should look for clues such as frequent visits for treatment of "accidents" or trauma, ecchymoses or injuries in various stages of healing on physical examination, and evidence of multiple old or recent fractures on radiographic studies.

*Frequency of injuries, rather than severity, is the strongest predictor of intimate partner violence.*

Certain types of injury should also prompt consideration of abuse as the etiology. Spiral wrist fractures or fingertip contusions on normally protected areas, such as inner arms or thighs, often indicate forceful grabbing. Pattern injuries, areas of central clearing surrounded by lines produced by the impact of an object, are characteristic of battering and may indicate the specific weapon that produced the injury. For example, imprints of baseball bats, fly swatters, combs, and shoe soles leave distinctive markings. According to some forensic pathologists, the most common pattern injury is that produced by the human hand. Other suspicious injuries include rug burns; the semi-circular imprints of human bites; thermal injuries from cigarette burns, household appliances, or hot-water immersion; and nasal or orbital fractures. Finally, injuries that suggest a defensive posture or struggle on the part of the patient or inconsistencies between the patient's explanation of injury causality and the anatomic location or type of injury observed should also alert clinicians to the possibility of domestic assault.

The clinician should also assess the patient for signs of sprains and/or fractures. These include localized ecchymoses, swelling, stiffness, or pain; increased pain with weight-bearing or movement of the affected area; and evidence of "step-off" injuries, dislocations, point tenderness, or joint instability. Sprains and strains are diagnosed by mechanism of action and physical evaluation. Sprains are classified as grade I (minimal injury), grade II (some muscle fiber injury), and grade III (muscle fiber tear and joint instability).

# Treatment

The acute treatment of injuries related to intimate partner violence is by and large identical to standard trauma management with a few important exceptions. First, although pain medications and anxiolytics can be helpful to many women who have experienced recent trauma, health care providers should weigh the risks against the benefits. Over-sedation or medication side effects may impair the woman's capacity to make decisions, execute a safety plan, protect herself and her children, or utilize available escape options.

Second, shock, feelings of dissociation or emotional numbing, and physical pain can compromise a woman's ability to comprehend and recall information during the medical visit. Verbal instructions should generally be supplemented with written handouts that cover treatment plans, medication side effects, injury management, follow-up appointments, and referrals to domestic violence hotlines or shelters. Some experts caution, however, about the potential hazards of providing written information. For some women, the discovery of such handouts by their abusive partners may precipitate further violence or intensified coercion and isolation. Clinicians should therefore decide on an appropriate means of information provision and follow-up through discussion with the individual patient. If written discharge instructions are provided, they should avoid mentioning the cause of injuries.

Treatment of specific violence-related injuries conforms to guidelines for the management of traumatic injuries more generally. Ice and non-steroidal anti-inflammatory agents can reduce the swelling and inflammation associated with contusions and hematomas. Patients can use make-up to cover visible injuries but, unfortunately, hematomas can take weeks to resolve. Analgesics such as acetaminophen aid in pain relief.

# Referral and Follow-up

At the conclusion of the visit, clinicians and staff need to arrange for appropriate referral and follow-up. They should remember that intimate partner violence is a long-term process and that any intervention after an acute violence episode represents the initial step in the woman's ongoing care. Some issues, such as treatment of severe depression or the management of post-exposure HIV prophylaxis, require immediate identification and referral for close follow-up. Others, such as substance abuse, long-term housing assistance, or financial planning, may best be addressed during subsequent visits. At the very least, all women should receive the number of a

*Any intervention after acute violence represents the initial step in the woman's ongoing care.*

24-hour domestic violence hotline, the locations and numbers of local battered women's shelters, and appointments for medical and social work follow-up. Patients should be referred back to their primary care provider, and permission should be requested for the treating clinician to directly contact the primary care provider. This is especially crucial when dealing with abused adolescents because many fail to keep appointments for follow-up care (4). See Chapter 4 for information regarding referral services and resources.

## Documentation

It is imperative that clinicians document clearly and completely when caring for victims of intimate partner violence. If the abused woman decides to pursue legal remedies, her credulity may be called into question if corroborating information cannot be found in the medical record. The record should include a complete description of the assault with quotes, if possible, from the patient's own account. It should also incorporate pertinent details of the social and past medical history and of the patient's current emotional state. Likewise, it is important that the chart notes be clear and legible. Successful prosecution should never be compromised by sloppy record keeping. The physician will generally be called to testify in person only if the written record is unclear.

The medical record should clearly indicate that the patient reports the injuries were the result of intimate partner violence. Phrases such as "the patient alleges" or "claims" should be avoided because they imply that the clinician does not believe the patient's account. Instead, phrases such as "the patient states" or "the patient reports" can be used. The patient's account of what parts of her body were injured, who inflicted the injuries, what happened, where she was when it happened, and when it happened should be recorded. If the patient denies abuse, the clinician should also document whether the nature and location of the injuries are inconsistent with the patient's explanation for them. For example, the clinician should state not only that the patient attributes her black eye to walking into a door, but also why the injury in question is suggestive of abuse and how the injury might have been inflicted. The chart should also note the names and actions of any other parties who participate in the evaluation, including medical consultants, social workers, domestic violence staff, and/or investigating officers.

Additionally, clinicians should utilize a body map (Fig. 3-1) or color photos to describe and visually document all injuries. Before taking photographs, the clinician should explain the rationale for photographic documentation, ask the patient's permission, and have her complete a written consent form. In order to connect the injuries to the patient, photographs should consist of a full body photo (including the head) and close-ups of each injury (5). Photos should include a ruler or other scale to convey the injury's size. The clinician

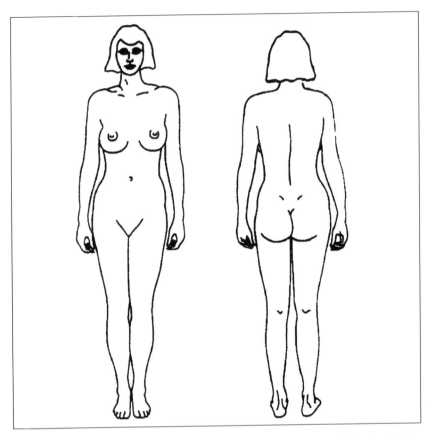

**Figure 3-1**  Body map to document injuries. (Adapted from Warshaw C, Ganley AL. Improving the Health Care System's Response to Domestic Violence: A Resource Manual for Health Care Providers. Family Violence Prevention Fund in collaboration with the Pennsylvania Coalition Against Domestic Violence.)

should place the patient's name and date on the back of each photograph and give the patient a full set for her records (provided doing so will not place her in more danger). Torn or blood stained clothing should be described, photographed, or preserved as corroborative evidence of physical trauma.

## Acute Sexual Assault

### Evaluation

Although the legal definition of rape varies by state, from a clinical perspective sexual assault is the use of force or threats to have sexual contact against

> ## Box 3-5    History-Taking After Sexual Assault
>
> * When and where the assault took place
> * All forms of sexual contact (including oral and anal contact)
> * All forms of injury
> * Mood
> * Pain or areas of discomfort
> * Patient behaviors after the assault (e.g., changing clothes, showering, bathing, douching, brushing teeth, enema use)
> * Previous episodes of sexual assault
> * Menstrual and sexual history
> * Contraceptive and/or STD prevention methods
> * Assailant's identity or description (if known)
> * Assailant's communicable disease status and risk factors (if known)
> * Assailant's use of weapons or other objects

the victim's will (see Chapter 1 for definitions of rape and other forms of sexual assault.) The incidence of reported rape has consistently increased since 1965, with lifetime prevalence estimates ranging from 6% to 22% (3). However, because of under-reporting, especially of partner rape, rates of sexual assault in the context of intimate partner violence remain uncertain.

### Approach
It is not the clinician's job to determine whether the charge of rape is valid. Rather, the clinician should evaluate and treat injuries, diagnose and manage sexually transmitted diseases and pregnancy, collect and preserve evidence, and protect against further physical and emotional consequences. Because of the need for accurate forensic evidence, as well as the myriad medical and mental health issues confronting survivors of sexual assault, most hospitals and clinics have developed specific sexual assault/rape protocols. Clinicians should check with hospital emergency department or acute care staff for locally mandated protocols. Community rape crisis centers and domestic violence organizations can also provide such information.

*It is not the clinician's job to determine whether a charge of rape is valid.*

### History
The medical interview should address all forms of sexual contact during the assault because up to one-third of sexual assaults include oral or anal penetration (Box 3-5). Physical evidence is rarely recovered more than 48 to 72 hours

after the event, although physical evidence of injury may persist for longer. Thus, the clinician should ascertain when the assault took place and use this information to guide evidence collection during the physical examination. The clinician should also inquire and document whether the patient changed, showered, bathed, douched, cleansed her mouth, or used an enema after the assault because these alter evidence retrieval. The history should include any previous episodes of sexual assault. The use of contraceptive and/or STD prevention methods as well as information pertaining to the assailant's communicable disease status and risk factors, if known, should likewise be determined. The clinician should also obtain the woman's menstrual and sexual history in order to assess her risk for pre-existing or rape-related pregnancy.

*Documentation*

A legal case, if pursued, will typically examine three issues: that sexual contact occurred, that it was nonconsensual, and that force or threat of force was used. Any sexual contact (e.g., vaginal penetration with the assailant's penis, with another body part, or with an object; oral or anal penetration; or other forced contact with genitalia) should be documented. If applicable, documentation should include evidence that contact was nonconsensual (e.g., patient's report that she struggled physically or verbally rebuffed the assault, or the patient's report that she was too frightened to resist or that her capacity to consent was impaired by intoxication). However, if the victim did not struggle, she should not be made to feel guilty or to feel that this implied consent. Likewise, it is important to diminish guilt in women who may feel that they brought this on themselves by being careless about their safety (walking alone at night, drinking too much and then being alone with the rapist) or by being sexually provocative on purpose. The use or threat of force, including the use of weapons or other objects, threats against children, etc., should be clearly recorded.

Although it is not the clinician's role to prove or disprove the patient's account, documentation of the event should facilitate, rather than impede, the patient's legal case should she decide immediately or later to pursue one. The clinician should thoroughly record the history, examination, and assessment in clear, non-technical terms so that a layperson can understand them. Abbreviations should be avoided. The medical chart should also note the patient's general medical condition and other evidence of trauma because such documentation provides legal corroboration of the assault. As always, photographs and body maps should be incorporated into the medical record. However, clinicians should remember that a well-documented diagram of physical injury can be more useful in legal proceedings than a poorly taken photograph.

# Physical Examination

There are often standard protocols and rape kits employed in the examination of sexual assault victims and staff trained in these protocols in each hospital. A typical rape kit might include instructions, a camera, specimen containers, tweezers for evidence collection, cotton swabs, and saline, among other things. Physicians should be prepared to follow standard protocols or work with trained staff because protocols may vary by state.

In order to avoid re-traumatization, the clinician should be particularly attentive to ensuring the woman's sense of safety and control during the physical examination. Once the clinician excludes life-threatening injury and ensures that the batterer is not present, he or she should ask whether the patient would like a medical assistant, domestic violence counselor, friend, or relative to be present during the examination. A chaperone may protect both the patient and the clinician, and some state medical societies recommend a chaperone for any pelvic examination regardless of the gender of the clinician. It is important for the patient to feel in control during the examination process. Before forensic evaluation, the patient should give her consent to examination, clothing and specimen collection, and photographs. Before beginning, the clinician should remind the patient that she is in control and can refuse or postpone any aspect of the evaluation. Orienting the patient to examination maneuvers and briefly explaining their rationale also help to assuage fear and discomfort. If after these steps the patient refuses any aspect of the examination, the clinician may attempt to modify potentially painful procedures (with the patient's permission) and/or reiterate their importance. Ultimately, however, the clinician should respect patient refusals and document them in the medical record (6).

The physical evaluation should include the entire body, as stated earlier. Clothing, especially if altered in the attack; debris such as grass, fibers, or weapon fragments; and bodily secretions like blood and semen should be collected, labeled, and preserved appropriately in containers according to instructions in the rape kit. Evaluation of bite marks by a forensic dentist may also prove helpful. Other potential bodily evidence includes debris under fingernails and saliva testing for acid phosphatase, which provides evidence of sperm deposition.

## Pelvic Examination

The examiner should begin by observing the external genitalia, including the pubic hair, urethra, and perianal area, for signs of injury or forced intercourse (bleeding, lacerations, swelling, hematomas, semen) or other trauma (cigarette or other burns, foreign bodies). The hymen or hymenal remnants should be evaluated and described. During the speculum examination, the examiner should look for similar evidence of trauma to the vaginal walls or cervix. The urethra, vagina, cervix, and rectum should be inspected for abnormal discharge, and samples should be obtained for wet mount, gram stain, culture, and DNA testing (see the Sexually Transmitted Diseases section below). Bimanual examination should focus on uterine sizing for potential pregnancy and signs of pelvic inflammatory disease, such as cervical motion tenderness and uterine or adnexal masses or pain. If examination reveals signs of peri-anal trauma or disease, the clinician should perform a digital rectal examination or anoscopy. Colposcopy may also be able to detect gynecological injury that was not visible without magnification.

### Semen Analysis

In cases of suspected sexual assault, careful examination and laboratory evaluation for semen and/or sperm comprise an essential part of the evaluation. Any areas of penetration or attempted penetration (oral, vaginal, anal) should be sampled with swabs and/or washings and tested for sperm, prostatic antigens, and DNA typing, if available through the rape kit protocol or a local laboratory. The clinician should examine wet preparations of swabs or washings under a 40x microscope for sperm. Although sperm are visualized after only 30% to 40% of sexual assaults with vaginal intercourse, the presence and motility of sperm may prove invaluable for estimating pregnancy risk and the timing of the assault. Motile sperm can be observed up to 6 (and rarely 12) hours after penetration, and non-motile sperm may be seen from 12 to 18 (and rarely up to 24) hours after intercourse. Two additional vaginal smears should be collected and dried for later use.

### Treatment of Trauma and Bleeding

Because the perineum is very vascular, lacerations may bleed profusely and large hematomas can develop. For any open wounds or lacerations, pressure should be applied to control bleeding. If hemostatis is difficult to maintain, further treatment options include the use of a vaginal pack to produce constant pressure on large lesions, repair of lacerations or tears with absorbable sutures, and/or ligation of bleeding vessels. In addition to the above, rapidly expanding hematomas may require surgical drainage and suturing. The clinician should remove, label, and preserve any foreign bodies. Injuries should be cleaned and repaired according to standard surgical procedure. Subsequent follow-up treatment may include pain medication and cold compresses to reduce swelling. Patients should also be educated regarding warning signs for secondary infections or sexually transmitted diseases. Consultation with a gynecologist may be indicated in the short-term or for follow up.

### Detection and Treatment of Sexually Transmitted Diseases

This section focuses on the management of acute STD exposures. However, clinicians should remember that patients may present long after the initial exposure, such as during routine PAP smears or when symptoms first appear. Although scant evidence exists regarding the risk of STD infection after sexual assault, the risk after an isolated incident is thought to be low (7). Nonetheless, because most sexual assaults involve unprotected sex, medical providers must incorporate STD detection and treatment into the acute gynecological evaluation.

DETECTION

As described above, external and internal examination both include inspection for signs of sexually transmitted diseases, such as ulcers or vesicles (suggestive of herpes, syphilis, chancroid, or lymphogranuloma venereum), papules or condylomata (suggestive of human papilloma virus or secondary syphilis), and pelvic lice. Even in asymptomatic patients, the clinician should routinely obtain cervical specimens for culture of *Neisseria gonorrhoeae* and culture or polymerase chain reaction (PCR) testing for *Chlamydia trachomatis*.

Options for chlamydia testing include culture of cervical secretions, PCR of cervical cells, or urinalysis with ligase chain reaction (LCR) for *C. trachomatis* DNA. The latter two methods exhibit high sensitivity and specificity with the use of proper specimen collection. All methods of chlamydia testing involve collection of the endocervical or urethral columnar epithelial cells infected by the organism. Thus, when performing cervical PCR testing, clinicians should first thoroughly clean off any remaining secretions from the cervical os. They should then place a second, non-wooden (because wood may be toxic to the organism) swab or endocervical brush inside the cervical canal, rotate the swab in the cervical os several times for a total of at least 20 seconds, and place it in the appropriate collection media. Alternatively, clinicians can utilize urine LCR testing. Again, proper sample collection is paramount; clinicians should instruct patients to collect only the first 10 cc of voided urine. If oral or anal penetration occurred, clinicians should also collect pharyngeal and/or anal cultures for *N. gonorrhoeae* by utilizing the same collection method as for cervical cultures to sample the posterior oropharynx and/or anal mucosa, respectively. In addition, clinicians should routinely collect samples of vaginal discharge for wet mount and culture of *Trichomonas vaginalis* and, if clinically indicated, wet mount and KOH for bacterial vaginosis and yeast.

If vesicles are present, the clinician should perform cultures for herpes simplex by opening an intact lesion, swabbing the lesion base, and sending the swab in viral medium for culture. Evaluation of genital ulcers should include culture for herpes simplex virus, as well as slides for gram stain and dark field microscopy for *Treponema pallidum*. In a patient with ulcers, the clinician should also consider slide preparation for direct immunofluorescence for *T. pallidum* and, especially in a patient with painful ulcers or supporative inguinal adenopathy, culture or PCR for *Haemophilus ducreyi*. The clinician should evaluate signs of urethral trauma and/or urinary tract infection with urinalysis and, if indicated, urine gram stain and culture.

In addition, the Centers for Disease Control (CDC) recommends collecting serum samples for syphilis, hepatitis B, and viral load and/or antibody testing for HIV (8). HIV testing should be done only after the clinician (or other appropriate health care worker) has discussed the rationale, risks, and benefits of HIV testing with the patient and obtained her written consent for testing. Such discussions should include an explanation of the medical rationale for viral load versus baseline antibody testing, the meaning of a positive or negative test, incidences of false-positive and false-negative test results, potential legal ramifications of HIV testing, availability of anonymous versus confidential testing, and options for post-exposure prophylaxis (PEP) (see discussion below). Although HIV viral load tests are quite accurate in most clinical situations, currently available tests exhibit false-positive rates of 5% to 10% among asymptomatic persons with low pre-test probabilities of infection. Consequently, most experts do not routinely advocate viral load determinations as part of standard PEP protocols. However, HIV sero-conversion in the context of sexual assault carries significant legal implications. Thus, despite the anxiety and potential harm engendered by a false-positive HIV test, we concur with the CDC recommendations that clinicians should discuss and offer HIV viral load and concurrent HIV antibody testing to make the diagnosis of primary infection for sexual assault survivors. Follow-up antibody testing should be performed as described below.

POST-EXPOSURE PROPHYLAXIS AND TREATMENT

Rates of follow-up after an initial medical evaluation for sexual assault may be as low as 50%. Many authorities therefore recommend routine prophylaxis for sexually transmitted disease after the acute event. Although the efficacy of prophylactic STD treatment after sexual assault is unknown, the CDC recommends empiric treatment regimens for bacterial vaginosis, trichomonas, chlamydia, and gonorrhea (Box 3-6) (discussion of HIV prophylaxis is presented below). The clinician should consider optimizing treatment adherence by using single-dose azithromycin for chlamydia treatment rather than the traditional 7-day course of doxycycline. Treatment options differ slightly for treatment of pharyngeal, urethral, and anal STDs. The patient should also receive vaccination for hepatitis B, with the first injection of the series occurring during the initial medical encounter. Hepatitis immune globulin need not be administered (7). In addition, the patient should receive risk reduction counseling regarding transmission of any sexually transmitted diseases (including HIV) that may have been acquired during the sexual assault (8). She may wish to include her sexual partner(s) in this counseling process.

Patients with genital ulcers should also be treated for ulcerative sexually transmitted diseases according to standard treatment guidelines. Women

---

**Box 3-6    Recommended Treatment Regimens for STD Prophylaxis or Treatment Following Sexual Assault***

---

Vaginal Infections

| Ceftriaxone | 125 mg IM × 1 dose (gonorrhea) |
| *plus* | |
| Metronidazole | 2 g PO × 1 dose (trichomonas) |
| *plus* | |
| Azithromycin* | 1 g PO × 1 dose, *or* |
| Doxycycline* | 100 mg PO bid × 7 days (chlamydia) |

Uncomplicated Pharyngeal, Rectal, or Urethral Infections

| Ceftriaxone | 125 mg IM × 1 dose, *or* |
| Ciprofloxacin† | 500 mg PO × 1 dose, *or* |
| Ofloxacin* | 400 mg PO × 1 dose (gonorrhea) |
| *plus* | |
| Azithromycin | 1 g PO × 1 dose, *or* |
| Doxycycline | 100 mg PO bid × 7 days (chlamydia) |

Treatment of Pregnant Women

| Ceftriaxone | 125 mg IM × 1 dose, *or* |
| Spectinomycin‡ | 2 g IM × 1 dose (gonorrhea) |
| *plus* | |
| Erythromycin base | 500 mg PO qid × 7 days, *or* |
| Amoxicillin | 500 mg PO tid × 7 days (chlamydia) |
| *plus* | |
| Metronidazole | 2 g PO × 1 dose (trichomonas) |

---

From Centers for Disease Control and Prevention. Guidelines for treatment of sexually transmitted diseases. MMWR. 1998;47:61-2, 74-5, 110.

* Doxycycline and ofloxacin are contraindicated in pregnant and lactating women. The efficacy and safety of azithromycin in pregnant and lactating women is uncertain.

† Contraindicated for pregnant and lactating women and women <18 years old.

‡ The efficacy of spectinomycin in pharyngeal infections is 52%, so this treatment regimen should be followed up by pharyngeal culture.

---

with findings suggestive of primary genital herpes should receive antiviral therapy and counseling. In cases where doubt exists as to the etiology of the ulcerative disease, clinicians should consider empiric treatment for syphilis and, in communities with significant prevalence of *H. ducreyi* infection, chancroid (7). For suggested treatment regimens, see Box 3-7. Under certain circumstances, the clinician should consider PEP for HIV after sexual assault; this is discussed below.

**Box 3-7    Recommended Treatment Regimens for Treatment of Ulcerative Sexually Transmitted Diseases***

Genital Herpes

| | |
|---|---|
| Acyclovir | 400 mg PO tid × 7–10 days, *or* |
| Acyclovir | 200 mg PO 5×/day × 7 –10 days, *or* |
| Famciclovir | 250 mg PO tid × 7–10 days, *or* |
| Valacyclovir | 1 g PO bid × 7 –10 days* |

Primary or Secondary Syphilis

| | |
|---|---|
| Benzathine penicillin G | 2.4 million units IM × 1 dose[†] |

Chancroid

| | |
|---|---|
| Azithromycin | 1 g PO × 1 dose, *or* |
| Erythromycin base | 250 mg IM × 1 dose, *or* |
| Ciprofloxacin | 500 mg PO bid × 3 days, *or* |
| Erythromycin base | 500 mg PO qid × 7 days |

From Centers for Disease Control and Prevention. Guidelines for treatment of sexually transmitted diseases. MMWR. 1998;47:19, 21, 31-3.

* Treatment duration can exceed 10 days if complete healing has not occurred.

[†] Alternative regimens for penicillin-allergic patients include doxycycline 100 mg PO bid × 4 days or tetracycline 500 mg PO bid × 4 days.

Follow-Up

The high no-show rates for follow-up after sexual assault make it imperative for clinicians to establish a therapeutic alliance during the initial encounter, to provide a clear plan for follow-up care, and to emphasize its importance. The clinician should make the patient an appointment for follow-up evaluation 2 to 3 weeks after the assault; ideally, the patient should return to the same clinician or her own primary care provider so that continuity of care can be ensured. (It is important for the clinician to obtain the patient's permission to contact the primary care physician.) At follow-up, the clinician should re-examine the patient and search for signs of persistent STD infection. This visit also provides an opportunity for confirming appropriate wound healing and excluding recurrent abuse. Any symptoms or signs of the latter should prompt re-testing, and possibly re-treatment, for chlamydia, gonorrhoea, ulcerative diseases, and/or blood-borne pathogens. Persistent symptoms may indicate medication non-adherence, misdiagnosis, antibiotic resistance, and/or immuno-suppression. If clinically indicated, patients should undergo repeat pregnancy testing. If initial results of HIV and syphilis testing are negative, patients should have repeat serologic testing at 6, 12, and 24 weeks (7).

POST-EXPOSURE PROPHYLAXIS FOR HIV

Although reports exist of HIV transmission after sexual assault, the risks of transmission after specific exposures during forced sexual contact are unknown. Evidence regarding the efficacy and safety of PEP for HIV infection is also lacking; however, non-randomized studies of AZT prophylaxis after percutaneous exposures among health care providers have demonstrated transmission risk reductions of 81% (9). Thus, in appropriate clinical situations, clinicians should provide HIV counseling and discuss prophylaxis options with victims of sexual assault. Although the window of maximum therapeutic efficacy remains unclear, data from animal studies suggest that prophylaxis is most effective during the first 1-2 hours after exposure (9). Most experts recommend against prophylaxis if the person presents more than 72 hours after exposure (9). Consequently, decisions regarding prophylaxis must be made during the initial medical encounter, despite the inopportune timing of such discussions in the immediate wake of an acute violence episode.

Decisions regarding HIV prophylaxis will depend on several factors: the assailant's known or estimated HIV status, the time elapsed between exposure and presentation, the type of exposure during assault (with the highest risks of transmission occurring during anal or vaginal penetration and oral penetration with ejaculation), patient factors that increase transmission (e.g., genital ulcers, tears, lacerations, or open wounds), underlying medical co-morbidities, existing or potential pregnancy, and the local epidemiology of HIV. Given the relative complexity, potential toxicity, and paucity of data regarding effectiveness and long-term outcomes of PEP in this setting, the patient's preferences and her motivation and ability to adhere to anti-retroviral treatment should also factor into the decision-making process.

There are no data about the risk of PEP in pregnancy. The risk of teratogenicity is highest in the first trimester, as with any medication. Because of this, it is important to evaluate the likelihood of exposure to HIV in weighing the risks and benefits of PEP during pregnancy, particularly during the first trimester. This is more commonly dealt with among health care workers who get needle sticks than with victims of sexual assault; in the former case, a great effort is made to test the index case (i.e., the patient whose blood was on the needle).

Patients who decide to undergo prophylaxis should receive education about proposed treatment regimens. As of December 2002, the recommended PEP antiviral regimen consists of either zidovudine 300 mg orally twice daily plus lamivudine 150 mg orally twice daily (also available in a single pill as combivir, one pill orally twice daily) for 28 days. Alternative regimens include stavudine 40 mg orally twice daily plus didanosine 200 mg orally twice daily (or 125 mg orally twice daily if the patient's weight is less than 60 kg) for 28 days. When the exposure is high-risk and the assailant is known to be HIV-infected, some recommend adding a non-nucleoside reverse transcriptase inhibitor or protease inhibitor, particularly if the assailant has advanced HIV disease, a high viral load, and/or current or previous anti-retroviral treatment. Ideally in such circumstances, prophylactic regimens should be based on the individual assailant's suspected viral resistance patterns and determined after consultation with an HIV specialist.

Patients should be monitored closely for medication adherence, drug toxicity, and symptoms or signs of acute HIV seroconversion. Clinicians can explore adherence issues by asking patients directly how and when they are taking their medications, what side effects they experience, and the frequency and timing of missed doses. Laboratory assessment should include complete blood counts and liver and renal function tests at baseline, at 2 weeks, and at 4 weeks. Serum should also be drawn for HIV antibody testing at baseline (to assess for pre-existing infection) and at 6, 12, and 24 weeks. Serum HIV RNA should also be drawn at baseline.

TREATMENT OF HIV

The clinical manifestations of primary HIV infection generally appear from one to several weeks after infection and consist of fever (greater than 80%), maculopapular rash (40% to 80%), pharyngitis (50% to 70%), lymphadenopathy (40% to 70%), and myalgias and arthralgias (50% to 70%) (10). In addition to obtaining HIV antibody and HIV RNA at baseline, individuals who develop symptoms of primary HIV infection should undergo repeat concurrent testing for HIV viral load and p24 antigen, as well as HIV antibody testing to confirm the diagnosis. With those patients who test positive, given the increasingly complex and changing nature of HIV pharmacologic regimens, clinicians should work in close consultation with and/or refer HIV-positive patients to physicians experienced in the management of HIV disease. Additional information and up-to-date management recommendations can be obtained from the HIV Hotline (888-HIV-4911 or http://pepline.ucsf.edu/PEP/pepnet.html), the California AIDS Hotline (415-863-2437), or the San Francisco AIDS Foundation (www.sfaf.org). In addition, the national PEP registry for non-occupational exposures can be reached by telephone at 877-HIV-1PEP.

*Pregnancy and Emergency Contraception*

Depending on the time of a sexual assault and its proximity to the patient's encounter with the medical provider, urine or serum pregnancy testing and/or emergency contraception should be offered. If the sexual assault took place more than 12 days before the medical evaluation, a urine pregnancy test can diagnose pregnancy with near perfect accuracy. If the rape occurred at least 7 days before the evaluation, the sensitivity of a quantitative serum β-HCG approaches 100%. Patients who have negative pregnancy tests but were assaulted during the previous 7 days or in whom a high clinical suspicion of pregnancy exists should undergo repeat testing at subsequent follow-up.

If the initial medical evaluation occurs within 72 hours of the assault, the woman should receive counseling about and prescriptions for emergency contraception, regardless of the timing of her menstrual cycle. Appropriate regimens include pre-packaged "morning after" pills or oral contraceptive agents plus an anti-emetic. The FDA has approved two commercial emergency contraception kits. The first method, Preven, contains a urine pregnancy test plus progesterone-estrogen combination pills. The more recent, Plan B, consists of a progesterone-only preparation, which results in a lower incidence of nausea, better adherence, and, consequently, higher efficacy. All exhibit high efficacy if used appropriately. For example, if used within 72 hours after intercourse, the regimen of two Ovral pills immediately and two pills 12 hours later is up to 98% effective at preventing pregnancy. Table 3-1 lists additional emergency

### Table 3-1   Emergency Contraception Regimens

| Regimen | Hormonal Content/Pill | Dose (No. of Pills)* | Pregnancy Rates (per 100) |
|---|---|---|---|
| No method | — | — | 8 |
| Plan B | 0.75 mg levonorgestrel | 1 | 1.1–2.9 |
| Preven | 50 µg ethinyl estradiol 0.25 mg levonorgestrel | 2 | 2–3.5 |
| Ovral | 50 µg ethinyl estradiol, 0.5 mg norgestrel | 2 white | Approximately 2 |
| LoOvral | 30 µg ethinyl estradiol, 0.3 mg norgestrel | 4 white | † |
| Nordette/Levlen | 30 µg ethinyl estradiol, 0.15 mg levonorgestrel | 4 orange | † |
| Levora | 30 µg ethinyl estradiol, 0.15 mg levonorgestrel | 4 white | † |
| Trilevlen, Triphasil | 30 µg ethinyl estradiol, 0.125 mg levonorgestrel | 4 yellow | † |
| Trivora | 30 µg ethinyl estradiol, 0.125 mg levonorgestrel | 4 pink | † |
| Alesse | 20 µg ethinyl estradiol, 0.1 mg levonorgestrel | 5 pink | † |
| Levlite | — | 5 pink | † |
| Ovrette | 0.075 mg norgestrel | All 20 | † |

* Take first dose immediately (within 72 hours of unprotected intercourse); repeat dose times one 12 hours later.
† Unknown.

contraception options. Some states have begun to make Preven and Plan B over-the-counter medications. Adolescents and women who experience ongoing sexual abuse and are consequently at continued risk for forced and/or unprotected sex should receive counseling about long-term contraception and offered methods that they can control and use without their partners' knowledge.

### Treatment of Psychological Outcomes

The psychological effects of sexual assault can be profound, ranging from emotional numbing, anger, guilt, and future relationship difficulties, to reactive depression, post-traumatic stress disorder, substance abuse, and suicide. However, many patients have delayed reactions to sexual assault and should consequently undergo screening for depression and other psychological effects both acutely and during subsequent follow-up.

The majority of sexual assault survivors experience significant adverse psychological outcomes. For example, in the initial months after sexual assault, up to 24% of women experience symptoms that meet the diagnostic criteria for depression, and up to 20% make suicide attempts. Twenty-five percent to 40% develop long-term sexual dysfunction, and 50% undergo separation from their partner or spouse in the initial 2 to 3 years after the assault (4,6). Post-traumatic stress disorder is a common sequela of sexual trauma and may persist for many years after the assault. Thus, the clinician should refer all such patients for mental health and primary care follow-up. In addition, the clinician should educate the patient that rape is an act of violence rather than one of sexual passion or desire and that no one deserves to be raped or sexually assualted. Specific strategies for reassuring and empowering the sexual assault survivor resemble those discussed in Chapter 2. These strategies include showing empathy and concern and diminishing the patient's sense of shame and guilt. Clinicians should not ask questions that sound judgmental, such as "What did you do to defend yourself?" or "What do you believe led to the sexual assault?"

> *Rape is an act of violence, not sexual desire.*

## Sexual Abuse of Minors

Although the management of adolescent sexual assault survivors shares many features of adult sexual abuse, several significant distinctions exist. These include high prevalence rates, greater risks of physical, emotional, and socioeconomic sequelae after assault, and the adolescent's legal status as a minor. Unfortunately, the highest incidence of sexual assault occurs during adolescence, where prevalence rates approach 15% (4). Given under-reporting, particularly of assaults by acquaintances, dates, or relatives, this figure probably underestimates the actual incidence of sexual abuse in this population.

An essential component of caring for adolescent survivors of sexual assault entails reinforcing that no one has the right to force them to have a sexual experience against their will, regardless of the social context (e.g., dating, family, or intimate relationship) or their own actions or behavior (e.g., attire, consent to kissing or foreplay, previous sexual experiences, or lack of "active" refusal). Adolescents, like adults, need to hear that sexual assault is an act of violence, not an expression of sexual desire.

In most cases, the parent or legal guardian should be present during the physical examination. Although the clinician should obtain informed consent from the adolescent for the examination, photos, and evidence collection, a parent or legal guardian should also sign consent forms, if feasible. However, if the minor needs acute treatment and a guardian is unavailable, the clinician should treat immediately. Moreover, before including any family, legal guardians, or friends, the clinician must ensure that they did not perpetrate or facilitate the assault.

*Before entrusting minors to family or friends, make sure they did not perpetrate the assault.*

Before the evaluation, the clinician, nurse, and/or qualified social worker should meet privately with the adolescent to ascertain whether the assailant has accompanied her to the visit, explore whom the patient trusts to be present during her evaluation, and obtain her permission before communicating information to and/or inviting participation from family members or legal guardians. Because of the legal ramifications involved in the medical treatment of minors (see the section on legal considerations below), the clinician should carefully document the adolescent's concerns and the rationale for not obtaining parental consent.

History, physical examination, and specimen collection should follow the outlines given above. Again, attention to the adolescent's safety and sense of control is of paramount concern. If appropriate, the clinician should utilize a pediatric speculum for the pelvic examination. Clinicians should use language that is appropriate to the patient's age and education to explain all procedures briefly, particularly with patients who have never previously undergone pelvic examinations.

Most consequences of adolescent sexual assault resemble those found in adults. For example, adolescents may exhibit increased medical disorders (chronic pain syndrome), psychiatric sequelae (depression, substance abuse, suicide), and behavioral problems (self-destructive behaviors). However, adolescents are at special risk for several medical and psychiatric sequelae. The presence of cervical ectropion probably places adolescent women at increased risk for contracting HIV and other sexually transmitted diseases, such as chlamydia and human papilloma virus. Adolescent women with a history of sexual assault also experience higher incidences of such eating disorders as bulimia nervosa. Given this population's high prevalence of sexual assault by family members and friends, adolescents frequently leave home to escape their abusers. Post-traumatic stress disorder may present differently in children and adolescents than it does in adults; for example, behavioral problems may be prominent (see Chapter 5). Such adolescents consequently face risks of homelessness, school drop-out, street violence, and prostitution, all of which have their myriad short-term and long-term sequelae. Suicide rates are also particularly high for adolescent survivors of sexual assault, with reports of suicide attempts in 20% of patients not referred to mental health specialists after an assault (4). We therefore recommend routine consultation with and referral to mental health providers for all adolescents who present after sexual assault.

Finally, because follow-up rates are low, children and adolescents must receive all education, treatment, protection information, and referrals at the time of acute presentation. Because parents may display reactions of guilt, anger, and helplessness, clinicians should also offer them support or resources and/or refer them to appropriate community organizations (see Chapter 4 and the Appendix).

## Mandatory Reporting and Other Legal Considerations

Clinicians must educate themselves about the reporting requirements for domestic violence/sexual assault in their state. At present, only two states (California and Colorado) have laws requiring the reporting of all domestic violence to local law enforcement. Other states mandate reporting of certain injuries incurred under specific circumstances, and a few have no reporting provisions at all. It remains to be seen if the possible unintended negative consequences of mandatory reporting laws (e.g., decreased detection rate secondary to victims' concerns about safety and confidentiality) outweigh their presumed benefit. Reporting laws pertaining to the sexual assault of adolescents also differ by state. Again, physicians should contact local legal experts regarding applicable legislation in their own jurisdictions.

Clinicians should also be aware of legal options available to the victim of violence. For example, a battered woman may choose to obtain a protection order (e.g., a restraining order or an emergency protective order) that requires the perpetrator to stay away from her residence, workplace, and/or person for a specified period of time. Women may also seek court orders that specify custody and visitation arrangements for children. Other legal options include legal separation, divorce, and child and spousal support. These may be particularly useful because batterers often use children to access and control their partners. Women may also elect to press criminal charges against the perpetrator, either immediately after the assault or after some deliberation. Pressing charges can lead to a range of emotions, from feelings of empowerment to feelings of fear, shame, guilt, or depression, especially if the woman does not prevail in court. Women often appreciate exploring these feelings with a mental health provider.

Physicians and other staff involved in the care of the patient may be required to appear in court to testify. Physicians should rely on the legal patient record of the patient's health. The patient's and/or clinician's attorney can typically brief the clinician on what to expect in court. Emotions related to the assault can affect the victim's presentation in court and even lead to inconsistent testimony. Accordingly, the clinician may need to testify to the victim's emotional state and its potential impact on her own testimony.

Concerns about requirements for obtaining parental consent before treating an adolescent add another layer of complexity to the management of sexual assault in this age group. In general, health providers cannot provide medical treatment to a non-emancipated minor without the permission of the parents or legal guardians. However, in most states, exceptions exist for the care of minors in cases of suspected child abuse or neglect. All states provide for the treatment of sexually transmitted diseases without parental consent, and federal privacy laws have secured the provision of contraception and family planning services to minors. Moreover, many states have legislation that specifically pertains to the management of adolescent sexual assault survivors. For example, under California law, an adolescent can consent to medical diagnosis, treatment, and evidence collection after sexual assault. However, clinicians must inform such a patient's parents or legal guardians unless the latter are suspected of perpetrating the abuse. Clinicians should also document any efforts to contact the patient's parents or guardians. Such regulations differ state by state; clinicians should consult with social workers or legal advisors at their local institutions for details of their state's specific regulations.

## Summary

Clinicians frequently come into contact with victims of intimate partner violence and sexual assault and should feel comfortable screening for violence and treating the acute symptoms of violence. Detection requires a high index of suspicion, a skillful medical interview, and a familiarity with the cardinal signs and symptoms of violence. Successful management depends on the clinician remaining attentive to the dynamics of power and control within the medical encounter, adopting an interdisciplinary approach, and "closing the loop" by referring the patient back to her continuity care provider. Careful documentation in the medical record, familiarity with local reporting requirements, and appropriate referral to other medical and community services are also key. Treating survivors of domestic violence and sexual assault should be a standard aspect of medical practice and medical education.

---

**Summary Box    Acute Intimate Partner Violence: Key Management Issues**

◊ Screen for violence routinely in the emergency department or urgent care setting.
  • Maintain a high index of suspicion for violence, especially if the clinical presentation includes injuries, nonspecific somatic symptoms, and/or psychological distress.
  • Assume that some patients may not disclose interpersonal violence.
◊ Establish a safe environment throughout the screening and evaluation.
  • Communicate empathy through reflective listening and validation.
  • Seek the patient's permission before examining her.
  • Partner with the patient to create a care plan.
◊ Evaluate the patient.
  • Examine for injuries (including evidence of multiple previous injuries).
  • Test for sexually transmitted diseases, including HIV.
  • Test for pregnancy.
  • Determine psychological distress (depression, post-traumatic stress disorder).
  • Determine current safety (risk of escalation of violence; risk of suicide).
◊ Treat injuries using standard trauma management with specific modifications.
  • Pain medications/anxiolytics if appropriate; however, bear in mind that oversedation or medication side effects may impair the woman's ability to make decisions and to execute a safety plan.
  • Shock may impair a woman's comprehension or memory of medical instructions.
◊ Document the examination clearly and in detail in the medical record.
  • Use the patient's own words to describe the situation.
  • Consider body maps and/or photographs.
◊ Arrange follow-up in primary care.
◊ Arrange appropriate referrals, e.g., mental health, social services, and legal services.
◊ Follow local law regarding reporting requirements.

---

**Summary Box    Acute Sexual Assault: Key Management Issues**

- Establish a safe environment for the evaluation.
- Take a detailed history (Box 3-5).
- Test for sexually transmitted diseases (including HIV), pregnancy, and semen (if within 24 hours of assault).
- Screen for depression, acute stress disorders, and suicidal ideation.
- Treat injuries.
- Consider prophylaxis for sexually transmitted diseases, HIV, and emergency contraception (within 72 hours of assault).
- Offer mental health referral (on emergency basis if indicated); offer referral to social services and legal services.
- Document clearly (e.g., diagrams, photographs).
- Schedule follow-up within 2-3 weeks after the assault (sooner if indicated).
- Act in accordance with local laws on reporting requirements.

---

## REFERENCES

1. Stark E, Flitcraft A. Woman battering. In: Wallace RB, ed. Public Health and Preventive Medicine. Stamford: Appleton and Lange; 1998:1231-8.

2. Egener B. Empathy. In: Feldman MD, Christensen, JF. Behavioral Medicine in Primary Care: A Practical Guide. Stamford, CT: Appleton and Lange; 1997:8-14.

3. Rose DS. Sexual assault, domestic violence, and incest. In: Stotlard N, Stewart D, eds. Psychological Aspects of Women's Health Care: The Interface between Psychiatry and Obstetrics and Gynecology. American Psychiatric Press; 1993:447-83.

4. Holmes M. Clinical management of rape in adolescent girls. Patient Care. 1999;4:42-63.

5. San Francisco Family Violence Council Health Care Committee. The San Francisco Domestic Violence Health Care Protocol: A Guideline for Practitioners. San Francisco: San Francisco Family Violence Council; 1997:8-9.

6. Hicks DJ. The patient who's been raped. Emerg Med J. 1998;11:106-20.

7. Centers for Disease Control and Prevention. Guidelines for treatment of sexually transmitted diseases. MMWR. 1998;47:RR-1.

8. Katz MH, Gerberding JL. The care of persons with recent sexual exposure to HIV. Ann Intern Med. 1998;128:306-12.

9. Centers for Disease Control and Prevention. Management of possible sexual, injection drug-use, or other non-occupational exposure to HIV, including considerations related to antiretroviral therapy. Public Health Service Statement. MMWR. 1998;47:RR-17.

10. Kahn JO, Walker BD. Acute HIV type I infection. N Engl J Med. 1998;339:33-9.

# CHAPTER 4

# Referral to Mental Health and Social Services

SUSAN M. FRAYNE, MD, MPH

GLENN N. SAXE, MD

PATRICIA ROBINSON, MSW, LICSW

The social, emotional, and economic forces that perpetuate violence can be enormous and beyond the scope of ordinary clinical practice. Additionally, primary care clinicians may be unfamiliar with interventions for the alleviation of post-traumatic distress (1-3). However, although primary care clinicians may experience feelings of powerlessness when treating patients who have experienced violence (4), they are actually in a powerful position to intervene. Once the clinician is aware of a patient's trauma history, he or she has three roles to play that are important to the patient's well-being and ultimate recovery: direct psychotherapeutic, biomedical, and facilitator roles (Box 4-1). The facilitator role is the focus of this chapter.

## Role of the Primary Care Provider

### Direct Psychotherapeutic Role

Primary care providers frequently underestimate the degree to which they directly participate in the patient's psychological healing. The opportunity for the patient to tell her story to an empathetic listener can help her to begin processing the traumatic event. This is the first step toward healing. Indeed, talking about the trauma is a cornerstone of the psychotherapy that mental health professionals offer to trauma survivors (5,6). Because medical providers are not trained psychotherapists, strategies for helping the patient to

---

**Box 4-1    Roles of Primary Care Provider in Alleviating Post-Traumatic Distress**

---

Psychotherapeutic
- Allow the patient to tell her story in a safe environment.
- Validate her experience ("I'm sorry that happened to you").
- Educate ("No one deserves to be hurt").

Biomedical
- Remain attentive to the power inequity of the patient-provider relationship.
- Make sure that exam/procedures are performed at the patient's pace.
- Elicit consent before touching the patient.

Facilitator
- Offer referral to mental health and other services.

---

feel comfortable telling her story while at the same time setting boundaries on the amount of detail she discloses in the medical setting are discussed later in this chapter. Additionally, validating, educational statements made by the clinician such as "I'm sorry that happened to you; no one deserves to be hurt" (7) can help the patient to begin to address her own feelings of guilt and self-blame. Validation by clinicians can have a particularly strong impact because clinicians are regarded as authority figures. Finally, the clinician can provide a safe, supportive environment in which the patient can tell her story. A safe environment can initiate a necessary change in beliefs commonly held by trauma survivors, some of which are that the world is a completely unsafe place, that no one can be trusted, and that she is an unworthy person (8,9).

These measures have several positive effects. They provide immediate and direct emotional first aid to the patient. They also foster an alliance that enhances the patient's comfort with referral for definitive mental health interventions. Even after mental health therapies have been initiated, a strong primary care relationship can serve as an anchor for the patient, who may have limited experience with long-term, positive, trusting relationships. Indeed, for some women, the primary care relationship may be the most consistent relationship ever experienced and can serve as a model for subsequent relationships. In such situations, the patient's simple act of showing up for regularly scheduled primary care visits represents a clinical success, even if she appears not to have made progress on other fronts. Thus, primary care providers are an integral part of the psychotherapeutic healing process.

## Biomedical Role

On more familiar territory, when performing physical examinations and medical procedures, knowledge of the trauma history enhances the provider's ability to alleviate suffering. Chapter 5 discusses approaches that can minimize the degree to which medical interventions are themselves traumatic to survivors of violence. Knowledge of the trauma history allows the health care provider to be particularly attentive to the possibility that it will affect response to medical treatments.

## Facilitator Role

Finally, primary care providers should not underestimate the power they have to refer patients for mental health services. Psychological concerns frequently present in the medical rather than the mental health setting and may go undetected (10,11). Patients may not self-refer for needed mental health care because of economic barriers (particularly in a managed care environment with primary care gatekeepers) or because of personal concerns (such as lack of knowledge about how to access care or about the potential benefits of therapy). The primary care provider's positioning to refer patients for mental health interventions magnifies his or her therapeutic potential. The rest of this chapter addresses logistics of referral.

# Who Needs a Referral?

Women who have experienced trauma may benefit from referral to two types of services: mental health services and trauma-specific services. Not every woman who has experienced violence in the remote or recent past will need to see a mental health specialist. Some women have already processed the trauma and integrated it into the fabric of their lives, either on their own or with the help of friends,

*Offer mental health consultation to all women with a trauma history.*

mental health professionals, or psychoeducational materials. However, because emotional suffering is often not clinically evident, we recommend that, in addition to screening for depression and post-traumatic stress disorder (PTSD) (see Chapter 2), mental health consultation be offered to all women with a trauma history. Patients with psychiatric conditions such as depression or anxiety may benefit from mental health referral, independent of whether or not the condition was caused by trauma (12). Referral becomes particularly important when the trauma is associated with complex conditions such as PTSD, dissociative disorders, eating disorders, or borderline personality disorder. Emergency referral is essential if the patient is acutely in danger of harming herself or others.

Social services specific to the trauma are helpful for many women, particularly those with ongoing violence exposure. For example, women in abusive relationships may benefit from information about shelters and legal services. Strategies for identifying such resources are described below.

# Barriers to Referral

Before considering how to refer patients to mental health, it is important to consider why patients might hesitate to accept referral and why clinicians might be uncomfortable raising the topic. Understanding barriers allows clinicians to surmount them.

## Patient-Level Barriers to Referral

There are a number of reasons patients might hesitate to accept referral to mental health services. Mental health care is stigmatized in our society; patients fear that they will be labeled as "crazy." Seeing a mental health provider may shake the patient's self-concept: instead of being a "person," she becomes a "mental health patient" and assumes a sick role with unique sociological meaning (13). This may be accompanied by feelings of loss of autonomy and control. If self-reliance is a key value for the patient, she may consider psychotherapy as a crutch. When the referral is for psychopharmacologic intervention, the patient may have a variety of different fears: addiction, "becoming a different person," side effects (e.g., sedation, sexual dysfunction), and jeopardizing job security (e.g., if the medication is detected on unannounced drug testing). Another fear is that any acknowledgement of the patient's weakness might heighten the risk of losing children to child protective services or to a partner suing for custody. Finally, there is a common misconception that psychic pain is not "real" pain, which may lead patients (and providers) to discount it. Indeed, the patient may not even recognize that she is suffering emotionally and instead may experience the post-traumatic emotion as a physical symptom (14,15).

Different patients have different reasons for being hesitant to accept a mental health referral. Because the reasons listed above are not exhaustive, a cornerstone of offering referral is exploring with the patient how she feels about referral. This is especially true if she expresses reluctance.

*Ask patient how she feels about mental health referral.*

## Provider-Level Barriers to Referral

Clinicians also need to be attuned to internal barriers within themselves that can thwart the referral process. Clinicians are not immune to the beliefs and fears raised above. As discussed in Chapter 6, exploration of these topics can elicit strong feelings in physicians. A physician's feelings of horror regarding violence may lead him or her to avoid the topic of trauma. Feelings of anger toward the patient, who may exhibit difficult behaviors in the clinical setting as part of her coping mechanism, may limit the clinician's enthusiasm about extending himself or herself on the patient's behalf. Feelings of fear may cloud the physician's decision-making.

The physician's reluctance to refer the patient to mental health can also stem from very natural countertransference reactions. The physician may feel like the patient's protector or rescuer. Such feelings are reinforced by patient pleas such as "You are the only one I have ever told, the only one I can trust, the only one who can help me"(16). The physician who accepts this assignment as rescuer may unintentionally reinforce countertherapeutic behaviors such as avoidance of expert mental health consultation.

In addition, clinicians may have knowledge gaps (e.g., believing that no effective therapies are available to treat psychological conditions or not knowing how to access mental health resources) or skills deficits (e.g., lack of experience in raising the topic of mental health referral with patients) (17). Additionally, in the current health care climate, time constraints can squelch any intentions to raise the topic of mental health care (4).

However, the time and effort invested in introducing the idea of referral and responding to the patient's concerns about referral may pay large dividends. Openness to the topic can lead to enhanced patient trust. The insights obtained can also inform a treatment strategy better targeted to the patient's situation. Just as allergen-induced asthma may be better treated by addressing allergen exposure than by prescribing bronchodilators, treatment for trauma-induced symptoms (e.g., depression, somatoform symptoms) may be best addressed by an approach that specifically addresses the trauma history rather than simply alleviates the symptoms. Indeed, physicians appear to be appropriately optimistic about their ability to provide services to women with a history of exposure to violence: more than 80% of physicians in one survey believed that they would be able to help survivors of physical and sexual abuse if such information were disclosed to them (18).

## Introducing the Concept of Mental Health Referral

Fortunately, making the referral can usually be accomplished quite efficiently. As with any medical procedure, the process of making a referral occurs most smoothly when the approach has been carefully planned and the skills needed to execute the procedure have been practiced. Informed consent is, of course, essential.

## General Strategies

Experiencing violence can lead to entrenched feelings of shame and low self-esteem (8). Shame about the need for mental health referral can compound these feelings. If the clinician is to avoid inflicting unintended pain, it is critical that he or she normalize the concept of referral. Simply alluding to other patients can provide comfort: for example, "Many of my patients have found that they felt much better after they saw one of our counselors." This can be followed by an explicit offer, framed in a way that makes it clear that the decision remains with the patient. For example, "Is that something you might be interested in?"

Putting the mental health referral offer into the context of the issues currently affecting the patient makes the likelihood higher that she will accept it. For example, before making the offer, it is helpful to find out what the patient's goals are for the clinic visit and to identify goals that the provider and patient share. It then becomes possible to weave the recommendation into the context of the patient's priorities. At the same time, it is important not to discount her current symptoms or to suggest that they are purely psychosomatic in etiology (19). It is not necessary to delay a mental health referral while awaiting results of tests designed to rule out medical conditions. For instance, for a patient presenting with fatigue, mental health evaluation can be presented as one aspect of a larger diagnostic and treatment plan: "I would like to evaluate you for several of the of the conditions that can cause fatigue. I would recommend that we get a blood test to be sure you are not anemic or low on your thyroid, and a consultation with a counselor to review whether aspects of your life that are causing stress could be contributing as well."

*Do not suggest that symptoms are purely psychosomatic.*

## Informed Consent

The mental health referral should occur with the patient's informed consent (Box 4-2). As the AMA Code of Ethics states, "the patient has the right to receive information from physicians and to discuss the benefits, risks, and costs of appropriate treatment alternatives," and, assuming she is

*Mental health referral requires informed consent.*

---

**Box 4-2     Elements of Informed Consent for Mental Health Referral**

---

Information
- What is the procedure?

  Explain what mental health treatment entails and what the expected duration could be.
- Why is the procedure indicated?

  Delineate clinical circumstances or symptoms for which referral is being made, including the ways that emotional distress appears to be interfering with health or well-being.

  Assure the patient that she is not crazy.
- What are its risks?

  Discuss the patient's concerns regarding stigma, employment implications, etc.
- What are its benefits?

  Discuss the ways in which mental health treatment can enhance health and well-being.
- What are its costs?

  Develop a treatment plan respectful of the patient's financial resources.
- What alternatives exist?

  Offer ongoing medical care irrespective of patient's decision and discuss other potentially beneficial approaches such as exercise, support from family and friends, and self-help books.

Consent
- Offer or even encourage referral, but do not pressure the patient.

---

competent, "the patient may accept or refuse any recommended medical treatment" (20).

Information comes in the form of patient education. The patient is empowered by knowing what a mental health professional does. A helpful first step is to explore what the patient already knows about counseling from exposure to the media, her own experiences, or the experiences of friends and family. This opens the door to discussion of any misconceptions she might have about mental health care. Common stigmas and misconceptions can be rectified once they are acknowledged. For example, "It used to be that people thought that if you went to a counselor, that meant you were crazy. Now we know that the majority of Americans experience major emotional suffering at some points during their lives that would benefit from medications or the help of a trained professional. Often counseling can be short term, just long enough to work through a difficult period." A straightforward approach can be taken with the patient if necessary by firmly stating, "You are not crazy."

The clinician can also ask the patient for her own hypotheses about how a history of exposure to violence appears to be affecting her current functioning (physical symptoms, emotional distress, social interactions, marital/partner/ parenting relationships, work-related functions). In this way, the clinician acknowledges the patient's personhood while at the same time alerting her to changes she may not have been able to see at close range. Knowing the patient's unique strengths facilitates this type of discussion. For example, "You mentioned that you have stopped painting. Having seen your portraits, I know you have a real gift. I am wondering if feelings of stress and low spirits are affecting you enough to keep you from doing something that you love?"

An explanation of the ways in which sequelae of trauma, such as depression, anxiety disorders, PTSD, and substance abuse, have a course outside of the patient's direct control can be comforting. This is especially true if the patient blames herself for the traumatic event, which is common (8), and for not being able to subsequently control her feelings. In explaining the degree to which these conditions are outside of her control, the clinician can also make a validating statement, acknowledging her resiliency and the ways in which she has been actively coping. For example, for a patient with major depression, the provider could say "I admire the way you have worked so hard to cope with this depression. You have managed to take two classes this past semester, despite the way you have been suffering. However, depression is a condition involving temporary changes in the levels of chemicals in the brain, and it usually does not go away just through force of will. Fortunately, with some extra support in this difficult time, combined with some medication, I expect that you will be feeling much better."

If the patient wishes, the family can also be involved in the education process, assuming they are not the perpetrators or facilitators of the violence (21). Trauma often leads to feelings of isolation and alienation, which can be reinforced by family and friends who share common societal misconceptions about mental health care. With education, family and friends can become allies in the therapeutic process.

Finally, the belief that psychic pain is not "real" pain should be challenged. Patients, like providers, may not recognize the profound effect of psychological distress on functional status and quality of life (22,23). To help a depressed patient understand the nature of psychological pain, a clinician could say, "Most people would take a pill for severe pain in their knee if they thought the pill could help. However, sometimes the same people deny themselves similar relief for the pain of depression, even though depression can hurt every bit as much as joint pain. In fact, for many people, depression can limit day-to-day functioning and enjoyment of life even more than joint pain does."

Patient consent to treatment is perhaps even more important than patient education. The woman who has experienced sexual assault or domestic violence has lived through the ultimate in nonconsensual acts: the violation of her very person. She may see herself as unworthy of self-determination and may feel particularly vulnerable when negotiating with health care providers, who are in a position of power. Therefore, in efforts to help, the clinician must guard against the temptation to push too hard by urging the patient to accept immediate referral to mental health. Such well-meaning attempts could miscarry. Several adverse outcomes are possible, even if the patient reluctantly accepts an intervention she does not desire. When a clinician becomes too forceful or intrusive with such things as referral, he or she can cause the patient to re-experience the emotions she felt during the violence for which she needs referral. In response, the patient may even flee from medical therapy. This latter outcome is particularly unfortunate because the primary care setting may be the only setting in which the patient will choose to receive care. Only the patient knows when she has had enough time to consider her options and enough time to develop trust in her health care team. The primary care provider's role is not to coerce the patient into seeing a mental health provider. The clinician empowers the patient by letting her reach her decision on her own terms, fully informed of her options.

> *Do not coerce the patient into seeing a mental health provider.*

## Where Should the Clinician Refer Patients?

The interface between medical and mental health services ideally should be seamless. Access to mental health professionals varies by clinical setting and patient insurance carrier. However, primary care providers should, if possible, establish connections with mental health providers, identifying providers to whom they feel comfortable referring patients. A personal endorsement by the referring clinician may improve the likelihood that the patient accepts the referral. In this way, when the need arises, referral can be expeditious.

The clinician can enlist the help of professionals from a variety of backgrounds. The prospect of seeing a mental health professional who will delve into traumatic memories that the patient has tried to suppress can be terrifying to the patient. Stabilizing the patient's post-traumatic symptoms with psychotropic medications is sometimes a critical first step, particularly when these symptoms overwhelm the patient's ability to communicate effectively or when the patient is acutely at risk of harming herself or others. Although primary care providers can prescribe psychotropic medications in straightforward cases, psychiatrists can provide particular support for the management of medication. Other mental health professionals (e.g., psychologists, psychiatric social workers, clinical nurse specialists) may similarly choose to emphasize stress reduction and modulation skills in the initial phases of therapy. These skills support subsequent trauma-specific psychotherapy, making it more tolerable to the patient. If indicated, trauma-specific psychotherapy may then occur in individual counseling sessions, in group therapy, or even in lay support groups.

Social workers can provide counseling (which may be perceived by the patient as less stigmatizing than counseling from a psychologist or psychiatrist), and they can identify appropriate community referral sites (see below). Clergy can provide accessible counseling consistent with the patient's specific religious beliefs. Finally, friends and family can be an important source of support, if the patient is comfortable disclosing to them. The patient's natural support system will typically confirm her values and beliefs and will either ratify or discourage any changes she is considering, such as whether to move to safety or remain in her current environment. Therefore, in discussions with the patient about her plans it is important to explore how her natural supports will respond.

There are some important caveats about selecting the person to whom the patient will be referred, however. First, not all mental health professionals or clergy have had specific training in the management of conditions seen in trauma survivors. This is particularly true for complex conditions such as eating disorders, dissociative disorders, and borderline personality disorder. There is a risk that a well-meaning but misinformed intervention could be counter-therapeutic or could even re-traumatize the patient, poisoning subsequent attempts to engage the patient in therapy. Therefore, the primary care provider should seek community resources with trauma counseling backgrounds. If there are no such resources in the local community, appropriate resources may be available in a nearby community. Alternatively, the local therapist may be open to gaining additional training in this area. Information about reputable training opportunities can be obtained through the International Society for Traumatic Stress Studies [www.istss.org] or the National Center for Post-Traumatic Stress Disorder [www.ncptsd.org] (see the Appendix). Given the high prevalence of violence against women, it would be beneficial for every community to have at least one resource with expertise in this field.

Second, expertise is necessary but not sufficient; the mental health provider needs to be a good communicator as well. The mental health professional should be someone who can be relied upon to remain in close contact with the primary care provider so that care can be coordinated.

Third, although family and friends can comprise a powerful patient support network, attempts to engage them in the therapeutic process can miscarry.

Family and friends have their own agendas and may have a variety of reactions to involvement. They may feel overwhelmed by the responsibility of supporting an acutely distressed patient, they may blame the patient for the events surrounding the trauma (especially if the violence was at the hands of another family member), or they may betray the patient's confidence to other family members. When the identified perpetrator is a family member, other family members may be caught between the patient and the alleged perpetrator in a loyalty bind. These possibilities should be reviewed with the patient before she decides whether or not to disclose to family or friends; often such discussions occur within the setting of ongoing psychotherapy. If the patient does decide to disclose to a family member or friend, she may elect to invite the family member or friend to a counseling session. That presents the therapist with the opportunity to provide psychoeducational interventions and begin to dispel trauma myths that the family member or friend may hold, which can undermine the therapeutic process. The mental health provider simultaneously can assess interpersonal family dynamics.

The clinician who is knowledgeable about community resources is in a strong position to help his or her patients directly by supplying practical information. He or she can also be helpful indirectly: making an effort to research resources assures the patient that concern for her is genuine, and it bolsters the therapeutic alliance.

A number of community resources are available to the patient (Table 4-1):

- *Hotlines:* The patient needs to be aware of hotlines that are available to provide emergency guidance. She should know that the hotlines listed in the Appendix can be accessed through the telephone service's

**Table 4-1    Community Resources for Patients**

|  | Counseling | Housing/Refuge | Legal Advocacy |
|---|---|---|---|
| Hotlines | X |  | X |
| Community-based counseling (private practice or in mental health centers) | X |  |  |
| Hospital-based programs | X | X | X |
| Drug/alcohol detoxification centers | X | X |  |
| Shelters | X | X | X |
| Legal advocacy programs (police, Victim's Witness Program) |  |  | X |
| Substance abuse programs | X |  |  |
| Treatment programs for batterers | X |  |  |

directory assistance line if the number is not available to her in an urgent situation. (She should of course be advised to call 911 or the local equivalent in emergency situations. Emergencies requiring a 911 call include immediate risk of injury to the patient or her children or the patient's own acute suicidal or homicidal ideation.) Hotlines vary in issues addressed (domestic violence, rape, child abuse, etc.), quality of advice provided (some are state funded and operated), hours of operation (some are available 24 hours a day, 7 days a week), and scope of services (provision of information, support, acute counseling, legal advice, or referral to local shelters).

- *Community-based mental health providers:* Mental health professionals in private practice or in mental health centers can provide counseling, and mental health centers may provide services on a free or sliding fee basis. Local detoxification and substance abuse treatment programs can also be very helpful if substance abuse is an issue.

- *Hospital-based violence programs:* Hospitals in larger communities often have their own battered women's, rape crisis, and violence prevention programs. These programs may have advocates, counselors, and even safe beds for overnight use.

- *Shelters/safe homes:* These provide temporary refuge to women who are fleeing a violent home situation. Their location is often secret, to prevent batterers from finding their victims. Each has its own rules about admission, length of stay, children, pets, and substance use. Some provide a direct link to additional services such as counseling, support groups, and legal aid. They may help a battered woman to develop a safety plan and consider transition into a new phase of life.

- *Legal advocacy programs:* Legal concerns can be a major barrier for a woman who wishes to leave her abusive partner. This is especially true if the batterer has threatened to seek custody of the children or refuse child support should she leave. It is also true if the victim has perpetrated violence (in retaliation or self-defense) or developed a substance abuse problem. The local police department often has a domestic violence or sexual assault unit, and the police can conduct on-site investigations, document investigation results, and remain on the scene until the victim is safe. They can also listen to the victim's concerns, offering her information or emergency referral (e.g., for medical care or to a safe house). Some police departments provide free cell phone service to battered women for use in case of emergency (such as a batterer violating a restraining order). Some police departments require officers to contact a hotline counselor, make a follow-up contact with the victim, and/or arrest the perpetrator. The Victims Witness Program, often located in the state district attorney's office, will assist with filing a restraining order.

- *Substance abuse programs:* Because substance abuse is common among survivors of violence, it may be necessary to refer the patient for substance abuse treatment. See Chapter 10 for more details.

- *Batterer programs:* Although discussion of them is beyond the scope of this chapter, programs are available to help batterers as well, with variable success rates (24). Some are comprehensive programs that are certified by the state. Others are more limited, primarily directed at anger management, and may not address the problem of battering in its entirety. Clinical Vignette 6 discusses treatment options for batterers in more detail.

## Locating Community Resources

There are many sources of information about community resources (Box 4-3). Clinicians who are hospital-based can contact their social work service, which typically makes referrals to community agencies and often maintains listings of contacts. Community relations staff at medical facilities also develop personal contacts at community agencies and can identify resources. Clinicians who are not hospital-based may be able to take advantage of programs developed at their local medical centers, which may be accessed through social

---

**Box 4-3    Sources of Information About Community Resources**

*Internal Sources*
- Social work service
- Community Relations department

*Community Sources*
- Local medical centers
- Local police departments

*Nationally Based Sources*
- Hotlines
  —National Domestic Violence Hotline (800-799-SAFE or 800-787-3224)
  —Rape, Abuse, Incest National Network (RAINN) (800-656-HOPE)

- Internet
  —Coalition on Domestic Violence (www.feminst.org/911/crisis.html)

work service. The local police department may also have access to information about resources, although the patient's name should not be disclosed without her informed consent except when legally mandated. Finally, state medical societies may be able to provide referral information. See the Appendix for specific referral resources.

If internal resources at the provider's facility are scarce, hotlines provide ready access to available resources. The National Domestic Violence Hotline can provide contact information on local resources. This hotline operates 24 hours a day in 50 states, the District of Columbia, Puerto Rico, and the Virgin Islands. Staffed by trained counselors, it provides crisis assistance, information about shelters, legal advocates, and mental health services. An additional resource for victims of rape or incest is the Rape, Abuse, Incest National Network (RAINN), which will automatically transfer the caller to the nearest rape crisis center, anywhere in the United States. Each affiliated rape crisis center provides confidential counseling and support. RAINN can also connect the caller with the specific state's Coalition on Battered Women.

In addition to hotlines, the Internet is an excellent source of information on domestic violence and sexual assault for clinicians seeking community referrals and patient education materials. A helpful place to start is the Coalition on Domestic Violence, which oversees a system of safe homes and shelters in each state and provides referral information. Additional information accessible through the Internet is included in the Appendix. (Of note, many communities have resources for men who have been battered or assaulted. The Coalition on Battered Women can inform the clinician of such local programs.)

## Adherence to Mental Health Referral

Acceptance of a mental health referral does not necessarily translate into arrival at a mental health provider's office. A woman's resolve may falter during the days or weeks intervening between primary care visit and mental health visit. Faced with the prospect of disclosing private information to a stranger, feelings of shame, vulnerability, and mistrust may overwhelm her desire for help.

A particularly helpful strategy is to capitalize on the momentum of a positive primary care visit. If a mental health professional can meet with the patient, even briefly, on the day of the primary care visit, the patient can determine that the mental health clinician is not a threatening person. Thus, the chances that she will follow up with a mental health referral increase. This is particularly true if the mental health provider can meet the patient in the more familiar primary care setting, at least for the brief introductory visit. The focus of this visit may be simply to orient the patient to therapeutic options available to her and what the assessment process will entail (25).

# What Happens When the Patient Presents to Mental Health Services?

When a woman with a trauma history is referred to a mental health professional (psychiatrist, psychologist, or licensed social worker), she will typically undergo an assessment phase followed by a treatment phase (psychotherapeutic and/or psychopharmacologic). An illustrative case is presented here, with a review of common approaches used during the assessment and treatment phases (Case 4-1).

---

CASE 4-1

---

*GR is a 32-year-old woman with a history of childhood sexual abuse referred to a hospital mental health clinic by her primary care doctor for help with ongoing suicidal ideation. The psychologist asks about her understanding of the reason for referral (her response, "My doctor sent me because I think about killing myself") and her expectations of the clinical encounter (her response, "I don't know if you can help me, but I can't go on like this"). The psychologist next attempts to fully characterize the primary mental health problem, which is suicidal ideation. GR thinks of suicide often and has on two occasions cut her arms superficially after feeling "overwhelmed." The clinician determines that this feeling is related to emotions of shame on the job ("I'm not good enough," "People don't like me"). Suicidal thoughts typically occur when GR feels her boss has spoken to her in a demeaning way and when she needs to make oral presentations. Historical assessment of these behaviors and emotions reveal that they began in early adolescence when she was sexually abused by her stepfather. GR reports that she felt intense shame and experienced suicidal ideation as a result of the demeaning way that her stepfather treated her. She was particularly ashamed when he would make public comments about her figure. On formal diagnostic assessment, GR meets the criteria for major depression and PTSD.*

*After determining that GR is at low risk for suicide, the psychologist explains to GR what the diagnostic assessment has revealed and how her trauma history may be contributing to her current symptoms. The psychologist recommends a course of outpatient psychotherapy and psychiatric referral for possible pharmacotherapy of depression and post-traumatic stress disorder symptoms. The psychologist describes what GR should expect from therapy: an initial phase in which she develops new skills (e.g., stress reduction techniques), followed, when she is ready, by a trauma-processing phase in which she learns new ways of coping with memories of her trauma.*

## Assessment Phase

As Case 4-1 illustrates, the mental health professional will usually clarify whether his or her understanding of the reason for referral corresponds with the patient's understanding and will explore the patient's expectations, hopes, and fears about the referral. Establishing a shared understanding of the goals of referral is a first step toward forming a therapeutic alliance.

Next, the mental health professional will try to develop a comprehensive understanding of the patient's primary mental health problems. This will typically require one to three sessions, each about an hour long. Sources of information include the referring clinician, the patient, and family members, if appropriate. This process starts with eliciting symptoms (e.g., suicidal ideation, anxiety, fatigue, avoidance, self-destructive behavior, nightmares, interpersonal difficulties, etc.) and characterizing them (e.g., frequency, precipitants, etc.). The mental health clinician will attempt to put these problems into the context of the patient's history of previous trauma (in childhood and adulthood) and characterize the patient's current social environment (regarding ongoing trauma, social support systems, etc.). This facilitates the identification of factors predisposing the patient to psychological symptoms and factors perpetuating or alleviating her symptoms. The clinician then formally assesses for the possibility of a major psychiatric diagnosis, which may be a consequence of previous trauma (e.g., PTSD, major depression, borderline personality disorder) or may be a pre-existing comorbidity complicating the response to the traumatic exposure (e.g., schizophrenia, dementia). Structured clinical instruments (e.g., paper and pencil tests) are sometimes used at this phase.

After completing this detailed psychological assessment, the clinician will usually share with the patient the formulation of her primary mental health problems. The treatment recommendations (psychotherapy and/or pharmacotherapy) will follow from the formulation. These recommendations are shared with the patient in a collaborative fashion so that the patient has as much control over the clinical encounter as possible because the patient may feel highly anxious about this discussion.

# Treatment Phase

It is beyond the scope of this chapter to fully describe treatments of psychological disorders for women exposed to violence. We give here a brief discussion of the different psychotherapy models developed for women with PTSD, the most common psychiatric disorder to occur after exposure to violence (6) (see Chapter 5 for a more detailed discussion of PTSD). We will then describe a variety of psychopharmacologic agents known to be effective for PTSD. Although the following descriptions outline fairly discrete treatments, in practice most mental health professionals use a combination of different psychotherapy approaches and will usually refer a patient with PTSD to a psychiatrist for psychopharmacologic evaluation.

## *Behavioral Approaches*

Behavioral approaches to PTSD are based on classical conditioning model theory: the traumatic event conditioned the woman to associate a variety of cues with certain emotional responses, which she re-experiences (in the form of PTSD symptoms) whenever exposed to these cues. For example, in the case above, GR's childhood trauma was associated with her stepfather's demeaning treatment of her, which often occurred in a public setting; as an adult, being treated in a demeaning way or having to give an oral presentation serve as cues that trigger her to experience PTSD symptoms (e.g., feelings of worthlessness and anxiety). A behavioral approach would attempt to diminish or extinguish this conditioned response by exposing the patient to these cues in the absence of the traumatic event. She might be asked to imagine the violence while in the safety of the therapist's office (imaginal exposure). Alternatively, she might be taken to the place where the violence occurred to be exposed to cues reminiscent of the trauma in the absence of the traumatic event (in vivo exposure). For example, in the case study above, GR might be asked to imagine her boss speaking to her in a demeaning way. By repeatedly imagining this interaction in a safe setting, the PTSD symptoms elicited by encounters with her boss gradually diminish. The patient would learn skills to help her regulate the intense emotions experienced as a result of PTSD. Numerous studies have documented the efficacy of exposure therapy to decrease PTSD symptoms and improve functional status (26,27).

## *Cognitive-Behavioral Approaches*

Cognitive-behavioral approaches are based on the theory that the traumatic event leads to unhelpful thoughts; these thoughts generate a cascade of extreme emotion and manifest as PTSD symptoms, which interfere with day-to-day functioning. For example, a woman who has been sexually assaulted may continually have thoughts such as "I'm going to be attacked" in situations where she is alone with a man; this may interfere with her ability to work effectively with men or to establish intimate relationships. In GR's case, thoughts like "I'm not good enough," "People don't like me," and "People think I'm a bad person" make her feel overwhelmed, which leads to self-cutting. The psychotherapist, in a safe and empathetic way, would challenge these thoughts and point out the ways in which they are unhelpful. In a cognitive-behavioral approach, the therapist would help the patient discriminate between situations that are safe and situations that are threatening. For example, in the case above, psychotherapy would particularly target how feelings of shame related to interpersonal scrutiny and interpersonal conflict are reminiscent of the feelings GR experienced during childhood abuse, and how the feelings of shame are driving the current suicidal ideation. GR may feel terrified about an upcoming presentation at work, saying "People will be looking at me and thinking I am dumb; I don't even deserve to be up there at the podium." Her therapist might challenge these thoughts and help her to learn to modify them by responding to her with "Do you remember your last presentation when you had similar thoughts, but afterward your co-worker came up and said he had learned something new from your presentation?" Cognitive behavioral approaches have been repeatedly demonstrated as effective for PTSD symptoms in women exposed to violence (28,29).

### Psychodynamic Approaches

Psychodynamic approaches are based on the theory that unconscious conflict and meanings associated with the traumatic event produce extreme emotions, which manifest themselves as PTSD symptoms. When using the psychodynamic approach, the therapist and patient explore the meanings of the experience of violence for the patient in her relationships with other people and, in particular, explore the conscious and unconscious links between the patient's current symptoms and conflicts that began in childhood. In GR's case, the therapist would in particular explore GR's feelings of shame and suicidal ideation in her current relations with authority figures and relate them to feelings that developed during incestuous experiences with her stepfather. This exploration would also focus on how the patient may experience feelings of shame and humiliation in her relationship with the therapist (transference). One important notion of the psychodynamic approach is that once the patient becomes aware of these feelings and how the feelings are related to previous trauma experiences, the patient has much more control over them. The effectiveness of psychodynamic approaches has not been documented as definitively as the effectiveness of behavioral and cognitive-behavioral approaches, however.

### Psychopharmacologic Approaches

Psychopharmacologic approaches are based on the theory that there are core biological processes associated with PTSD that can be remedied with psychopharmacologic agents (30,31). The agents that currently have the most empirical support are the selective serotonin reuptake inhibitors (SSRIs) such as fluoxetine (Prozac) and sertraline (Zoloft) (32,33). Other agents that have been demonstrated to be effective are the tricyclic antidepressants such as amitriptyline (Elavil) (34) and imipramine (Tofranil) (35) and the mono-amine oxidase inhibitors such as phenelzine (Nardil) (36,37). In practice, most patients with PTSD are treated with an SSRI, sometimes in combination with a benzodiazepine.

## When the Patient Declines Referral

There is, of course, the chance that even an informed patient will decline mental health referral when initially offered. Sometimes such a decision is consistent with the clinical impression: the patient appears not to be experiencing current trauma-related distress. However, at other times the clinician is concerned that the patient is actively suffering emotional distress but has declined mental health referral. In this case, several approaches can be productive (Box 4-4).

First and most important, the clinician should emphasize that if the patient ever changes her mind about mental health care in the future, she is welcome to raise the issue. Often a patient returns requesting referral at a later date, either because she is in more acute distress or because she has developed more trust in the provider: the time feels right to her. By introducing the possibility of counseling at an initial visit and reiterating the offer periodically at follow-up visits, the primary care provider has opened a door. The patient will decide when she is ready to step through it.

---

**Box 4-4    Approaches to Patient Who Declines Mental Health Referral Despite Objective Evidence of Emotional Distress**

- Assure her that she can request referral in the future.
- Clarify her reasons for declining referral; correct misunderstandings.
- Explore her views about how past trauma is affecting her life.
- Offer ongoing follow-up but make limits of own expertise clear to patient.
- Consider a clinical session in which a mental health provider joins the patient and primary care provider.
- Provide limited psychotherapeutic and/or psychopharmacologic intervention in primary care setting.
- Promote nonpharmacologic approaches (e.g., progressive muscle relaxation, exercise, nutrition, work therapy, alcohol/drug avoidance).

Next, the clinician needs to make sure that he or she understands the patient's rationale for declining referral (13), so any misconceptions can be corrected. The clinician can ask how much the patient's symptoms bother her, whether she feels she would benefit from counseling, what other measures she feels would help her, what her attitudes toward taking medication are, and what experiences she has had (or friends and family have had) with mental health professionals. The clinician can also explore the degree to which she is aware of her own feelings and determine whether she subscribes to a belief that emotional distress can have physical manifestations. However, in patients with symptoms felt secondary to a somatization disorder, it is important to be aware that telling patients that their symptoms are caused by psychological forces may not have the desired therapeutic effect. Although the recognition and treatment of somatization disorder is beyond the scope of this book, it is important for primary care providers to be versed in the clinical management of somatization disorder because this condition is so common in trauma survivors (38).

If the patient does not want to go to a mental health professional, she may be willing to have a mental health provider come to her (39), if such services are available. In some clinical settings, particularly hospital-based settings, social workers are available to provide these services. If a primary care setting feels safer or less stigmatizing to her, the patient may appreciate an offer to have a one-time joint visit with a mental health provider in the primary care provider's office. Meeting the mental health provider may assuage her doubts and lead to a willingness to pursue formal referral. Even if this does not happen, the clinical contact puts the mental health provider in a better position to be helpful to the primary care provider in ongoing case conferences.

The primary care provider needs to make it clear to the patient that a recommendation for counseling does not represent abandonment and should assure the patient that he or she will continue to evaluate her, tend to her physical health needs, and provide ongoing support for emotional issues as well. However, a primary care provider untrained in psychological interventions for trauma survivors should be cautious not to overstep the bounds of his or her expertise. Although relationship-building and validation of feelings about traumatic experiences are inherently therapeutic, attempts to actively counsel the patient could go awry despite the best and most compassionate intentions. Psychotherapy involves talking, but it is a specifically goal-directed style of talking, and one that requires years of training to master. The provider should be aware of his or her limitations as a counselor and should make sure that the patient understands any limitations of this kind as well. When psychological issues begin exceeding the primary care provider's comfort level, he or she should be honest and inform the patient that more expert input is available than he or she is able to provide.

There are, however, a number of interventions the primary care provider can take to reduce psychological distress in patients. Most primary care providers are comfortable with psychopharmacologic interventions for common and uncomplicated psychiatric conditions such as depression and anxiety. These medications can help stabilize patients by reducing their emotional symptoms, although the patient must be monitored for atypical responses to medications or lack of response, which would necessitate referral to a psychiatrist. With training, primary care clinicians can successfully provide limited psychotherapy (40,41). Additionally, basic stress-reduction skills such as progressive muscle relaxation (42) can be taught in the primary care setting. Patient education materials or nurse-run seminars could foster such skills. Self-help books can also be a valuable psychoeducational tool. Other nonpharmacologic measures such as exercise, nutrition, work therapy, and alcohol avoidance may have a positive emotional effect on the patient as well. Stabilizing the patient's emotional distress enhances her functional status and may help her to feel less overwhelmed by the possibility of committing to psychotherapy.

If the patient's trauma history appears to be impairing her psychosocial functioning and she is not seeking therapy, the primary care provider would be well advised to seek professional input. By presenting the case to a mental health expert, the primary care provider can explore options that will optimize his or her effectiveness. The mental health expert can give advice about managing the patient within the primary care setting and can help with strategies that may facilitate eventual referral. Additionally, because caring for patients who have experienced violence and/or are experiencing psychiatric distress can be personally and professionally challenging for the clinician (see Chapter 6), mental health input can be personally reinvigorating for and supportive of the clinician.

## Organizational Systems that Facilitate Referral

It is important to establish systems of care for addressing the needs of trauma survivors, so that when the need arises resources can be quickly mobilized (Box 4-5).

Whichever organizational system is adopted, specific interventions can facilitate the patient's movement to and from the mental health care setting. At some sites, the social worker is the first point of contact, or the intake assessment is performed by one mental health clinician who then refers the patient to a different clinician for ongoing care. Hand-outs and brochures in the waiting room and in the clinician's office describing the range of mental health services available can help normalize and streamline

## Box 4-5    Organizational Systems That Facilitate Mental Health Referral

The program adopted at a particular facility should be consistent with the resources, philosophy, and clinical needs of the institution. The fundamental principle behind all of the following model systems is that the care of women who have survived violence must be interdisciplinary and collaborative.

*Model 1*

In the most elaborate model, mental health and primary care providers work side by side in a single clinical unit (Read JP, Stern AL, Wolfe, J, Ouimette PC. Use of a screening instrument in women's health care: detecting relationships among victimization history, psychological distress, and medical complaints. Women and Health. 1997;25:1-17; Jackson G, Gater R, Goldberg D, et al. A new community mental health team based in primary care: a description of the service and its effect on service use in the first year. Br J Psychiatry. 1993;162:375-84). Patients perceive the system as holistic. Providers identify themselves as members of a single team and have ample opportunities to share perspectives and offer each other support for challenging management issues. This is probably the most desirable approach, especially for women with severe trauma-related sequelae and heavy health care utilization. Such an approach appears to increase referral rates for psychiatric symptoms (Jackson et al), although its impact on long-term outcomes has not been established. Our own experience with this model has been so powerful that we encourage other health care systems to give it serious consideration.

*Model 2*

Medical and mental health services are available within a single building (e.g., a medical center) but not in adjoining office space. Interdisciplinary approaches to care are still feasible with this arrangement but require some planning. It may be helpful to identify one or two counselors and psychiatrists willing to serve as the major recipients of referrals. It then becomes feasible for this small group of primary care providers and mental health providers to remain in close contact with each other around the management of their shared patients. They may choose to hold regular case conferences to ensure communication, facilitate coordinated treatment planning, and provide opportunities to teach and support each other.

*Model 3*

Many primary care clinics have no on-site mental health providers. This model poses the most challenges. To ensure coordinated care for patients attending such clinics, the primary care clinician must make an extra effort to identify psychiatrists and other mental health professionals in the community to whom they feel comfortable referring patients and with whom they can easily communicate. Because patients may choose any mental health professional from geographically heterogeneous locations in the community, telephone and written interactions are particularly important for maintaining coordinated care. In particular, sending a written consultation to the mental health provider (and requesting a return written report) may improve the quality of the initial evaluation.

the referral process, while decreasing the patient's anxiety about what to expect. The primary care provider can offer the patient the use of his or her phone to call the mental health provider or ask if she would like the therapist to contact her, rather than expecting the patient to make the first call on her own.

Finally, it is worthwhile to invest in crisis preparedness education. Primary care providers should be versed in the management of psychiatric emergencies. Support staff and security officers should also receive training for crisis situations in the management of patients who have experienced trauma. For example, anyone responding to a psychiatric crisis needs to understand that restraints, although occasionally necessary, can retraumatize women by triggering memories of previous assaults. Likewise, providers need to be aware that a patient may enter a dissociative state when faced with extreme stress, which may explain combative, bizarre, or withdrawn behaviors (see Chapter 5). They also need to recognize that a woman in crisis may be particularly reassured by the presence of a familiar and trusted health care provider (such as a nurse, a primary care physician, or a mental health clinician). Involving longitudinal care providers in emergency care can help to de-escalate a crisis situation. Explicit procedures for addressing a mental health crisis should be available to all personnel (Box 4-6). To the maximum extent possible, the response to a psychiatric crisis should be a team effort, and one that has been carefully choreographed in advance.

---

**Box 4-6   Elements of a Psychiatric Crisis Plan for Primary Care Providers**

- Defines types of situations that constitute a psychiatric emergency (e.g., suicidal ideation, homicidal ideation, acute risk of victimization, patient or family disrupting clinic operations).
- Delineates roles of involved staff (e.g., medical providers, mental health providers, nonclinical staff, hospital security staff).
- Specifies how patient's immediate safety will be ensured.
- Specifies how provider's and staff's immediate safety will be ensured.
- Notes how involuntary commitment (if needed) will proceed.
- Explains how the patient will be transported to definitive care.
    (E.g., If the patient is suicidal, she will need to be escorted to definitive care [even if it is in the same building], and commitment documentation may need to be completed before transport.)
- Outlines steps to be taken to avoid retraumatizing the patient (e.g., policies regarding use of restraints).

# Summary

Primary care providers are well positioned to address the psychological and social sequelae of violence, particularly if they have identified a responsive referral network and instituted a team approach to care. National attention to the magnitude of the violence problem has led to the development of extensive hospital-based and community-based resources, many of which are easily accessible to clinicians. Clinicians can and should offer their patients referral to mental health services and to other community services. The approach to referral should be supportive, normalizing, and non-coercive. A strong pre-existing relationship between primary care providers, mental health providers, social workers, and community services will greatly benefit women presenting with sequelae of past trauma.

## REFERENCES

1. Fontana A, Rosenheck R. Effectiveness and cost of the inpatient treatment of posttraumatic stress disorder: comparison of three models of treatment. Am J Psychiatry. 1997;154:758-65.
2. Foa EB, Meadows EA. Psychosocial treatments for posttraumatic stress disorder: a critical review. Annu Rev Psychol. 1997;48:449-80.
3. Davidson JR. Biological therapies for posttraumatic stress disorder: an overview. J Clin Psychiatry. 1997;58:29-32.
4. Sugg NK, Inui T. Primary care physicians' response to domestic violence: opening Pandora's box. JAMA. 1992;267:3157.
5. Foa EB. Trauma and women: course, predictors, and treatment. J Clin Psychiatry. 1997;58:25-8.
6. Foa E, Keane T, Friedman M, eds. Effective Treatments for PTSD: Practice Guidelines from the International Society for Traumatic Stress Studies. New York: The Guildford Press; 2000.
7. Koss M. The Health Burden of Rape: Keynote Address at the Women Veteran's Health and Issues of Sexual Trauma Conference, San Diego; 1994.
8. Herman J. Trauma and Recovery. New York: Basic Books; 1992.
9. McKegney CP. Surviving survivors: coping with caring for patients who have been victimized. Prim Care. 1993;20:481-94.
10. Perez-Stable EJ, Miranda J, Munoz RF, Ying YW. Depression in medical outpatients: underrecognition and misdiagnosis. Arch Intern Med. 1990;150:1083-8.
11. Lefevre F, Reifler D, Lee P, et al. Screening for undetected mental disorders in high utilizers of primary care services. J Gen Intern Med. 1999;14:425-31.
12. Conway T. The internist's role in addressing violence: a review of current recommendations and a model for intervention. Arch Intern Med. 1996;156:951-6.
13. Kleinman A, Eisenberg L, Good B. Culture, illness, and care: clinical lessons from anthropologic and cross-cultural research. Ann Intern Med. 1978;88:251-8.
14. Walker EA, Katon WJ, Roy-Byrne PP, et al. Histories of sexual victimization in patients with irritable bowel syndrome or inflammatory bowel disease. Am J Psychiatry. 1993;150:1502-6.

15. Saxe GN, Chinman G, Berkowitz R, et al. Somatization in patients with dissociative disorders. Am J Psychiatry. 1994;151:1329-34.

16. Crane M, Mather S. Team approach to treatment and referral of female sexual trauma survivors. Federal Practitioner Supplement. 1998;15:14-15.

17. Rodriguez MA, Bauer HM, McLoughlin E, Grumbach K. Screening and intervention for intimate partner abuse: practices and attitudes of primary care physicians. JAMA. 1999;282:468-74.

18. Friedman LS, Samet JH, Roberts MS, et al. Inquiry about victimization experiences: a survey of patient preferences and physician practices. Arch Intern Med. 1992;1152: 1186-90.

19. Morse DS, Suchman AL, Frankel RM. The meaning of symptoms in 10 women with somatization disorder and a history of childhood abuse. Arch Fam Med. 1997;6:468-76.

20. AMA Council on Ethical and Judicial Affairs. Code of Medical Ethics. Chicago: American Medical Association; 1997.

21. Alpert EJ. Violence in intimate relationships and the practicing internist: new "disease" or new agenda? Ann Intern Med. 1995;123:774-81.

22. The Counselling Versus Antidepressants in Primary Care Study Group. How disabling is depression? Evidence from a primary care sample. Br J Gen Pract. 1999;49:95-8.

23. Covinsky KE, Fortinsky RH, Palmer RM, et al. Relation between symptoms of depression and health status outcomes in acutely ill hospitalized older persons. Ann Intern Med. 1997;126:417-25.

24. Gondolf EW. Patterns of reassault in batterer programs. Violence Vict. 1997;12:373-87.

25. Gorroll A, May L, Mulley A. Primary Care Medicine: Office Evaluation and Management of the Adult Patient, 3rd ed. Philadelphia: JB Lippincott; 1995.

26. Keane T, Fairband J, Caddell J, Zimering R. Implosive (flooding) therapy reduces symptoms of PTSD in Vietnam combat veterans. Behavior Therapy. 1989;20:245-260.

27. Keane TM, Kaloupek DG. Imaginal flooding in the treatment of a posttraumatic stress disorder. J Consult Clin Psychol. 1982;50:138-40.

28. Foa EB, Rothbaum BO, Riggs DS, Murdock TB. Treatment of posttraumatic stress disorder in rape victims: a comparison between cognitive-behavioral procedures and counseling. J Consult Clin Psychol. 1991;59:715-23.

29. Resick PA, Schnicke MK. Cognitive processing therapy for sexual assault victims. J Consult Clin Psychol. 1992;60:748-56.

30. Charney DS, Deutch AY, Krystal JH, et al. Psychobiologic mechanisms of posttraumatic stress disorder. Arch Gen Psychiatry. 1993;50:295-305.

31. van der Kolk BA, Herron N, Hostetler A. The history of trauma in psychiatry. Psychiatr Clin North Am. 1994;17:583-600.

32. van der Kolk B, Dryfuss D, Michaels M, et al. Fluoxetine in posttraumatic stress disorder. J Clin Psychiatry. 1994;55:517-522.

33. Davidson J, Foa E. Diagnostic issues in posttraumatic stress disorder: considerations for the DSM-IV. J Abnorm Psychol. 1991;100:346-355.

34. Davidson JRT, Kudler HS, Saunders WB, et al. Predicting response to amitriptyline in posttraumatic stress disorder. Am J Psychiatry. 1993;150:1024-1029.

35. Burstein A. Treatment of posttraumatic stress disorder with imipramine. Post-Traumatic Stress. 1984;25:681-7.

36. Davidson JRT, Walker JI, Kilts C. A pilot study of phenelzine in the treatment of posttraumatic stress disorder. Br J Psychiatry. 1987;150:252-5.

37. Demartino R, Mollica F, Wilk V. Monoamine oxidase inhibitors in posttraumatic stress disorder: promise and problems in Indochinese survivors of trauma. J Nerv Ment Dis. 1995;183:510-15.

38. Courtois CA. Adult survivors of sexual abuse. Primary Care. 1993;20:433-46.

39. Levy S, Pollak J, Walsh M. Primary care psychology: current status and future prospects. Ann Behav Sci Med Ed. 1994;1:43-8.

40. Brody DS, Lerman CE, Wolfson HG, Caputo GC. Improvement in physicians' counseling of patients with mental health problems. Arch Intern Med. 1990;150:993-8.

41. Brody DS, Thompson TL 2nd, Larson DB, et al. Strategies for counseling depressed patients by primary care physicians. J Gen Intern Med. 1994;9:569-75.

42. Gorroll A, May L, Mulley A. Primary Care Medicine: Office Evaluation and Management of the Adult Patient, 3rd ed. Philadelphia: JB Lippincott; 1995.

# CHAPTER 5

# Ongoing Management of Patients with Post-Traumatic Stress Disorder

GLENN N. SAXE, MD

SUSAN M. FRAYNE, MD, MPH

Unique and sometimes challenging issues can arise in the provision of medical care to women who have experienced interpersonal violence. In some women, past trauma may lead to ongoing psychological consequences, such as post-traumatic stress disorder (PTSD). PTSD can influence a woman's interaction with others, including health care providers. PTSD is common enough that all medical providers will eventually encounter it in a patient under their care (1). Although other psychological consequences of interpersonal violence, such as depression, suicidality, anxiety disorders, and eating disorders, are also common, their medical management is reviewed elsewhere (2-8) and is not a focus of this chapter.

This chapter reviews the clinical presentation of women with PTSD caused by a history of interpersonal violence and outlines a clinical approach to their medical care needs. After defining PTSD and complex PTSD, we examine the clinical presentation for each and discuss the management of both in the medical setting. Specifically, we focus on core symptoms of PTSD (re-experiencing traumatic memories, avoidance, emotional arousal, numbing) and associated symptoms that can be seen with complex PTSD (dissociative symptoms, relationship difficulties, affect dysregulation, somatization, and harmful behavior) (9-11). Finally, we recommend a clinical management approach for primary care providers based on psychological theories about the impact of traumatic events upon a woman's functioning.

# Clinical Presentation in the Medical Setting: An Overview

## Post-Traumatic Stress Disorder

PTSD is the most common mental health problem associated with traumatic events, although other problems such as major depressive disorder are also common (see Chapter 1). PTSD is a complex and multiply determined psychiatric disorder involving dysregulation of biological, behavioral, cognitive, and interpersonal systems after a traumatic event (11-13) (see Box 2-12 in Chapter 2 for complete DSM-IV criteria for a diagnosis of PTSD). People with PTSD have been exposed to an event that involved the threat of death or serious physical injury to themselves or to someone else. The traumatic event is experienced with "intense fear, helplessness, or horror" (criterion A) (9), and individuals with PTSD develop a number of well-documented psychiatric symptoms in its aftermath.

These symptoms fall into three categories (9). First is the *re-experiencing* of the trauma through nightmares, flashbacks, and intense distress at reminders of the trauma (criterion B). Second are *avoidance and numbing* symptoms (criterion C). Patients with PTSD will avoid people, places, and activities that are reminiscent of the traumatic experience because they may precipitate traumatic flashbacks. The third major category of symptoms is a heightened level of *emotional arousal* (criterion D) that leads to symptoms such as irritability, difficulty concentrating, and an exaggerated startle response. Traumatized patients spend a great deal of time thinking about the threat of recurrent trauma and will go to great lengths to ensure their own safety. Trauma resulting from violence can alter a woman's world view, leading her to see the world as an unsafe place and people as inherently bad and to believe that the violent experience was her own fault. These symptoms and beliefs color her interpersonal interactions, including those she has with medical providers.

The symptoms of PTSD can occur after a broad range of traumas such as assaults, accidents, disasters, combat, severe illnesses, and injuries (1,14). Trauma appears to be more likely to lead to PTSD in women than in men, although this finding may reflect differences in the types of traumas suffered by women and men (1,15). Women have a much higher prevalence of sexual assault, which appears to be the type of trauma most likely to lead to PTSD.

## Complex Post-Traumatic Stress Disorder

The "core" symptoms of PTSD (re-experiencing trauma through memories, avoidance, numbing, increased arousal) described above are sometimes complicated by "associated features": dissociative symptoms, severe relationship difficulties, problems with affect regulation, somatization, and aggressive or self-destructive behaviors. These symptoms will be described in detail in the following sections. The core plus associated symptoms together form a syndrome that has been labeled *complex PTSD* (9,10,16). The mnemonic "TRAIN CRASH" is a useful way of remembering these two components of PTSD (17), where "TRAIN" refers to the core symptoms of PTSD and "CRASH" refers to the associated features seen in complex PTSD (Box 5-1).

The associated symptoms of PTSD almost always occur in the setting of a history of chronic trauma in childhood (10,11). Physical abuse, sexual abuse, and emotional abuse or neglect occurring during this critical developmental phase can lead to particularly severe and pervasive responses that persist into adulthood. Trauma in childhood affects adult psychopathology in three ways. First, an individual's personality develops during childhood. Chronic personality problems like borderline personality disorder can result from childhood experiences of trauma, leading to an array of maladaptive behaviors. Although not discussed in detail here, borderline personality disorder shares a number of features with complex PTSD. Second, a person's style of coping with stress is largely learned during childhood. However, coping mechanisms learned in the setting of childhood abuse may not translate well to the adult world. For example, a child may learn to dissociate during sexual abuse in order to distance herself from painful emotions and physical sensations. However, if as an adult she dissociates during difficult interpersonal interactions, she may jeopardize relationships or even her own safety. Third, children learn functional or dysfunctional styles of interpersonal interactions from their adult role models. If a child's caregivers are physically abusive, she learns that people are not to be trusted and that violence is the only way to resolve conflict.

---

**Box 5-1    Criteria for Complex PTSD: "TRAIN CRASH"**

Core Symptoms
T  –  Traumatic event
R  –  Re-experiencing
A  –  Avoidance
I  –  Increased arousal
N  –  Numbing of responses

Associated Symptoms
C  –  Consciousness alterations (dissociation)
R  –  Relationship difficulties
A  –  Affect dysregulation
S  –  Somatization
H  –  Harmful behavior (aggressive, self-destructive)

---

Thus, women exposed to chronic abuse in childhood receive powerful messages that they carry into adulthood. These learned behaviors influence their relationships with others, including health care providers.

## Core Symptoms of Post-Traumatic Stress Disorder: Implications for Medical Care

### Re-Experiencing Traumatic Memories in the Medical Setting

Encounters with the medical setting can lead patients to re-experience memories of past traumas. Characteristics of a provider (e.g., gender, race, vocal qualities, personality type, cologne) may remind the patient of her assailant. Additionally, there is a power differential inherent in the provider-patient relationship, and this may be reminiscent of the power differential in the assailant-victim relationship. Characteristics of the health care setting may also remind the patient of the setting in which the trauma occurred. For example, a small examination room may remind a woman of a closet in which she was locked during childhood, or an examination table may remind her of a bed upon which she was sexually assaulted. Events occurring in a medical setting are also very likely to elicit traumatic memories. For example, touching that occurs during a physical examination or procedure may bring back memories of a previous trauma. This is particularly true if the body parts being examined were involved in the assault (e.g., pelvis, rectum, mouth, or breasts, depending on the type of sexual assault); if the examination is more invasive (e.g., ear-nose-throat, dental, genitourinary, or colorectal procedures); if the examiner must be physically close to the patient for the examination (e.g., for funduscopic examination); or if the procedure involves loss of control for the patient (e.g., if a procedure is being performed behind her back or behind drapes, or if she is physically or chemically restrained for the procedure).

Such trauma memories elicited by the clinical setting can lead to a variety of extreme feelings, including powerlessness, helplessness, loss of control, shame, guilt, self-loathing, anger, and rage. The patient may not be consciously aware of these feelings and may not be able to discuss them. Sometimes, in response to overwhelming emotions, a patient may dissociate, becoming disoriented to time and place (or even person) and may acutely believe that she is back in the context of the traumatic event.

### Clinical Approach

The ideal approach to such emotions experienced in the clinical setting is to prevent them from occurring in the first place. The primary means of preventing post-traumatic emotions is to help the patient have as much control over the clinical encounter as possible. It is particularly important that the patient understand the ground rules: 1) she does not have to answer any questions that she is not comfortable answering, and 2) the clinical encounter can be stopped at any time. The clinician must also respect these ground rules. Additionally, the clinician should identify the patient's most important concerns and anxieties about the clinical encounter and work with her to address these concerns.

> *To prevent post-traumatic emotions, the patient must have as much control over the clinical encounter as possible.*

Clinical approaches to the patient who is re-experiencing traumatic memories in the medical setting are summarized in Table 5-1.

ADDRESSING PATIENT CONCERNS

By understanding the patient's agenda, anxieties, and concerns, the clinician can anticipate situations that may precipitate post-traumatic emotions. For example, a patient with a history of childhood sexual abuse may be very frightened of invasive procedures like pelvic examination, colonoscopy, and

**Table 5-1    Re-Experiencing Traumatic Memories in the Medical Setting**

| Description | Clinical Approach |
|---|---|
| The clinical setting can elicit trauma memories, especially procedures involving: | Prevent the traumatic memory from occurring by giving the patient control over the clinical encounter. Informed consent is critical: |
| • Examination of part of her body that was involved in the assault (e.g., pelvis, mouth)<br>• Invasiveness (e.g., dental, colorectal)<br>• Physical proximity of the examiner (e.g., funduscopic examination)<br>• Patient's loss of control (e.g., physical restraint, chemical restraint) | • Explain the examination or procedure before she changes into a gown.<br>• Let her know that she does not have to consent to the examination or procedure and that she can withdraw her consent at any time.<br>• Find out what her concerns are ("Is there anything about this procedure that worries you?").<br>• Anticipate the possibility that a procedure or examination may be difficult for the patient and brainstorm with her about interventions that might make the procedure less frightening.<br>• Alert the patient's psychotherapist about the upcoming procedure.<br>• Using nonthreatening terms, explain what is happening throughout the procedure.<br>• Request consent before each new phase of the examination.<br>• If the patient requests that a procedure be terminated, *stop* immediately. |

even dental work. Sometimes this will require a number of sessions to determine the patient's specific concerns, to offer her options, and to plan for how the procedure can be best tolerated.

The clinician should ask open-ended questions to find out what the patient's concerns are: "Is there anything about this procedure that worries you?" The clinician should also elicit the patient's ideas about what might make her feel less uncomfortable. Examples of specific questions to ask to discover the patient's concerns and wishes are given in Box 5-2.

Spending this time with a patient exploring her concerns powerfully communicates caring, concern, and willingness to respect her needs and priorities. The messages inherent in these communications are contrary to the messages she received as an abused child and will serve to increase trust and to minimize the likelihood that the clinical encounter will elicit post-traumatic memories.

If the patient is in psychotherapy, it is essential that she address concerns about medical procedures with her psychotherapist and that the medical

---

**Box 5-2    Eliciting Patient Concerns and Wishes**

Patient Concerns and Anxieties
- "Do you have any worries about the procedure?"
- "Are you worried that being examined will bring back memories of past trauma?"
- "Do you have any concerns about being sedated for the procedure?"

Patient Wishes
- "Do you want to have a friend or family member [or perhaps a member of the clinic staff who is already known to her] present for the procedure?"
- "Do you want to listen to music or a relaxation tape on headphones during the procedure?"
- "Do you want to tour the procedure room in advance and meet the technicians who will be assisting?"
- "Would you be more comfortable if we left the office door open?"
- "Do you want sedation for the procedure?"*

---

\* Note that a decision to pretreat with a benzodiazepine before a procedure should be made with the patient's full participation. Although sedation can often be therapeutic, in some circumstances it can trigger memories of trauma. For example, if the assailant sedated the patient with drugs or alcohol to facilitate her toleration of childhood sexual abuse, the clinician's act of suggesting that she take medication can bring back memories of her abuser's insistence that she accept sedation. Also, in this instance, while sedated, she will feel the way she did while being abused, through the process of state-dependent memory.

provider keep the psychotherapist apprised of upcoming medical interventions that are likely to be disturbing for the patient. The therapist can work with the patient on a regular basis to anticipate difficulties and to generate strategies that will maximize her sense of control. The therapist and primary care clinician should share information and support each other's work. This type of communication between clinicians involved in the patient's care can help the patient to feel more in control.

REQUESTING PATIENT CONSENT
The clinician should request the patient's consent to perform a procedure while she is still dressed, and only after she has received information about what the procedure will entail and what its risks and benefits are, and only after all her questions have been answered. She must not feel coerced into consenting to a procedure. Once the patient consents to a procedure, she needs to understand her right to withdraw her consent at any time, and the provider must respect that right.

*The patient has the right to withdraw consent to any procedure at any time.*

In addition, throughout the examination or procedure, the clinician should request consent periodically (e.g., before moving from the heart examination to the breast examination he or she could ask, "May I perform your breast exam now?") and should explain what he or she is doing, especially if the patient cannot see the examiner. Efforts should be made to use the least threatening terms possible (18). For example, clinicians can refer to the "bills" (not the "blades") of the speculum, and "foot rests" (not "stirrups"). The patient can be asked to "let your knees drop apart" rather than "spread your legs." The clinician should speak in a calm, un-rushed, gentle voice. If the patient asks that the procedure be stopped, it is imperative that the clinician do so immediately (or as soon as it is safe to do so).

## Avoidance

Individuals with trauma histories can lead very restrictive lives. Patients may become so fearful that the traumatic event will recur (or even that a painful memory of the traumatic event will recur) that they avoid all situations and people that remind them of it. Because aspects of the medical setting can bring back memories of the traumatic event, patients will often avoid clinical encounters. Even patients who desperately need medical attention may stay away from clinicians for long periods of time. Patients who do present for care may avoid discussing certain topics. For example, a patient may not disclose that she is having rectal bleeding because she is terrified that this disclosure will lead to a rectal examination, which in turn will elicit frightening memories of her trauma. This avoidance can put patients at medical risk. It is important to determine how to help patients with trauma histories get the medical attention that they need without overwhelming them with trauma-related emotion.

### Clinical Approach

Working with a patient who avoids medical treatment can lead to a difficult clinical dilemma. To aggressively insist that the patient present for treatment can be perceived as intrusive and the clinician perceived as frightening. This may lead the patient to flee treatment. Alternatively, to not actively recommend that the patient receive the medical care that she needs may be perceived by the patient as neglectful. The clinician is also at medical-legal risk if he or she does not clearly recommend standard treatment. Thus, the patient's avoidant behavior can place the clinician between the untenable poles of appearing (from the patient's perspective) to abuse the patient (by insisting on medical care) and appearing to neglect the patient (by not insisting on medical care). This dilemma is not uncommon. The clinician must provide a clear explanation of recommended interventions but do so in a way that the patient will not perceive as intrusive. For example, "I know you are reluctant to have a blood test today. However, with the vomiting you have been having, I am concerned that you could have a low potassium level. If your potassium is low, we can easily treat it with a pill. However, if untreated, low potassium can even lead to death. Therefore, can we discuss your concerns about having the test and brainstorm about what might make it less difficult for you to go through with it?" If the patient refuses emergency interventions in this setting, the clinician must seek psychiatric consultation to assess competency and make sure the patient's avoidant behavior does not reflect passive suicidality through a process of traumatic re-enactment (19). It will rarely be required that a patient will need a guardian appointed or will need an involuntary hospitalization because of avoidance of medical care. When it seems that these maximally intrusive options may be necessary, they need to be considered carefully by medical and psychiatric providers as a team.

Optimally, such "show-downs" are prevented in the first place by helping the patient to decrease her avoidant symptoms. This is best accomplished by helping to increase her feelings of control within the clinical encounter, by identifying her concerns, working with her agenda, and intensively communicating care and concern. Pharmacologic treatment of anxiety may also help to decrease her avoidant symptoms (20).

Systematic desensitization techniques (21) can be used in cases of severe anxiety (with input from a psychotherapist) to help the patient minimize her

**Table 5-2    Avoidance**

| Description | Clinical Approach |
| --- | --- |
| Medical encounters can elicit painful memories of trauma. The patient may seek to protect herself by<br>• Avoiding clinical encounters (e.g., failing to show for scheduled appointments)<br>• Failing to disclose important medical history (e.g., if afraid that disclosure will lead the clinician to recommend an invasive examination) | • Allow the patient to be in control of the clinical encounter.<br>• Anxiolytics can help with anxiety.<br>• Systematic desensitization can decrease severe anxiety about clinical encounters.<br>• If the patient declines urgently needed care, make sure she clearly understands the implications of her decision; then seek psychiatric consultation to assess competency and suicide risk. |

avoidance of medical settings or interventions. These techniques require exposure to the avoided medical procedure in a stepwise way. For example, in the case of a patient who avoids a pelvic examination, the clinician can construct a continuum of exposure to the pelvic examination that gradually increases in intensity. The first session is spent talking about the examination. During the second session, the patient views the speculum and other instruments. At the third session and with the patient's consent, the examination occurs. However, one must bear in mind that avoidance of medical treatment or failure to disclose important medical history can occur regardless of the degree of skill, care, or concern of the clinician. Clinical approaches are summarized in Table 5-2.

## Emotional Arousal

An increased state of emotional arousal is common in patients with PTSD and may intensify as a result of anxiety experienced in the health care setting. A woman with a trauma history may startle easily, jumping when a telephone rings. She may seem distracted and have difficulty concentrating on the clinician's medical instructions. She may be hypervigilant about threats to her person. For example, she may be afraid to drive into the city where the clinic is located if she perceives urban areas as dangerous. Her fears may also extend to other perceived threats, such as concern that physical symptoms she is experiencing could be attributable to cancer.

*Clinical Approach*

The clinician can take a number of steps to decrease the patient's symptoms of increased emotional arousal. Most important is to minimize the risk that she will experience the clinical encounter as reminiscent of her previous trauma, as discussed above.

The clinical environment should be safe and soothing: quiet, peaceful music playing in the waiting room, comfortable chairs, adequate temperature control in the examination room, avoidance of loud or rushed speech or technical terms, and minimization of telephone calls and other interruptions during the clinical encounter can all help. Also, feeling in control of the clinical encounter (e.g., by being offered options and by not being pressured to submit to physical examinations and procedures, as previously described) will help lessen the patient's anxiety and startle reactions.

Poor concentration directly interferes with quality medical care: a distracted patient may forget to provide important information to her clinician and may not remember her provider's instructions. The steps described above to decrease levels of anxiety will help the patient to concentrate. However, additional steps can be taken to minimize its risk. For example, if the clinician senses that the patient was distracted when describing the history of present illness, he or she can query her again on important elements of the history later in the clinical encounter, when she may feel more relaxed and attentive. The clinician can also reflect his or her observations back upon the patient: "You seem a little distracted right now. A lot of patients feel nervous at the doctor's office. Are you feeling uneasy?" If the patient's answer is affirmative: "Is there anything I can do to make you more comfortable?" Asking patients to repeat back instructions can ensure that the information was heard, if this can be done in a manner that does not humiliate the patient. For example, "I just gave you a lot of information, and I know it was pretty complicated. Can you tell me what your understanding is of what I just said, so I can make sure that I explained it clearly?"

*Give patients written instructions and educational materials.*

Finally, after screening for literacy (22), clinicians are strongly urged to give patients written instructions and written patient education materials to supplement the information they provide verbally.

Strong fears (e.g., fear of cancer, fear of infectious diseases) are also more easily addressed when they are understood in the context of increased levels of arousal and hypervigilence. Trauma-related feelings of terror may become displaced: physical symptoms may be a new perceived threat to the patient. It is important to find out what worries the patient (e.g., "Many people have ideas about what could be making them feel ill. Have you had any ideas about what might be causing your symptoms?"). This makes it possible to target education about the condition appropriately. Making it clear to the patient that her concerns are being taken seriously and clearly explaining how the clinical findings inform the clinical assessment can help reassure her. Clinical approaches are summarized in Table 5-3.

**Table 5-3    Emotional Arousal**

| Description | Clinical Approach |
| --- | --- |
| Exaggerated startle response and hypervigilance | • Create a safe, calm clinical environment.<br>• Allow patient to feel in control of the clinical encounter (e.g., offering her choices, not pressuring her to agree to procedures). |
| Poor concentration | • Re-query about important elements of the medical history later in the interview, when the patient feels less anxious.<br>• Ask the patient what might make her feel more comfortable.<br>• Request that the patient repeat instructions to ensure she understood them.<br>• Provide the patient with a written list of instructions. |
| Strong fears | • Find out what worries the patient.<br>• Make it clear that her concerns are being taken seriously.<br>• Let her know how the clinical findings inform the differential diagnosis.<br>• Treat underlying anxiety pharmacologically, if appropriate. |

## Numbing

Patients with PTSD may cope with distressing feelings by wrapping themselves in an emotional cocoon. They may exhibit a restricted range of emotions. For example, they may not be able to express affection towards others. At the extreme, they may temporarily dissociate (see below). This can interfere with the clinician's sense that he or she has successfully connected with the patient.

*Clinical Approach*

The medical provider can be reassured that the patient's tendency to be emotionally distant or aloof is another manifestation of her PTSD, not a reflection upon the clinician's communication style. For patients with PTSD, the ability to develop caring relationships often comes only after extended psychotherapy. Medical providers can serve as excellent role models for patients, allowing them to have an experience with a safe, well-bounded, supportive, and trusting interpersonal relationship. This relationship can serve as a template that allows the patient to practice skills that will serve her well in other future relationships. Clinical approaches are summarized in Table 5-4.

# Complex Post-Traumatic Stress Disorder: Implications for Medical Care

A subset of women who have experienced violence will develop not only the core symptoms of PTSD but also the associated symptoms. When the core and

**Table 5-4    Numbing**

| Description | Clinical Approach |
|---|---|
| • Emotional distance and/or restricted range of emotions | • Prepare for the possibility that it may take months or years until the patient feels safe enough to interact freely. |
| • Lack of "connection" between patient and provider | • Continue to provide the patient with a safe, supportive professional relationship, which will serve as a model for her future relationships. |

associated symptoms occur together, they are often referred to as complex PTSD (10,11,16). Complex PTSD is almost always associated with a history of severe, repetitive abuse in childhood. This section describes major presentations of complex PTSD and discusses how medical providers can respond to them.

## Dissociative Symptoms

Dissociation is "a disruption in the usually integrated functions of consciousness, memory, identity, or perception of the environment. The disturbance may be sudden or gradual, transient or chronic"(9). Anyone can have dissociative episodes, such as "spacing out" in a stressful moment. However, dissociative episodes are more common in patients with PTSD and may be more striking in nature (23,24). For example, the patient may become suddenly distant and rigid, staring into space and not responding to her name, or she may appear disoriented, crying or speaking about remote events as if they were currently occurring. She may even seem to assume a different persona, for example, speaking in a different tone of voice and with a different accent and affect. In patients with the complex form of PTSD, dissociative episodes can recur in a pathological pattern that qualifies as a dissociative disorder. The dissociative disorders include dissociative fugue (in which the patient suddenly travels to an unexpected place and is confused about her own identity), dissociative amnesia (in which the patient forgets information that is emotionally laden because it is reminiscent of previous trauma), and dissociative identity disorder (formerly known as multiple personality disorder, in which the patient experiences herself as another person[s]). These problems are not rare (23-25) and, as with other symptoms of PTSD, may be triggered by the clinical encounter. It is helpful for the clinician to anticipate dissociative episodes by screening for a history of dissociation. Screening questions include "Are there periods of time you cannot account for?" and "Have you ever found yourself somewhere and didn't know where you were or how you got there?"

*Clinical Approach*

When the patient dissociates, the major interventions are to re-orient her and to address the triggering emotion (typically fear). To re-orient her, the clinician should communicate in a calm but assured voice such information as where the patient is (name of hospital, clinic, etc.), who the patient is with (name of clinician), and why she is there (e.g., to give her

> *Re-orient patient who dissociates by calmly explaining where she is, why she is there, and that she is safe.*

relief from the symptoms she has been experiencing) (23). To assure her that she is safe, the clinician can tell her directly that she is safe, and the clinician should stop touching her (e.g., if dissociation occurred in the middle of an examination). Although a clinician may feel inclined to reach out to comfort the patient, it is generally best not to touch someone while she is dissociating because she may misinterpret the sensation. In most instances this verbal re-orientation or "grounding," combined with efforts to make her feel safe, will be enough to help the patient to leave her dissociative state.

Regardless of any clinical intervention during a dissociative state, this state is usually self-limiting within a few minutes. Although the clinician may find this painful to observe, it must be remembered that patients with PTSD live their lives entering and exiting post-traumatic states of emotion. Dissociation is one of the ways they cope with strong emotions.

After the patient has regained control, the clinician should normalize the event. He or she may give the patient an objective description of what occurred ("You became confused for a little bit") and should let her know that many people experience dissociation ("Many people experience this when they are in a stressful setting"). If the patient does not respond to re-orienting and the episode does not appear to be self-limiting, a psychiatric consultation may be in order. Chronic dissociative disorders are an indication for psychiatric consultation because they typically reflect complex psychopathology. Clinical approaches to the patient experiencing a dissociative episode in the clinical setting are summarized in Table 5-5.

## Relationship Difficulties: Traumatic Re-Enactments in the Clinician-Patient Relationship

Individuals with histories of trauma can have interpersonal difficulties that complicate the clinical encounter. Because the ability to develop and sustain effective interpersonal relationships is a major developmental task of childhood, women from abusive and neglectful families of origin may have learned dysfunctional interaction styles. Children who are victims of child abuse repeatedly have their trust violated. However, in a family in which child

**Table 5-5    Dissociation**

| Description | Clinical Approach |
|---|---|
| In an acute dissociative episode, in response to a strong emotion (typically, fear), the patient may<br>• Suddenly become rigid<br>• Stare into space and not respond to her name<br>• Appear disoriented, crying or speaking about remote events as if they were currently occurring<br><br>Chronic dissociative disorders include<br>• Dissociative fugue<br>• Dissociative amnesia<br>• Dissociative identity disorder | • Re-orient the patient (where she is, who is with her, why she is there).<br>• Assure the patient that she is safe.<br>• If dissociation occurs during a medical procedure, stop the procedure.<br>• Do not touch the patient while she is dissociating, even in an attempt to comfort her.<br>• Chronic dissociative disorders reflect significant impairment and require psychiatric consultation. |

abuse occurs, it is not uncommon for the abuser to be perceived as helpful in other, nonabusive, situations. There is great confusion in the survivor of child abuse about who is safe and who is dangerous, who helps and who hurts. Women with such childhood experiences may be inclined to form similarly disturbing relationships with caregivers throughout life (10,26,27), and this has direct relevance in the medical setting.

One result of these childhood experiences is that women may learn to trust too little. In the clinical setting, this may lead the patient to be wary of following her doctor's advice. She may refuse needed interventions or fail to disclose critical information because of mistrust of the clinician or fear that the clinician will harm her. Sometimes a patient's consent to perform a procedure paradoxically represents mistrust: she may worry about retaliation and abandonment from the clinician for declining recommendations, leading her to agree to an unwanted test.

Alternatively, patients may trust too easily and thus become vulnerable to continued violations. In this instance, patients may be repeatedly victimized by other people. Although the cause of revictimization is unknown, it may be related to difficulties discerning safe, interpersonal boundaries because of boundary violations and poor role models in childhood (10,26). At the extreme, this problem makes patients with histories of child abuse vulnerable to boundary violations from clinicians, including sexual abuse (28). However, there are many less extreme ways that excessive trust can also become manifest in even the most caring of clinician-patient relationships. Patients can be so trustful of clinicians that they consent to procedures and treatments without fully considering the risks and benefits or before they are psychologically prepared to go through with them. Similarly, patients may consent to unwanted treatments because they worry about offending the clinician. They may also over-idealize their clinicians ("You're the only doctor I can trust"), setting themselves up for disappointment and feelings of betrayal when, as will inevitably happen, the clinician does not live up to this unrealistic ideal.

Closely related to difficulties with trust are issues of caring. Because many patients with histories of child abuse have intense emotions regarding basic notions of care, and because care is central to the clinician-patient relationship, this relationship is ripe for the re-creation of these emotions. In this "traumatic re-enactment," the patient re-enacts early life relationships in her current relationship with the clinician. Traumatic re-enactments commonly occur around issues of treatment. The patient may want a particular treatment (e.g., an opioid pain medication) or test (e.g., an MRI) that the clinician considers not to be indicated. Alternatively, the clinician may recommend a treatment, test, or referral that the patient does not want to accept. An ordinary clinical negotiation can escalate into a traumatic re-enactment for some patients who come from an abusive background. The clinician must walk a fine line between abusing the patient (e.g., by insisting on treatment) or neglecting the patient (e.g., by failing to treat). This complex psychodynamic phenomenon is illustrated in the following clinical case studies.

CASE 5-1

*Mrs. Jones is a 28-year-old woman with a history of childhood sexual abuse who has insulin-dependent diabetes mellitus. She has been Dr. Smith's patient for 3 years. Mrs. Jones is notoriously non-adherent to her insulin regimen and has begun to show early signs of vascular complications related to diabetes. Dr. Smith has gently encouraged Mrs. Jones to take her insulin regularly. Mrs. Jones frequently struggles with Dr. Smith about this plan and has accused her physician on a number of occasions of trying to "control" her. Dr. Smith frequently considers more vigorous confrontation regarding compliance but never clearly informs Mrs. Jones about the medical consequences of her behavior. Dr. Smith notices feelings of relief whenever Mrs. Jones cancels her appointment. Six months after her last visit, Dr. Smith is informed that Mrs. Jones had been admitted to the emergency room after being found in an unresponsive state. When Dr. Smith visits her in the hospital, Mrs. Jones angrily accuses Dr. Smith of abandonment: "You did not call me for months!"*

*Ms. Norton is a 38-year-old woman with a history of childhood sexual abuse. She has had three previous psychiatric hospitalizations for suicide attempts. She sees Dr. Barnes every 2 months for vague physical complaints, the cause of which is unknown. During these visits she frequently hints at suicidal ideation while cautioning Dr. Barnes: "I trust you. You would never send me back to the psych ward." Dr. Barnes feels awkward during these exchanges and never pursues them, focusing instead on the presenting complaint. Ms. Norton now tells Dr. Barnes that she recently purchased a handgun and put the barrel in her mouth the previous evening "to see what it would feel like." She refuses to answer any of Dr. Barnes' questions about her suicidal risk (responding instead with accusations: "I know what you're up to. You want to put me in the hospital.") and angrily leaves the office. Dr. Barnes calls security, who are forced to restrain Ms. Norton in a violent struggle in the lobby. Ms. Norton is brought to the emergency department and placed in four-point restraints. She is heard yelling that Dr. Barnes had her "gang-raped in front of everyone."*

These examples illustrate how earlier traumatic relationships may become re-created in the clinical setting. In Case 5-1, Dr. Smith at first finds herself walking the untenable tightrope between appearing to the patient to be abusive (by being controlling) and appearing to be neglectful (by failing to be a rescuer). Then Dr. Smith falls toward the neglective side, ultimately being accused by the patient of abandonment.

In Case 5-2, Dr. Barnes is walking the same tightrope. She distances herself from the patient (and from the feelings engendered by the patient's suicidal hints) by focusing on the presenting medical complaint and neglecting to pursue the suicidal hints. The patient, finally, expresses her suicidal ideation in a way that Dr. Barnes cannot ignore but in a way that attempts to disempower Dr. Barnes. Dr. Barnes then feels compelled to implement extreme controlling measures.

Of note, the psychiatric literature often refers to the concept of traumatic re-enactment in terms of "transference" and "countertransference"[26]. Transference occurs when the patient assigns the characteristics of a person from her past upon the clinician (for example, her abusive father or her mother, who tried to protect her from her father). Countertransference occurs when the clinician assigns the characteristics of a person from his or her own past (the clinician's child, for example) onto the patient.

## Clinical Approach

Traumatic re-enactments are among the most difficult of clinical problems. These situations arouse intense feelings in both the patient and the clinician. They can cloud clinical judgment and lead to boundary violations that are potentially hazardous to both patient and clinician. Nevertheless, traumatic re-enactments are not necessarily signs of treatment failure and can, in a way, be seen as an indicator of closeness in the clinician-patient relationship (patients tend to develop traumatic re-enactments with people whom they care about). Therefore, the following paragraphs contain recommendations designed to minimize the frequency and intensity of traumatic re-enactments.

At their core, traumatic re-enactments reflect great anxiety on the part of the patient about basic notions of care (e.g., "Does she care about me?" "Does she like me?" "Can I trust her?"). Sometimes behaviors that appear highly provocative can be seen as tests of whether the clinician cares sufficiently. During a traumatic re-enactment, the clinician should assess whether basic notions of care are at stake. In Case 5-1, Mrs. Jones, for example, is noncompliant and does not present to appointments for months. Her noncompliance may be a test of whether Dr. Smith cares about her ("If the doctor really cares she will call and insist that I get treatment"). It might have been helpful for Dr. Smith to be more active in her recommendations for treatment while communicating to the patient the difficulties of providing this treatment: "You need treatment and I will worry about your health if you don't get this treatment. I really want to help you but find it difficult because every time I suggest treatment you say I am controlling. How can we work on getting you the care that you need without you feeling controlled?"

Traumatic re-enactments may engender very uncomfortable feelings in clinicians. Not uncommonly, clinicians may experience feelings of anger, fear, helplessness, guilt, and shame during traumatic re-enactments. These feelings can influence clinician behavior. For example, clinicians may react to feelings of helplessness by distancing themselves from patients, and they may retaliate against a patient who makes them feel helpless and ashamed by humiliating the patient. Clinicians may respond to internal feelings of guilt by overextending themselves for the patient, perhaps extending a visit beyond the normally allotted time or agreeing to see the patient after hours. Unfortunately, such clinician behaviors may lead to further exacerbation of traumatic re-enactments. It is very important for clinicians to be aware of these feelings and to question the degree to which they are influencing clinical judgment. It often helps to review such cases with colleagues. Treating such patients within a clinical team is ideal because emotions related to the care of the patient can be discussed and strategies for addressing them can be identified.

Maintenance of interpersonal and professional boundaries is critical (29). Occasionally, traumatic re-enactments are motivated by the patient's desire to have a non-professional relationship with the clinician ("if she cared she would let me call her at home"). It is essential that the clinician maintain established boundaries. See Chapter 6 for a discussion of how providers can care for themselves and Clinical Vignette 1 for additional discussion of boundary issues.

Mental health consultation and referral is usually helpful when traumatic re-enactments occur. A mental health professional can work with the patient to address the complex psychological underpinnings of traumatic re-enactment. The mental health consultant can also serve as a sounding board for the clinician, who may want guidance about how to manage ongoing traumatic re-enactments.

As discussed earlier, struggles often arise around whether a patient should receive a particular intervention. This situation may also lead to traumatic re-enactments with a patient. This is because the clinician is likely to feel the need to exert strong pressure on the patient to agree to urgently needed treatment, which may remind the patient of the strong pressure her abuser used upon her. This situation requires psychiatric consultation. Clinical approaches are summarized in Table 5-6.

*If patient declines urgently needed medical care, immediate psychiatric consultation is advised.*

## Table 5-6　Relationship Difficulties

| Description | Clinical Approach |
|---|---|
| The patient may re-enact traumatic early life relationships in her relationship with the clinician. For example:<br>• Trusting too little or too much<br>• Looking at the clinician as an abuser or a rescuer<br>• Attaching special meaning to the caring nature of the professional relationship<br><br>The provider may unintentionally enter into this traumatic re-enactment, crossing established boundaries. For example:<br>• Seeing himself or herself as a rescuer or hero, as the only one who can help the patient<br>• Retaliating against the patient with demeaning statements<br>• Avoiding the patient (e.g., not returning phone calls) | • Be attuned to strong feelings towards a particular patient (e.g., anger, helplessness, pride, guilt) and question whether they are influencing clinical judgment.<br>• Discuss the case with colleagues who are not entwined in the clinical relationship and who can thus give objective suggestions.<br>• Maintain professional boundaries.<br>• Refer the patient to a mental health professional to address the complex psychological underpinnings of traumatic re-enactment, and to help her move toward healthier relationships.<br>• While pushing the patient too hard to accept a needed medical intervention may make her feel "abused" by the clinician, it is at the same time important to communicate very clearly why the procedure is needed.<br>• If the patient declines urgently needed treatment, a psychiatric consultant can assess competency and suicidality. |

## Affect Dysregulation

Patients with complex PTSD may have particular difficulty with affect regulation, i.e., maintaining an affect appropriate to the context (11,30). During what seems like a neutral conversation, the patient may explode in anger or break down in tears. The display of emotions may seem disproportionate to the precipitant. Angry outbursts may have a particularly damaging effect upon clinician-patient relationships and may in turn impair the clinician's ability to deliver effective care.

*Clinical Approach*
The clinician may be annoyed or frustrated by such emotional displays by the patient and may dread seeing the patient's name on the day's list of appointments. Nevertheless, because clinicians are ethically bound to provide high-quality care to every patient, some coping strategies for the clinician are in order. First, it is often helpful to talk about one's feelings with a trusted colleague. This provides an opportunity for the clinician to vent in a safe environment, rather than risking the possibility that his or her frustration will boil over in the clinical encounter, emotionally harming the patient and/or the clinician-patient relationship. A mental health colleague may be particularly well positioned to provide valuable problem-solving insights. Second, a clinician's anger often dissipates when he or she bears in mind that the patient's poor interpersonal interaction style represents part of the pathology of her disease and is not fully in her own control. Third, it can be helpful to identify an "empathetic hook," some characteristic of the patient that the clinician can admire, perhaps the fact that she is raising two children on her own, or the fact that she enjoys classical music, or even her persistence in advocating for herself in the clinical encounter. Keeping this strength in mind can help the clinician to see the patient more empathetically, reframing even difficult clinical encounters.

Interventions that help the patient to control her affect will make the clinical encounter more positive for both patient and provider. Acutely, medical providers can avoid escalating the situation by speaking in a calm voice, echoing the patient's words so she knows she has been heard, and apologizing (if appropriate). Because anxiety often underpins outbursts of anger or grief, the clinician should explore and address any underlying fears. The clinician can refer the patient to a mental health provider for anxiolytics and/or counseling (e.g., anger management skills), which will help the patient to more successfully modulate her affect. This will allow her to interact more effectively with her medical provider, as well as with other people in her life. Because patients often feel humiliated once the passion of the moment has passed and recognize that their outbursts interfere with a number of relationships, they typically appreciate the opportunity to learn such skills. However, mental health referral is best offered in a moment of calm, rather than in the midst of an outburst.

Medical providers must be familiar with strategies for screening for acute suicidal or homicidal ideation (6). When there is a concern about possible suicidality or homicidality, the clinician should seek immediate psychiatric consultation for safety assessment and to determine whether emergency hospitalization is required. Again, it is important to remember that involuntary hospitalization will be particularly traumatic for a survivor of interpersonal violence. Therefore, before resorting to involuntary hospitalization, the involved clinicians should first see if the patient will agree to be admitted voluntarily. To increase the chances that this will happen, the patient should be given the opportunity to express her concerns about hospitalization and these concerns should be addressed if possible. The clinician should also clearly explain why hospitalization is needed (i.e., stress that the goal is to help her and ensure her safety, not to harm her) and what hospitalization would involve. As has been emphasized previously, the patient will feel less frightened and will experience less traumatic memories if she has some control over the situation. Although it is not possible to offer an acutely suicidal patient a choice between admission and discharge, it is at least possible to offer her a choice between involuntary admission and voluntary admission. If after this attempted negotiation the admission must be involuntary, use of physical restraints should be avoided unless essential to ensure the patient's safety. Clinical approaches are summarized in Table 5-7.

**Table 5-7    Affect Dysregulation**

| Description | Clinical Approach |
|---|---|
| Emotional lability (e.g., sudden outbursts of anger or tearfulness) can<br>• Interfere with the patient-provider relationship<br>• Frustrate, upset, or alienate the clinician<br>• Distress the patient | • Avoid escalating the situation acutely; speak in a calm voice and make it clear that the patient has been heard.<br>• Talk with a colleague about the feelings engendered by the patient's outbursts; this allows the clinician's feelings to be ventilated in a safe environment, where they will not harm the patient.<br>• Recognize that the patient's strong feelings are part of the pathology of her condition and are not fully within her control.<br>• Identify an "empathetic hook," some characteristic of the patient that can be admired.<br>• Refer the patient to a mental health provider for psychotherapy and/or anxiolytics to help her modulate her affect.<br>• Seek emergency psychiatric consultation if the patient may be suicidal or homicidal. |

## Somatization

Somatization involves the presence of physical symptoms in the absence of known organic etiologies or out of proportion to the known etiology. Box 5-3 outlines the DSM-IV criteria for somatization disorder. In addition to somatization disorder, there are several other somatiform disorders that can be seen with greater frequency in patients with PTSD, including conversion disorders (31,32).

As Chapter 1 describes, women with a history of experiencing violence are likely to have several chronic or episodic physical symptoms and medical conditions. These can be caused by somatization disorder (33) or by a number of other competing physiologic mechanisms (e.g., neuroendocrine dysregulation). It is beyond the scope of this chapter to fully describe the causes and treatments of somatiform disorders, but individuals with histories of trauma, particularly those with complex PTSD (32), are at higher risk for somatization. In addition to physiologic mechanisms, for women who have been victims of violence, two important psychological mechanisms for development of physical symptoms include 1) the communication of distress through somatic symptoms, and 2) the representation of traumatic experiences in somatic symptoms.

First, somatic symptoms can serve as a means to communicate distress (31). For children who are abused or neglected, the expression of physical symptoms and the visits to the doctor may have been their only experiences with caring authority figures. Such powerful early life experiences can color the means by which individuals seek help for the rest of their lives. It is important to understand that the individual often is not consciously aware that this is the motivation for her behavior. There can be great hope on the part of patients that the doctor will remove the distress by solving the physical problem. The underside of this hope is, of course, the inevitable disappointment when the distress is not removed and the physical problems are not clearly solved.

Second, in some cases, traumatic experiences not consciously remembered are experienced as physical sensations in the body: "the body keeps the score" (31). For example, a woman sexually molested as a child may experience chronic vaginal pain. A woman who was strangled may report chronic difficulty swallowing. This phenomenon, called "body memory," has been described for centuries and was an important component of the initial conceptualization of hysteria (32).

### Clinical Approach
A team approach that integrates primary care with mental health care is ideal in the management of somatization disorder. As in the case of traumatic re-enactments, responding to somatization can easily place the clinician between the untenable poles of abusing and neglecting the patient. To aggressively

## Box 5-3    DSM IV Criteria for Somatization Disorder*

A. A history of many physical complaints beginning before age 30 years that occur over a period of several years and result in treatment being sought or significant impairment in social, occupational, or other important areas of functioning

B. Each of the following criteria must have been met, with individual symptoms occurring at any time during the course of the disturbance:

(1) *Four pain symptoms:* a history of pain related to at least four different sites or functions (e.g., head, abdomen, back, joints, extremities, chest, rectum, during menstruation, during sexual intercourse, or during urination)

(2) *Two gastrointestinal symptoms:* a history of at least two gastrointestinal symptoms other than pain (e.g., nausea, bloating, vomiting other than during pregnancy, diarrhea, or intolerance of several different foods)

(3) *One sexual symptom:* a history of at least one sexual or reproductive symptom other than pain (e.g., sexual indifference, erectile or ejaculatory dysfunction, irregular menses, excessive menstrual bleeding, vomiting throughout pregnancy)

(4) *One pseudoneurological symptom:* a history of at least one symptom or deficit suggesting a neurological condition not limited to pain (conversion symptoms such as impaired coordination or balance, paralysis or localized weakness, difficulty swallowing or lump in throat, aphonia, urinary retention, hallucinations, loss of touch or pain sensation, double vision, blindness, deafness, seizures; dissociative symptoms such as amnesia; or loss of consciousness

C. Either (1) or (2):

(1) After appropriate investigation, each of the symptoms in Criterion B cannot be fully explained by a known general medical condition or the direct effects of a substance (e.g., a drug of abuse, a medication)

(2) When there is a related general medical condition, the physical complaints or resulting social or occupational impairment are in excess of what would be expected from the history, physical examination, or laboratory findings

D. The symptoms are not intentionally produced or feigned (as in Factitious Disorder or Malingering)

---

* Adapted from Diagnostic and Statistical Manual of Mental Disorders. Washington, DC: American Psychiatric Association.

investigate every physical complaint of a patient with somatization disorder can lead to enormous medical intrusions on the patient and can be perceived as abusive. The clinician risks inflicting iatrogenic harm. To not investigate these complaints can be perceived as neglectful. It is easy to dismiss these symptoms as "psychiatric" and miss important medical diagnoses. Patients readily sense this: "My doctor thinks my problem is all in my head."

Clinicians must develop a sensible balance: investigating symptoms when appropriate (remembering that patients with somatization disorder do develop other diseases just like any other patient) and reassuring patients when investigation is not warranted (34). Understanding the communicative nature of the physical complaints can help the clinician form an appropriate response. In other words, symptoms can diminish when patients feel that their concerns are seriously considered and that they are working with a clinician who cares for and about them.

*Somatiform symptoms cause real suffering and should be addressed.*

Clinicians can find somatization disorder very frustrating to treat (35). Evaluations can take a great deal of time and may seem to have a low yield. It is important not to respond punitively or dismissively to the patient because this will only make somatic symptoms worse (by communicating to the patient that she is not cared for). Although there may not be a physiologic basis for her symptoms, her suffering is very real and should be validated. For example, "I'm sorry that you have been feeling bad lately. It sounds like it has been very hard on you." Even though physicians may dread the long list of symptoms that patients with somatization disorder bring to a visit, frequent, scheduled visits (with development of written contracts, if necessary, to minimize unscheduled visits) can have a positive effect. This makes the patient feel more secure that she will not be abandoned and that her concerns are being taken seriously. She learns that she does not have to beg for help.

*Frequent appointments can have a positive effect on patients with somatization disorder.*

Although increased primary care contact often decreases somatiform symptoms, mental health referral, surprisingly, may be less effective, depending on how it is framed. Just as it is usually not helpful for a medical provider to suggest to the patient that her symptoms may be psychologically based, patients usually do not respond well to a mental health referral for the purpose of treating somatization disorder: they typically do not see a connection between their physical symptoms and their underlying emotional state and thus feel that the referral to mental health suggests that their clinician does not believe that their symptoms are real. However, a mental health referral directed at helping the patient cope with the stress of chronic illness or at helping to

**Table 5-8    Somatization**

| Description | Clinical Approach |
| --- | --- |
| Somatic symptoms not readily explained by known physiologic processes. Psychologic factors include<br>• Somatic symptoms, which can represent a means to communicate distress<br>• A traumatic experience not consciously remembered, which may be experienced as a physical sensation in the body | • Take the patient seriously: her suffering is real, and she will be devastated if she feels that "My doctor thinks my problem is all in my head."<br>• Validate the patient's experience and communicate care: "I am sorry that you have been feeling bad lately."<br>• Schedule primary care visits at a frequent, regular interval independent of symptoms, with a written contract (if necessary) to minimize the use of unscheduled or telephone contact.<br>• Remember that patients with somatiform disorders can develop physiologic illnesses.<br>• At the same time, avoid excessive diagnostic evaluations, particularly invasive tests, which may lead to iatrogenic harm.<br>• Consider mental health referral to help the patient cope with chronic physical symptoms or to treat her PTSD; referral to treat the somatization disorder itself is typically not acceptable to the patient. |

alleviate her PTSD symptoms may be well received. As her PTSD is treated and her anxiety level and coping skills improve, the patient's somatiform symptoms may also start to decrease. After extended psychotherapy, she may come to a point at which she and her therapist can begin to explore the possible connection between somatic symptoms and dissociated memories of child abuse. Clinical approaches to the patient with somatization are given in Table 5-8.

## Harmful Behavior

Patients with histories of trauma can engage in behavior that harms them. Self-mutilation is the prototype of such self-destructive behavior. For example, the patient may ritually cut herself (not necessarily with any suicidal intent) or burn herself. Eating disorders (including anorexia nervosa and bulimia) (36) and substance abuse are other forms of harmful behavior commonly seen in trauma survivors. Suicide is the most extreme self-destructive behavior and has increased prevalence in women who have been traumatized. Primary care clinicians need to be skilled in the assessment of risk and in understanding the motivations for such behavior. There are two primary motivations for self-destructive behavior in patients with trauma histories: 1) the regulation of emotion and 2) the communication of distress.

As described earlier, patients with PTSD can fluctuate between extremes of intense emotion and numbing of emotional responses. Self-destructive behavior, particularly self-mutilation, can be motivated by a desire to relieve these extreme emotions. Patients who self-mutilate often say that they feel calmer during and after the behavior. Bulimics also may feel that induced vomiting can relieve internal stress. Substance abuse has an obvious potential to soothe. Occasionally, patients in a state of emotional numbing (such as is seen in borderline personality disorder) mutilate to feel "real" or "alive."

Patients may also engage in harmful and self-destructive behavior in order to communicate distress to others. Frequently, children who live in abusive and neglectful families feel they need to communicate in extreme ways to elicit care. Self-destructive behaviors can be seen as examples of extreme expressions of the need for care, related to an expectation that care will not be forthcoming. The example of Ms. Norton in Case 5-2 illustrates such extreme behaviors. Ms. Norton may have believed that she needed to tell Dr. Barnes that she put a handgun barrel in her mouth in order to get the physician's attention.

### Clinical Approach

Whether the patient is engaging in self-destructive behavior to modulate extreme emotions or to communicate distress, this problem should be an important focus of individual psychotherapy with a therapist knowledgeable about complex PTSD. However, in making the referral to mental health, the medical provider must be cautious not to shame the patient. Normalizing statements can be helpful. For example, "Many women who have experienced violence like you will hurt themselves [or make themselves vomit or take drugs] as a way of coping with their painful memories. However, because these behaviors put your health at risk, I recommend that you see a counselor to help you to work toward safer coping mechanisms." Once the patient is in ongoing psychotherapy with a mental health clinician, the medical provider can discuss with the patient safer ways of regulating emotion or communicating distress. This can be therapeutic for the patient also because it expresses a willingness to help her when she is in distress.

*When referring patient to mental health providers, keep her from feeling ashamed.*

In addition to referring the patient for psychological intervention, the medical provider must remain attuned to the medical consequences of self-destructive behavior. Patients who cut themselves are at risk of infection and bleeding, and it is important that their tetanus vaccination status be up to date. Without condoning the behavior, the medical provider should determine whether the patient uses sterile instruments to cut herself (just as providers ask injection drug users about use of sterile needles).

Patients with eating disorders can have a host of physiologic complications, including electrolyte disturbances, dehydration, dental erosion, esophageal

---

**Box 5-4    Suggested Elements for an Eating Disorder Management Contract**

---

- Frequency of visits with medical, nutrition, and mental health providers
- Monitoring plan (e.g., weight, orthostatic vital signs, laboratory tests)
- Parameters for mandatory increase in visit frequency
- Parameters for hospitalization
- Other patient responsibilities (e.g., keeping a food log)

---

rupture, osteoporosis, and sudden death. Although it is beyond the scope of this book to review the management of eating disorders (8,37), a few important elements deserve mention. First, the team managing the patient's care should include not only medical and mental health providers but also a nutritionist. The nutritionist can encourage the patient to keep a food and fluid intake log and can assesses the patient's adequacy of calorie, fluid, and nutrient intake. This log should also include a record of any bulimic activity, exercise patterns, and the use of diet pills, laxatives, and diuretics. In addition to reviewing the patient's log, the medical provider should also monitor for physiologic complications, such as weight loss, dehydration, electrolyte disturbances, osteoporosis, and hypoglycemia, and determine the need for emergency hospitalization. This may require frequent visits (e.g., weekly) if the patient's eating disorder symptoms are active. When hospitalization occurs and is involuntary, the patient will almost certainly experience it (initially) as revictimization, and traumatic re-enactments will probably ensue. Therefore, it is critical that the patient's mental health provider participate in the admission process.

Explicit patient-provider contracts are extremely useful for patients with eating disorders, particularly if they have a trauma history. Contracts should be developed jointly between the medical provider, the mental health provider, the nutritionist, and the patient; all parties should receive a written copy of the contract. Potentially important elements of a contract are outlined in Box 5-4.

The management of alcohol abuse and other substance use disorders is covered in detail in Chapter 10. The dual diagnosis of PTSD and substance abuse can be particularly serious (38) and refractory to treatment. Clinical approaches to patients with various harmful behaviors are summarized in Table 5-9.

## Team Approach to Care

As was discussed in Chapter 4, a team that includes medical and mental health providers is particularly well positioned to coordinate the complex health care needs of women with PTSD related to previous interpersonal violence.

**Table 5-9     Harmful Behavior**

| Description | Clinical Approach |
|---|---|
| Patients with a trauma history may engage in harmful behaviors including<br>• Suicide attempts<br>• Self-mutilation<br>• Eating disorders<br>• Substance abuse<br><br>The motivations for these behaviors include<br>• Regulation of emotion<br>• Communication of distress | • Refer patient to mental health provider as an emergency if the patient poses an acute danger to herself or others.<br>• Women with eating disorders who are at increased risk of death (e.g., women with very low body mass index) may require emergency psychiatric consultation even in the absence of expressed suicidal ideation.<br>• When making a non-emergency mental health referral, normalizing statements can be helpful.<br>• Although harmful behaviors always require attention, they do not necessarily require emergency intervention if the patient's life is not in immediate danger. |

Regardless of whether a clinician has access to such systems of care, it is important to be aware of the effect that medical and mental health care can have upon each other.

Medical care can lead to an exacerbation of mental health symptoms; for example, medical procedures can cause intense psychological distress. Conversely, mental health care can lead to an exacerbation of medical problems. Trauma memories intentionally explored in the mental health setting may increase emotional distress, which can in turn increase risky behaviors. For example, while a woman is going through trauma processing she may need to describe very disturbing aspects of the trauma with her therapist. In response to her emotional distress, she may increase behaviors like smoking, using alcohol or drugs, self-mutilating, or bulimia. Ongoing communication between medical and mental health providers can help to prevent such deterioration. Chapter 4 explores approaches to coordination of care.

## Summary

Post-traumatic stress disorder can raise complex management issues in the medical setting. Because the health care environment can elicit memories of previous trauma, clinicians must take steps to make sure that the patient feels safe and in control. This can decrease the risk that she will avoid medical care or develop symptoms of hyperarousal. If, despite efforts to prevent them, traumatic memories occur during a clinical encounter and the patient dissociates, the clinician should seek to reorient the patient and reassure her that she is safe. Because the patient can unconsciously slip into re-enactments of previous traumatic relationships, and because the patient-clinician relationship can be destabilized by the patient's difficulty with affect regulation, a team approach to care that addresses interpersonal aspects of the patient-provider relationship can be helpful. Somatiform symptoms often decrease when the patient is seen on a frequent, scheduled basis in the medical outpatient setting and when the physician acknowledges that the patient's suffering is real and involuntary. Clinicians should not give the patient the impression that her symptoms are "all in her head." Given the extreme distress typically underlying self-destructive behaviors such as self-mutilation, suicidality, and eating disorders, as well as their potential lethality, referral to a psychotherapist is almost always indicated when these behaviors are present. Such concrete strategies can improve interactions between the previously traumatized patient and her clinician and thereby lead to improved quality of care.

## REFERENCES

1. Kessler RC, Sonnega A, Bromet E, et al. Posttraumatic stress disorder in the National Comorbidity Survey. Arch Gen Psychiatry. 1995;52:1048-60.
2. Depression Guideline Panel. U.S. Department of Health and Human Services, Public Health Service, Agency for Health Care Policy and Research. Depression in Primary Care: Vol 1. Detection and Diagnosis. Clinical Practice Guideline Number 5. April 1993. AHCPR Publication 93-0550.
3. Depression Guideline Panel. U.S. Department of Health and Human Services, Public Health Service, Agency for Health Care Policy and Research. Depression in Primary Care: Volume 2. Treatment of Major Depression. Clinical Practice Guideline Number 5. April 1993. AHCPR Publication 93-0551.
4. Levenson J, ed. Depression. Philadelphia: American College of Physicians; 2000.
5. Hirschfeld RM, Keller MB, Panico S, et al. The National Depressive and Manic-Depressive Association consensus statement on the undertreatment of depression. JAMA. 1997;277:333-40.
6. Hirschfeld RM, Russell JM. Assessment and treatment of suicidal patients. N Engl J Med. 1997;337:910-5.
7. Brody DS, Thompson TL, II, Larson DB, et al. Strategies for counseling depressed patients by primary care physicians. J Gen Intern Med. 1994;9:569-75.
8. Walsh JM, Wheat ME, Freund K. Detection, evaluation, and treatment of eating disorders: the role of the primary care physician. J Gen Intern Med. 2000;15:577-90.
9. American Psychiatric Association. Diagnostic and Statistical Manual of Mental Disorders, 4th ed. Washington, DC: American Psychiatric Press; 1994.
10. Herman J. Trauma and Recovery. New York: Basic Books; 1992.
11. van der Kolk BA, Pelcovitz D, Roth S, et al. Dissociation, somatization, and affect dysregulation: the complexity of adaptation to trauma. Am J Psychiatry. 1996;153:83-93.
12. Charney DS, Deutch AY, Krystal JH, et al. Psychobiologic mechanisms of posttraumatic stress disorder. Arch Gen Psychiatry. 1993;50:295-305.
13. Shalev AY, Bonne O, Eth S. Treatment of posttraumatic stress disorder: a review. Psychosom Med. 1996;58:165-82.

14. Breslau N, Davis GC, Andreski P, Peterson E. Traumatic events and posttraumatic stress disorder in an urban population of young adults. Arch Gen Psychiatry. 1991;48:216-22.

15. Saxe G, Wolfe J. Gender and posttraumatic stress disorder. In: Saigh P, Bremner J, eds. Posttraumatic Stress Disorder: A Comprehensive Text. Boston: Allyn and Bacon; 1999:160-79.

16. van der kolk B, van der Hart O, Marmar C. Dissociation and information processing in posttraumatic stress disorder. In: van der kolk B, McFarlane A, Weisaeth L, eds. Traumatic Stress: The Effects of Overwhelming Experience on Mind, Body, and Society. New York: Guilford Press; 1996:303-27.

17. Saxe GN, Wolfe J. Posttraumatic stress disorder. In Yee E, Baillie S, et al, eds. Women's Primary Care Guide. Washington, DC: Department of Veterans Affairs; 2001.

18. Wallis LA, Tardiff K, Deane K. Changes in students' attitudes following a pelvic teaching associate program. J Am Med Womens Assoc. 1984;39:46-8.

19. Herman JL, Perry JC, van der Kolk BA. Childhood trauma in boderline personality disorder. Am J Psychiatry. 1989;146:490-5.

20. Marmar C, Foy D, Kagan B, Pynoos R. An integrated approach for treating posttraumatic stress. In: Oldham J, Riba M, Tasman A, eds. American Psychiatric Press Review of Psychiatry. Vol. 12. Washington, DC: American Psychiatric Press; 1993:239-73.

21. Foy D, ed. Treating Post-Traumatic Stress Disorder: Cognitive Behavioral Strategies. New York: Guildford Press; 1992.

22. Parker RM, Baker DW, Williams MV, Nurss JR. The test of functional health literacy in adults: a new instrument for measuring patients' literacy skills. J Gen Intern Med. 1995;10:537-41.

23. Putnam F. Diagnosis and Treatment of Multiple Personality Disorder. New York: Guildford Press; 1989.

24. Saxe G, van der Kolk BA, Berkowitz R, et al. Dissociative disorders in psychiatric inpatients. Am J Psychiatry. 1993;150:1037-42.

25. Ross CA. Epidemiology of multiple personality disorder and dissociation. Psychiatr Clin North Am. 1991;14:503-17.

26. McCann LI, Pearlman LA. Psychological Trauma and the Adult Survivor: Theory, Therapy, and Transformation. New York: Brunner/Mazel; 1990.

27. van der Kolk BA. The compulsion to repeat the trauma. Psychiatr Clin North Am. 1989;12:389-411.

28. Kluft R, ed. Incest Related Syndromes of Adult Psychopathology. Washington, DC: American Psychological Association Press; 1990.

29. Gabbard GO, Nadelson C. Professional boundaries in the physician-patient relationship. JAMA. 1995;273:1445-9.

30. van der Kolk BA, Fisler RE. Child abuse and neglect and loss of self-regulation. Bull Menninger Clin. 1994;58:145-68.

31. van der Kolk BA. The body keeps the score: memory and the evolving psychobiology of posttraumatic stress. Harv Rev Psychiatry. 1994;1:253-65.

32. Saxe GN, Chinman G, Berkowitz R, et al. Somatization in patients with dissociative disorders. Am J Psychiatry. 1994;151:1329-34.

33. Morse DS, Suchman AL, Frankel RM. The meaning of symptoms in 10 women with somatization disorder and a history of childhood abuse. Arch Fam Med. 1997;6:468-76.

34. Kaplan C, Lipkin M, Jr., Gordon GH. Somatization in primary care: patients with unexplained and vexing medical complaints. J Gen Intern Med. 1988;3:177-90.

35. Hahn SR, Kroenke K, Spitzer RL, et al. The difficult patient: prevalence, psychopathology, and functional impairment. J Gen Intern Med. 1996;11:1-8.

36. Laws A, Golding JM. Sexual assault history and eating disorder symptoms among white, Hispanic, and African-American women and men. Am J Public Health. 1996;86:579-82.

37. Kearney-Cooke A, Striegel-Moore RH. Treatment of childhood sexual abuse in anorexia nervosa and bulimia nervosa: a feminist psychodynamic approach. Int J Eat Disord. 1994;15:305-19.

38. Hoff RA, Rosenheck RA. Long-term patterns of service use and cost among patients with both psychiatric and substance abuse disorders. Med Care. 1998;36:835-43.

# CHAPTER 6

# Bearing Witness: The Effect of Caring for Survivors of Violence on Health Care Providers

GLENN N. SAXE, MD

JANE M. LIEBSCHUTZ, MD, MPH

ELIZABETH EDWARDSON, MD

RICHARD FRANKEL, PHD

Almost all health care professionals will eventually treat patients who have experienced violence and other traumatic events. Although clinical encounters with such patients are usually rewarding, they can lead to difficulties for clinicians. This chapter addresses those difficulties: how they arise, how they affect clinical encounters, and how they affect clinicians personally. It also offers suggestions for clinicians to consider in order to improve their effectiveness in treating women who have histories of violence while at the same time maintaining their own emotional stability and health.

## Hearing the Patient's Story: The Concept of Bearing Witness

Clinicians are witnesses. Bearing witness means making empathetic contact with another human being. It means lessening the burden by being with and listening to the patient. Implicit in the notion of bearing witness, however, is the burden of tolerating what one hears and sees. Clinicians may be the first person in a patient's life to be notified of previous abuse and trauma, and the humanity in each clinician cannot help but be touched and affected by such disclosures. The way that bearing witness affects each clinician varies. Although physicians may have expert clinical training, they are first and foremost human beings who will respond to another person's horror in human ways. The deleterious consequences that sometimes occur for the clinician treating patients who have experienced violence are natural responses, but they must be recognized and managed so the clinician can maintain his or her health while successfully caring for patients with a trauma history.

## Consequences of Bearing Witness

Some of the most common deleterious consequences that bearing witness can have upon clinicians, as outlined in Table 6-1, are hopelessness, fear, anger, confusing feelings of sexual arousal, and boundary violations.

### Hopelessness

Clinicians treating patients with traumatic stress see its relentless nature. Sometimes interventions fail, and sometimes referrals to mental health professionals do not help the patient. The patient who is a trauma survivor commonly gives up hope that her memories of the trauma will ever stop replaying in her mind. Treating a patient who is losing hope can have a profoundly negative impact on the clinician, who will respond to the patient in ways consistent with his or her own background and psychology. Feelings of hopelessness are extremely hard to bear, particularly for health care professionals who, as a group, are strongly motivated to help people and like to see positive results from their efforts. The clinician may begin to lose hope, too, believing that the patient will not get better. In such situations, clinicians may withdraw from the patient and be less alert to such symptoms as suicidal ideation. As clinicians lose hope, they may avoid appointments with the patient because the hopelessness and sense of failure that arise as a result of seeing the patient are hard to tolerate.

**Table 6-1   Consequences of Bearing Witness**

| Consequence | Description |
|---|---|
| Hopelessness | Feeling that clinical intervention will not be effective and that the patient will never get better |
| Fear | Feeling of being personally unsafe and anxious as a consequence of understanding what the patient has experienced |
| Anger | Feeling of anger that is a consequence of the way in which the patient's experience challenges the clinician's belief in a just world |
| Sexual arousal | Sexual feelings that develop as a consequence of hearing the patient's story |
| Boundary crossings | Non-therapeutic enactment of the aforementioned feelings with the patient |

Clinicians' hopelessness in relation to particular patients can begin to infiltrate other aspects of their practice and personal life. The clinician may start to see patient care more broadly as hopeless and harbor thoughts of restricting his or her practice or quitting medicine completely. Major depression may also develop, with its characteristic global despair infecting all areas of the clinician's professional and personal life.

Alternatively, a clinician's personal life can influence his or her ability to care for trauma survivors. For example, a clinician experiencing the burden of his or her own illness, divorce, or other family difficulties may not have the emotional resources to do what it takes to bear witness and properly treat a patient. At such times, the clinician may be particularly vulnerable to the feelings that tend to arise when bearing witness, such as fear and hopelessness.

### Fear

Trauma assaults one's sense of living in a safe and predictable world. When clinicians work with patients who have experienced violence, it challenges and sometimes shatters the clinician's own belief in a safe and predictable world. The act of bearing witness to horror naturally leads to the concern of "What does it mean for me?" Clinicians frequently will ask themselves questions consciously or unconsciously: "Am I safe?" "Are my children safe?" "Can this happen to me or someone in my family?" It is not uncommon for clinicians to have nightmares about events similar to those their patients experienced, and they may begin to avoid situations and people their patients are afraid of. For example, a clinician who works with a patient who was sexually assaulted in a dark parking lot may develop a range of anxiety symptoms related to sexual assault and barren parking lots.

Similarly, the clinician may experience intrusive memories of the patient's story. Such memories may disturb the clinician's normal interpersonal interactions, including family dynamics and sexual function. These thoughts may also interfere with the clinician's sleep, leading to fatigue and irritability. The anxiety experienced with vicarious intrusive memories is a result of making empathetic contact with the patient. "Vicarious traumatization," the development of one's own post-traumatic symptoms through one's relationship with another who has these symptoms, is probably the most accepted term for this phenomenon (1).

### Anger

Trauma not only shatters the sense of a safe world, it also shatters the sense of a just world. This sense of justice or fairness is powerfully ingrained in people, and challenges to it may lead to feelings of profound anger. Clinicians may find themselves feeling angry at the perpetrator, at the patient, at political or legal authorities, or even at God in order to preserve their sense of fairness.

*Clinicians may find themselves feeling angry at the patient.*

Sometimes the clinician may respond angrily to a patient's hopelessness ("You're not trying hard enough," "You don't want to get better," "You like the attention"), or they may find themselves having such thoughts as "She should have known better," "How could she be so careless," and even "She deserved it." Because clinicians are trained to be dispassionate and even-handed, feeling angry in these cases may cause them to feel uncomfortable with themselves and even to question their own clinical competence. Again, it must be recognized that such feelings are human accompaniments to bearing witness to horror.

### Sexual Arousal

Among the most uncomfortable feelings that can arise in the process of bearing witness is sexual arousal related to hearing details about a patient's sexual assault. Such feelings can elicit great shame in the clinician. Clinicians may worry about exploiting the patient to gratify their own sexual feelings and about their own mental health because of the shame and discomfort that can accompany these feelings. Human sexuality is extremely complex, and voyeuristic, sadistic, and masochistic emotions can partly comprise its nuances. If such feelings are causing significant shame for the clinician, and, certainly, if there are concerns about acting on these feelings with a patient, then personal consultation with a mental health professional is warranted. Otherwise, it may suffice to know that these feelings are natural human responses to empathizing with another human being.

### Boundary Violations

Blurring and violation of boundaries sometimes occurs when bearing witness. For example, acting on a sexual feeling with the patient is obviously a gross violation of professional ethics (2). More subtle boundary violations are common, however (3). It is particularly important to note when behavior toward a patient deviates from one's usual clinical practice because this is a clue that a boundary violation may be occurring. For example, clinicians may find themselves spending more time with the patient than is usual or seeing patients at unusual times and locations (3a). They may also prescribe non-standard treatments or treatments outside of their area of expertise in an effort to meet the patient's requests. To maintain boundaries it may be necessary for the clinician to refer certain patients to mental health providers for detailed screening and history taking.

*Deviation from one's usual professional behavior should be noted by the clinician.*

## Special Problems for Health Care Professionals Who Have Themselves Experienced Trauma

The prevalence of childhood abuse, sexual assault, partner abuse, and elder abuse in medical students and practicing physicians has only recently been explored. Initial data suggest that the prevalence in health care providers is comparable to the prevalence in the general population. In one study of medical students and medical faculty, 13% of respondents reported at least one form of physical abuse and/or forced sexual activity by a partner in their adult life; 15% reported physical and/or sexual abuse as a child; and 24% reported physical and/or sexual abuse in their lifetime. Stratified by gender, 24% of the women reported physical and/or sexual abuse as an adult, whereas 6% of the men reported abuse as an adult (4). Twelve percent of responding faculty and medical students at one university reported a history of sexual abuse in their lifetimes (6% as a child, 7% as an adult) (4). The prevalence of post-traumatic stress disorder (PTSD) in medical students and staff who have experienced violence is unknown but is likely to be fairly common (presumably the same as in the general population) because many individuals who have experienced assault (particularly sexual assault) develop PTSD (5).

The process of bearing witness is likely to be particularly complicated for medical staff and trainees who have been personally exposed to trauma or who have PTSD (6). Such individuals are more than witnesses; they are themselves survivors of terrible events. The practitioner's own post-traumatic symptoms can be triggered by hearing the patient's story, which can make his or her experience with the patient more immediate

*A practitioner's own post-traumatic symptoms may be triggered by a patient's story.*

and severe, even if the provider has previously recovered from PTSD. The practical suggestions described below are applicable to all clinicians but particularly to those with personal histories of trauma.

## Practical Suggestions for Clinicians

Practical suggestions for increasing personal well-being and clinical effectiveness are given below. They are summarized in Table 6-2.

### Take Care of Yourself and Lead a Balanced Life

The likelihood of providing inappropriate care or violating boundaries increases if clinicians are not caring for their own personal needs. For example, clinicians may skip meals, fail to exercise, and live in a state of chronic sleep

**Table 6-2    Practical Suggestions for Clinicians**

| Suggestion | Description |
|---|---|
| Lead a balanced life | Attend to personal care, health, and activities that enhance feelings of well-being. |
| Recognize trouble | Be vigilant for warning signs that work is compromising clinical effectiveness and personal well-being. |
| Psychotherapy | Work with a trained psychotherapist, which can be very helpful when there is difficulty managing feelings as a consequence of work (or anything else). |
| Group support | Seek out activities and contacts with other clinicians who are engaged in similar work. |
| Consultation or supervision | In situations of difficulty, ask for advice: *Never worry alone.* |
| Training opportunities | Take advantage of the many training opportunities available to enhance clinical skills. |

deprivation. They may use alcohol or drugs to blunt strong feelings elicited by working with patients who have experienced violence. They may also immerse themselves in work to the exclusion of friends, social engagements, life partners, and social support. The absence of personal support can lead clinicians to become overly invested in their patients, which can

*Clinicians who immerse themselves in their work can become overly involved with their patients.*

in turn leave them particularly vulnerable to strong feelings engendered by patients who have experienced violence. The overall effects upon clinicians' personal lives can be wide-ranging and significantly disruptive or harmful.

However, there are many ways to care for oneself. The basics are important: adequate sleep, nutrition, and exercise. In addition to increasing physical stamina (and by extension, emotional stamina) and serving as an outlet for stress, exercise can provide a social environment in which clinicians can interact with people not associated with the stressful work environment, such as a yoga class, a health club, or a hiking club. Also important for clinicians is to have their own primary care physician who can provide them with preventive care.

Cultivating a spiritual life can also act as a buffer against the difficulties of caring for victims of violence. Organized religious communities, music, creative writing, art, social activism, and an active appreciation of nature are various options for creating, strengthening, and maintaining a spiritual foundation.

### Recognize When You Are in Trouble

Clinicians may experience a variety of emotional complications as a result of treating patients who have experienced violence. These problems tend to develop and present insidiously, and changes to the emotional state and daily routine initially manifest themselves in subtle ways. Avoiding a particularly disturbing patient or seeing such a patient after hours is one example of how a troubled clinician may change his or her usual routine. Because of the insidious nature of this kind of emotional disturbance, it is difficult to recognize when interactions with patients become problematic and therefore important to be vigilant when treating patients who are survivors of trauma.

One clear indication that a problem is developing or has already developed is that family members, friends, or colleagues express concern about the clinician's behavior or emotional state. Detachment and feelings of numbness are strong indications of a problem, in addition to yelling at a patient, recurrent conflicts with colleagues, increased use of alcohol or other drugs of abuse, and frequent crying. When a clinician does have his or her own personal trauma history, it is likely that dealing with certain patients will trigger disturbing feelings. Even if the clinician has already processed the disturbing feelings that resulted from his or her own past trauma, they may reappear, especially when treating a patient who has experienced violence, and need to be addressed again. It is important for clinicians who have experienced violence to be vigilant of their own emotional state and to seek help if and when they find themselves becoming disturbed.

*Psychotherapy*
Psychotherapy is an important option for many clinicians who need help processing the emotions engendered by caring for patients. In every health care setting, physicians care not only for patients who have experienced violence but also for sick, vulnerable, and dying patients. Interactions with patients in the heightened emotional states of such conditions demand that the physician bear witness to the individual's experience. This is especially true when caring for patients who have experienced violence. Over time, the cumulative residue of bearing witness to patients' illness, loss, and violence experiences can affect even psychologically healthy clinicians. Psychotherapy can help the physician process the emotions encountered as part of his or her emotionally challenging job. It can also help the physician understand the personal meaning of his or her reactions to patients and patient experiences and strengthen him or her as a clinician and as a person.

There are a variety of mental health professionals and styles of psychotherapy. For the clinician seeking such help, it is important to research the options before choosing a mental health professional. For example, it is useful to conduct a brief phone interview with potential psychotherapists to ask about their practice style and expectations. It can also be useful to have an in-person, single session with a few different psychotherapists to determine the best fit.

## Use Group Support: The Interdisciplinary Team

Some of the feelings that naturally develop within a therapeutic relationship with patients who have experienced violence are unsettling and confusing.

*Sharing feelings with colleagues can help both the clinician and the patient.*

Outside of formal psychiatric training, there is rarely explicit training of the primary care physician to identify and process these feelings. It is therefore easy for clinicians to feel isolated when dealing with serious clinical problems, so sharing the burden with others can help clinicians process their feelings and consequently improve treatment approaches to the patient.

For clinicians who want to delve deeply into the patient-physician relationship, the American Academy of Physicians and Patients (www.physician-patient.org ) organizes CME workshops throughout the year. Another option, Balint groups, started by Michael Balint, a British psychiatrist, are peer-support groups based on the premise that case-based discussions of patients facilitated by a psychiatrist are useful to general practitioners (7).

An ideal setting is a multidisciplinary group of providers who meet regularly to discuss difficult cases. The group might include physicians, nurses, and mental health professionals such as social workers, psychologists, and psychiatrists. Discussion of difficult cases provides support for the physician and helps create a team plan for patient care, which is one of the cornerstones of caring for women with severe mental health sequelae of violence (see Chapter 5 for details on caring for women with PTSD).

## Seek Out Consultation or Supervision for Patient Management

Although support groups are very helpful for clinicians, especially if they are managing a personal emotional burden, such groups may not be available or may not solve all the issues directly related to patient care. In this case, consulting a mental health professional, a supervisor, or a learned colleague for advice or guidance regarding care of the patient is an important option. Mental health referral for the patient should also be considered (see Chapter 4). Consulting a colleague or mental health practitioner may be particularly useful for both clinician and patient when the clinician's own anxiety is aroused by a clinical situation such as a patient's suicidal ideation or actions. Occasionally, a clinician who has a personal trauma history may decide that it is best to refer a particular patient to another provider for trauma-related care because that patient's history stirs up too many personal memories for the clinician. Consultation with a peer or supervisor may help facilitate such a decision when necessary, to the benefit of both clinician and patient.

*Take Advantage of Training Opportunities*

A clinician's fund of knowledge about a particular issue can influence his or her level of comfort and satisfaction when caring for patients with a history of violence. A recent study showed that physicians who have taken a workshop on domestic violence in the past 12 months have more confidence and more frequently inquire about domestic violence in their patients (8). Education opportunities include workshops at national meetings, such as, for internists in particular, annual meetings of the American College of Physicians-American Society of Internal Medicine (www.acponline.org) and the Society for General Internal Medicine (www.sgim.org). These organizations often offer workshops on interpersonal violence in which one can discuss issues related to treating patients who have experienced violence. The Family Violence Prevention Fund (www.fvpf.org) is also a useful resource for training opportunities for health professionals. See the Appendix for additional resources.

# Summary

Clinicians who work with patients who have experienced violence have the opportunity to successfully treat their patients and enjoy the rewards of such success. However, the process of bearing witness to the trauma of patients can also have a number of deleterious consequences. Helplessness, fear, anger, and confusing feelings of sexual arousal can be difficult for clinicians to withstand and manage. Clinicians with their own trauma histories may be particularly vulnerable. Self-care, psychotherapy, group support, education and training, and consultation with peers and supervisors should all be utilized to ease the burden and enhance clinical effectiveness of clinicians treating patients with a history of trauma.

## REFERENCES

1. McCann L, Perlman LA. Vicarious traumatization: a framework for understanding the psychological effects of working with victims. J Trauma Stress. 1990;3:131-49.
2. Council on Ethical and Judicial Affairs, American Medical Association. Sexual misconduct in the practice of medicine JAMA. 1991;266:2741-5.
3. Peterson MR. At Personal Risk: Boundary Violations in Professional-Client Relationships. New York: WW Norton; 1992.
3a. Frankel RM, Williams S. Sexuality and professionalism. In: Feldman MD, Christensen JF, eds. Behavioral Medicine in Primary Care: A Practical Guide. New York: McGraw-Hill/Appleton & Lange; 1997.
4. deLahunta EA, Tulsky AA. Personal exposure of faculty and medical students to family violence. JAMA. 1996;275:1903-6.

5. Kessler RC, Sonnega A, Bromet E, et al. Posttraumatic stress disorder in the national co-morbidity survey. Arch Gen Psychiatry. 1995;52:1048-60.

6. Carbonell JL, Figley CR. When trauma hits home: personal trauma and the family therapist. J Marital Fam Ther. 1996;22:53-8.

7. Scheingold L. A Balint seminar in the family practice residency setting. J Fam Pract. 1980;10:267-70.

8. Elliott L, Nerney M, Jones T, Friedmann PD. Barriers to screening for domestic violence. J Gen Intern Med. 2002:17:112-6.

# Special Considerations

# CHAPTER 7

# Mistreatment of Older Women

CALVIN H. HIRSCH, MD

The mistreatment of older women occurs frequently, and clinicians may encounter its victims in all medical settings, from primary care clinics to the nursing home. Without a heightened awareness of the problem, the consequences of abuse can be mistakenly attributed to the effects of chronic disease or age-related changes. The recognition of abuse, followed by appropriate clinical interventions, may help to decrease the emotional and physical morbidity it engenders.

This chapter reviews the definitions and epidemiology of elder abuse, provides clues and suggestions for its detection and management, and describes how to report it in a manner that assists Adult Protective Services (APS) and law enforcement in their investigations.

CASE 7-1

*Mrs. Roberts is a 74-year-old widow. She shares her home with her brother and sister-in-law, who allegedly moved in to help take care of her. Although Mrs. Roberts' diabetes mellitus and hypertension are poorly controlled, and she has been recently diagnosed with mild-to-moderate dementia, her brother and sister-in-law refuse to accompany Mrs. Roberts to the clinic on her scheduled visits or take responsibility for administering her medications.*

*Mrs. Curtis is a 68-year-old hemiparetic woman admitted to the hospital for acute pyelonephritis. After Mrs. Curtis returns home, an aide from the home health agency notices blood on her diaper and faint bruises on her wrists. Mrs. Curtis initially refuses to talk about these findings but eventually confides to the visiting nurse that, once or twice a week, her husband ties her to the rails of her hospital bed and rapes her. She admits to living in fear of him. Nevertheless, she refuses any intervention from APS, stating she does not want to be placed in a nursing home.*

*Mrs. Dennis is a 71-year-old woman caring for her 76-year-old husband, who has advanced Alzheimer's disease. He is ambulatory only with assistance, foul-mouthed, and often combative during personal care and feeding. Afraid of being punched, Mrs. Dennis leaves her husband in his soiled clothing and diapers for up to days at a time and infrequently attempts to bathe him. Her two sons, who live hours away, have not been supportive and have criticized her for wanting him placed in a nursing home. When Mr. Dennis is brought to the emergency department because of a change in mental status, the nurses find a cachectic, filthy, malodorous man with a stage IV pressure ulcer over the sacrum and extensive maceration of the skin of the inner thighs. The emergency department admits him and notifies APS, whose investigation leads them to ask the district attorney to bring charges of criminal neglect against Mrs. Dennis. After the sons refuse to take responsibility for their father, the county conserves Mr. Dennis and authorizes his transfer to a skilled nursing facility. The district attorney agrees to drop the charges against Mrs. Dennis but not before she has spent several thousand dollars in attorney's fees. The incident causes her estrangement from her children.*

As these cases illustrate, abuse of older women can involve complexities associated with age and illness. In Case 7-1, abuse consisted of the exploitation of a demented sister to obtain free housing while neglecting her medical needs. The victim of Case 7-2 dreaded the unwanted and painful sexual advances of her husband but feared nursing home placement more. In Case 7-3, the wife was first victimized by her demented husband, then punished by APS and the legal system. Although in most cases like this APS would instead help the wife to access resources to care for her husband, such scenarios are sometimes seen. Because of financial constraints, isolation, illness, disability, and defenselessness, older victims may have fewer options, and those options, such as institutionalization, may be perceived as worse than the abuse itself.

*Older women may have fewer, and worse, alternatives to a violent home setting.*

## Definitions

### Elder Abuse and Neglect

*Mistreatment* can be defined as the physical or sexual abuse, neglect, psychological abuse, or financial exploitation of an older adult (Box 7-1). In most states, the definitions and laws governing elder mistreatment are extended to dependent adults, defined as nonelderly individuals whose physical or mental impairments render them incapable of carrying out normal activities without the help of others. Inconsistencies in the definitions used by elder abuse researchers have contributed to a lack of standardization in the statutory definitions used by states to govern reporting and prosecution.

*In most states, laws governing elder mistreatment extend to dependent adults.*

Conceptually, *physical abuse* incorporates acts of violence, such as hitting and slapping; the infliction of injuries; unwanted sexual contact; and inappropriate mechanical restraint or restraint accomplished by intentional misuse of sedating medication. This definition applies to any perpetrator, whether or not the abuser is related to the victim and regardless of the victim's degree of

---

**Box 7-1    Spectrum of Elder Mistreatment**

- Physical abuse
- Sexual abuse
- Neglect
- Psychological abuse

- Financial exploitation
- Self-neglect
- Domestic violence

disability. *Neglect* refers to the failure of the primary caregiver to adequately meet the care needs of a dependent adult, such as failing to provide adequate food, hydration, clothing, or shelter, or failing to help the older person receive medical care. *Psychological abuse* involves efforts to inflict emotional harm through intimidation, threats, or derogatory language. Ignoring the elder and violating the older person's civil rights by isolating him or her from visitors, telephone calls, or mail represent an extension of emotional abuse. *Financial exploitation* involves the misappropriation of an elder's money or property through embezzlement, fraud, or outright theft.

*Self-neglect*, considered by many authorities and states to be a special category of elder mistreatment, refers to the inability of an individual to perform essential self-care tasks, such as obtaining food, clothing, shelter, or medical care, because of a physical or mental impairment.

## Domestic Violence

Domestic violence is one of the forms that elder mistreatment can take. Long-standing patterns of spousal abuse do not come to a halt simply because a couple reaches old age, yet comparatively little research has investigated domestic violence in the elderly. Once a victim attains the age statutorily defining status as a senior citizen (usually age 65), the reporting and management of domestic violence become incorporated into the reporting laws and services designed for elder abuse. Some experts have complained that the concept of power and control, which is considered central to interventions for the younger domestic violence victim, becomes overshadowed by the dominant explanatory paradigms for elder mistreatment, such as caregiver stress, when the domestic violence victim is old. They argue that this conceptual shift hampers the ability of APS to adequately address the older domestic violence victim's need for protection and support (1). Available data suggest that many abused older spouses are, in fact, frail. A comparison of 22 cases of elderly spouse abuse with 53 cases of elder abuse by adult children revealed that abused wives were more likely to suffer from longstanding physical abuse, to be in worse health, to be more dependent in their activities of daily living, and to be lonely and reliant on their spouses for companionship (2). Thus, domestic violence can be a particularly severe, and etiologically distinct, form of elder mistreatment.

# Epidemiology

Reported data on the incidence and prevalence of elder mistreatment likely represent the tip of an iceberg because the true figures remain concealed by lack of recognition and the reluctance of elders to reveal abuse out of shame, denial, fear of reprisal, or concern about the invasion of privacy. Lachs et al (3) reviewed 11 years of referrals to Connecticut's Ombudsman on Aging. From these referrals, they extrapolated a 6.4% prevalence of abuse among the senior population of New Haven. Self-neglect was the most commonly reported type (73%), followed by neglect by others (17%). Two large-scale, cross-sectional surveys of elders in Boston (4) and Canada (5) found that 3% to 4% of seniors admitted to experiencing some form of abuse (excluding self-neglect) after the age of 65. Among survey respondents, 0.5% to 2% acknowledged physical abuse, and 0.4% reported being neglected. The 1996 National Elder Abuse Incidence Study estimated a low prevalence of 1.3% among non-institutionalized persons over age 60 (6). This figure, which includes self-neglect, has been criticized for relying heavily on substantiated referrals to APS and probably underestimates the true prevalence because of under-detection and under-reporting. The surveys suffer from recall bias and the omission of data for the most dependent and cognitively impaired elders. Of note, elderly men and women appear equally likely to be victims of mistreatment.

The epidemiology of abuse perpetration has also been explored. In the Boston prevalence study, spouses emerged as a significant proportion of the perpetrators of abuse, with spouses more likely to commit physical abuse than other relatives. Among perpetrators, men appear more likely to commit physical abuse, while women are more likely to be neglectful.

## Elder Abuse as a Chronic Illness: Health Effects

Elder abuse, like domestic violence, tends to occur chronically over months to years and may have different manifestations, sometimes resulting in recurrent medical crises. The frequency and intensity of the abuse may escalate over time (7), increasing the risk of serious medical consequences. The consequences of abuse and neglect also include excess hospitalizations and visits to the emergency department. Lachs et al (8) found that 42 (23%) of 182 confirmed elder abuse victims living in the greater New Haven, Connecticut area had at least one visit to the emergency department attributable to abuse during a 5-year period. During 13 years of follow-up, older victims of abuse were found to have a three-fold greater risk of dying compared to unabused seniors, after adjustment for age, sociodemographic factors, and co-morbidity (9).

## Recognizing Elder Abuse: A Clinical Approach

For many dependent elders, a scheduled visit to the primary care physician is the only outing away from home and the only opportunity for abuse to be

*For many dependent elders, a scheduled doctor visit is the only opportunity for abuse to be detected.*

detected. Unfortunately, despite the prevalence of elder mistreatment, physicians all too often attribute the medical consequences of abuse to aging or underlying disease processes. To detect elder mistreatment, a clinician must be aware of the risk factors (Box 7-2), especially the presence of dementia. The clinician must also be alert to clues in the history and physical examination that indicate possible abuse (Box 7-3). Finally, because elder mistreatment can occur in the absence of risk factors or physical clues, the clinician must directly screen for abuse (Box 7-4). The next four sections describe these important steps in detail.

---

**Box 7-2    Risk Factors for Elder Mistreatment by Caregivers in the Community Setting**

- Excessive dependence of the elder on caregiver for activities of daily living
  - ➤ Resentment by caregiver for giving too much, getting back too little
  - ➤ Particularly common in setting of dementia
- Caregiver dependence on elder (housing, financial support)
- The stressed-out caregiver
  - ➤ Poor pre-morbid quality of the relationship
  - ➤ External stressors (job, family, finances)
  - ➤ Lack of social support
  - ➤ Emotional burden
  - ➤ Depression
  - ➤ Increasing care needs of a demented relative
- Psychopathology in the caregiver
  - ➤ Substance abuse
  - ➤ Sociopathic personality
  - ➤ Hostility toward elder
  - ➤ Authoritarian and rigid toward others
  - ➤ Financial exploitation of elder
- History of family violence (child or spousal abuse)
- Sociocultural/environmental
  - ➤ Inadequate housing
  - ➤ Resentment and anger from elder over decline in stature within family
  - ➤ Demanding personality of elder
  - ➤ Cultural sanctions against seeking help outside family

Adapted from Jones JS, Holstege C, Holstege H. Elder abuse and neglect: understanding the causes and potential risk factors. Am J Emerg Med. 1997;15:579-83.

## Box 7-3    Clues for Possible Elder Mistreatment

- Caregiver-patient interactions
  - ➤ Tension or indifference between caregiver and patient
- Caregiver behaviors
  - ➤ Absent for appointment of cognitively impaired elder
  - ➤ Fails to visit patient in hospital
  - ➤ A history of "doctor hopping" (taking the elder to multiple different doctors)
  - ➤ Poor knowledge of patient's medical problems
  - ➤ Excessive concern about costs
  - ➤ Attempts to dominate medical interview
  - ➤ Verbal abuse or hostility toward elder during encounter
  - ➤ Hostility toward health care provider
  - ➤ Evidence of substance abuse or mental health problems
  - ➤ Evidence of financial dependence on elder
- Elder behaviors
  - ➤ Fearfulness toward caregiver
  - ➤ Flinching
  - ➤ Reluctance to make eye contact
  - ➤ Diagnosis of dementia with history of disruptive behavior
  - ➤ In demented person, unexplained resistance to, or fear of, physical touch, removing clothes, toileting, bathing of private parts
  - ➤ Depression, anxiety, insomnia
- Suspicious physical signs
  - ➤ Reluctance to answer questions about a suspicious physical finding or illness
  - ➤ Implausible or vague explanations for injuries given by caregiver or patient
  - ➤ Multiple bruises or bruises at different stages of healing
  - ➤ Bruises in unusual locations
  - ➤ Pattern injuries (injuries in the shape of the object used to inflict them, such as bite marks, cigarette burns)
  - ➤ Evidence of old injuries not previously documented
  - ➤ Broken nose, teeth
  - ➤ Radiographic evidence of old, misaligned fractures
  - ➤ Poor hygiene
  - ➤ Subtherapeutic levels of drugs
  - ➤ Patient lacking his or her eyeglasses, dentures, or hearing aid

Adapted from Kleinschmidt KC. Elder abuse: a review. Ann Emerg Med. 1997;30:463-72; and Lachs MS, Pillemer K. Abuse and neglect of elderly persons. N Engl J Med. 1995;332:437-43.

---

**Box 7-4    Screening Questions for Mistreatment in Elders**

- General lead-in questions
  - ➤ "Do you feel safe where you live?"
  - ➤ "Who helps you with the things that you have trouble doing yourself?"
- Physical abuse
  - ➤ "Are you afraid of anyone at home?"
  - ➤ "Have you ever been slapped, punched, or kicked?"
  - ➤ "Have you ever been tied down, or locked inside in your room or house against your will?"
  - ➤ "Has anyone forced you to have sexual contact against your will?"
- Neglect
  - ➤ "Are you made to wait a long time for food or medicine?"
  - ➤ "Have you been left alone for long periods?"
  - ➤ "When you need assistance, do you have trouble getting someone to help you?"
- Psychological abuse
  - ➤ "Are you yelled at?"
  - ➤ "Have you been threatened with punishment or placement in a nursing home?"
  - ➤ "Are you kept isolated from friends or other relatives?"
  - ➤ "Do you get the 'silent treatment' at home?"
  - ➤ "Do you have frequent disagreements with [principal caregiver]?"
  - ➤ "When you disagree, what happens?"
- Financial exploitation
  - ➤ "Who handles your checkbook and pays the bills?"

Adapted from Kleinschmidt KC. Elder abuse: a review. Ann Emerg Med. 1997;30:463-72; and Lachs MS, Pillemer K. Abuse and neglect of elderly persons. N Engl J Med. 1995;332:437-43.

---

## Risk Factors for Abuse and "Double Direction" Violence

Assessing a patient's risk for abuse begins with an understanding of the patient's degree of dependence. This is best ascertained through a systematic assessment of the patient's functional and cognitive status. In a cohort study of older adults from New Haven, Connecticut followed for 9 years, functional dependence and cognitive impairment independently predicted confirmed elder abuse after adjusting for age, gender, race, income, and other risk factors. Persons who developed cognitive impairment

*Assessing risk for abuse begins with understanding the patient's degree of dependence.*

during the 9 years of follow-up were more than twice as likely to be abused than those impaired at baseline and five times more likely to be abused than cognitively intact participants after controlling for age, gender, race, and income (10). Thus, dementia emerges as a major risk factor for elder mistreatment.

In addition to dependency of the elder, caregiver stress was identified in early studies as a principal risk factor, leading to the development of respite programs and caregiver support groups. Subsequent research pointed to the economic dependency of the abuser on the elder (e.g., for housing and financial support), especially if the abuser was an adult child, while downplaying the role played by the older adult's functional impairments. Studies suggested that abusers were more likely to have past or present psychiatric problems, a history of alcohol or drug abuse (7,11), and underlying personality disorders (12). Abusive caregivers, in general, have been providing care longer, have been caring for patients with more severe impairment, have a higher perceived burden of caregiving, have more depressive symptoms, and have had a worse pre-morbid relationship with the patient, compared to non-abusers.

It is important to recognize that the cognitively impaired elder is not only at increased risk of being the victim of abuse but is also at increased risk of being the perpetrator of abuse. Up to 12% of the caregivers of demented adults commit acts of physical violence toward the patient, but one-third are themselves the recipients of abuse from the patient (13). Abuse of the demented elder often starts with abuse by the demented elder. This can lead to a cycle of "double direction" violence. Violent and threatening behavior occurs in one-fifth to one-quarter of dementia patients (14), usually at the more advanced stages, and is highly correlated with angry verbal outbursts. Agitation and anger can be triggered by para-

*Ask the caregiver whether the demented elder has hurt him or her.*

noid delusions or misperceptions of reality or may be provoked by actions taken by the caregiver, such as impatiently dragging the patient to the toilet to change a soiled diaper. The clinician should explicitly ask the caregiver whether the demented elder has hurt him or her or use a simple, standardized screening instrument, such as the Neuropsychiatric Inventory (15).

An extreme example of abuse of caregivers by demented elders is homicide (16). Access of the demented patient to firearms and other weapons (even kitchen knives) substantially increases the risk of accidental injury or death of the patient, caregiver, and others. Sixty percent of the households of patients attending a memory disorders clinic in the southeastern United States possessed a firearm; 25% of these households kept them loaded (17). In cases of suspected elder abuse, as well as in suspected domestic violence, the clinician should routinely inquire about the presence and accessibility of weapons and recommend their removal from the home.

## Assessment of Decisional Capacity

The physician may need to render an opinion about the patients' decisional capacity, either to identify patients at risk for abuse or in the course of helping to stop abuse. Early dementia may affect reasoning, judgment, insight, and other forms of executive functioning before deficits in short-term memory become obvious. These patients may retain their ability to carry out many aspects of daily living, and maintenance of social graces, presentable appearance, and verbal fluency may mask their dementia during a routine medical encounter. In addition, many patients fail to recognize, or are in denial of, their cognitive deficits at this stage. These individuals are susceptible to financial abuse, especially schemes aimed at persuading them to part with their money. In a primary care practice, it is not uncommon for the patient to share information with the physician that should raise a suspicion of financial abuse and, as a corollary, concern over the patient's ability to exercise sound decision-making.

Mrs. Roberts, the 74-year-old victim in Case 7-1, consistently denied that there was anything wrong with the way her brother and sister-in-law treated her, or that she had any significant medical problems. The determination of cognitive impairment, based on a Mini-Mental score of 21 out of 30 (18), confirmed the impression that she was unable to manage her medical conditions and facilitated the appointment of her youngest daughter as conservator. However, the American legal system would consider Mrs. Roberts legally competent until proven otherwise in a court of law. An elder or dependent adult is allowed to make decisions that may threaten health and safety as long as that individual is deemed competent. (It should be emphasized that the legal competency of an adult may not alter the responsibility of the clinician to report suspected abuse.) By extension, APS generally emphasizes self-determination and freedom over safety. Mrs. Curtis' preference to remain at home despite repeated sexual abuse by her husband (Case 7-2) similarly raised doubts about her decisional capacity. However, a psychiatric evaluation found her to be cognitively intact and fully aware of the consequences of her decision. After counseling about her options, her refusal of an intervention by APS was honored, and she was allowed to remain at home.

Decisional capacity consists of four major components: 1) cognition (attention, information processing, and executive functioning), 2) reality testing (lack of delusions and hallucinations), 3) absence of a mood disorder affecting decision-making (e.g., severe depression), and 4) the ability to understand the nature of what is being considered and the potential consequences of the decision (Table 7-1). In general, decisional capacity is not considered an all or nothing trait. Most states and courts recognize that loss of decisional capacity in one domain (e.g., finances) does not preclude decision-making ability in another (e.g., where the patient chooses to live).

**Table 7-1    Decisional Capacity: Testing for the Four Components**

| Component | Contents | Methods for Testing |
|---|---|---|
| Cognition | Attention and information processing | Mini-Mental State Exam (18) (Table 7-2) |
| | Executive functioning: insight and judgement | Behavioral clues<br>• Impulsiveness<br>• Insisting on living alone when not able to meet self-care needs |
| | Executive functioning: reasoning (abstract and problem-solving) | Clock drawing (19) (three-step command)<br>• Draw a clock<br>• Fill in the numbers<br>• Set the time to 10 minutes past 11<br>Behavioral clues<br>• Difficulty making decisions<br>• Lack of originality in thinking (e.g., copying decisions of others)<br>Ability to describe similarities and differences<br>• "How are a car and a plane similar?"<br>• "How are sugar and vinegar different?"<br>Logical reasoning<br>• "What would you do if you arrived in a strange city and needed to locate a friend?"<br>• "What would you do if you came home and found the kitchen flooded?"<br>• "What would you do if you were stranded at the airport with only one dollar?" |
| | Executive functioning: organization and planning | • Clock drawing (19)<br>• Difficulty performing multi-step tasks, e.g.,<br>  • Difficulty anticipating consequences<br>  • Difficulty preparing a meal<br>  • Difficulty following a recipe |
| Reality testing | Lack of delusions or hallucinations | Behavioral/historical clues (from patient/informant) |
| Lack of mood disorder affecting decision-making | Lack of depressive symptoms | Geriatric Depression Scale (20) (Box 7-5) |
| Understanding nature and consequences of decision | Insight and judgement | Evidence of understanding<br>• "If you continue to live alone, how will you get your needs met?"<br>• "What will happen if you decide to have/not have this operation?" |

Primary care and other medical clinicians should have the ability to screen for decisional capacity, although difficult cases may require a referral to a neurologist, psychiatrist, or psychologist for mental status testing. The Mini-Mental State Exam (18) (Table 7-2) tests most areas of cognition except executive function. These include attention and concentration, calculation, orientation, registration, comprehension, language, and constructional ability. Executive functioning consists of insight, judgment, reasoning, organization, and planning. Clues to impaired executive function include poor planning and organization (e.g., running out of medications before seeking a renewal), the inability to anticipate consequences, trouble making a decision, impulsiveness, poor insight, and lack of originality in thinking (e.g., copying the decisions of others). Abstract reasoning can be tested by asking the patient about similarities and differences between entities (e.g., the similarity between a car and a plane, the difference between sugar and vinegar). The clinician can screen for impaired logical reasoning by asking the patient what he or she would do in a particular circumstance. For example, what might she do if stranded at the airport with only one dollar? What would he do if he came home and found the kitchen flooded with water? What would she do if she arrived in a strange city and needed to locate a friend? Observing the patient draw a clock, fill in the numbers, and set the time (e.g., to ten minutes past eleven) offers the clinician insight into organizational and planning skills, abstraction, the ability to follow a multi-step command, and visuo-spatial skills (19). Thought process impairment (delusions or hallucinations) may be identified during the course of conversing with the patient or through an informant. Clinicians can screen for depression in the elderly using the Geriatric Depression Scale (Box 7-5) (20).

## Clues to Mistreatment

An attentive clinician can often detect clues suggesting possible elder mistreatment (see Box 7-3). Injury patterns often resemble those seen in acute domestic violence (Chapter 3). The caregiver's behavior may suggest indifference or hostility. He or she may fail to accompany the patient to a clinic visit or fail to supply the patient with needed eyeglasses, dentures, or hearing aids. Subtherapeutic drug levels may be a marker of neglect. Observed interactions between caregiver and patient may be problematic, or the patient may appear frightened or depressed. The presence of any such clues should prompt further inquiry into the possibility of mistreatment.

## Screening

In addition to screening for decisional capacity, identifying other risk factors for elder mistreatment, and watching for clues suggesting abuse, clinicians

## Table 7-2   Mini Mental State Examination

| | Max. Score | Actual Score |
|---|---|---|

**Orientation**
- What is the (year) (season) (date) (day) (month)?    (5)    ___
- Where are we: (state) (county) (town or city) (hospital) (floor)?    (5)    ___

**Registration**
- Name 3 common objects (e.g., "apple, table, penny"): Take 1    (3)    ___
  second to say each. Then ask the patient to repeat all 3 after
  you have said them. Give 1 point for each correct answer.
  Then repeat them until he/she learns all 3. Count trials and
  record. Make sure patient hears you. Trials: _____

**Attention and calculation**
- Count serial 7's backwards from 100. Give 1 point for each    (5)    ___
  correct answer. Stop after 5 answers. Alternatively, spell
  "WORLD" backwards. One point for each correct letter.
  (100 93 86 79 72 or D-L-R-O-W).

**Recall**
- Ask for the 3 objects repeated above. Give 1 point for each    (3)    ___
  correct answer. (NOTE: Recall cannot be tested if all 3 objects
  were not remembered during registration.)*

**Language**
- Point to, and have patient name, a "pencil" (or "pen") and    (2)    ___
  "watch."
- Repeat the following: "No ifs, ands, or buts."    (1)    ___
- Follow a 3-stage command: "Take a paper in your right hand,    (3)    ___
  fold it in half, and put it on the floor."†
- Display in large letters: "CLOSE YOUR EYES" and ask the    (1)    ___
  patient to read and obey the command.
- Ask the patient to write a sentence (must be a full sentence    (1)    ___
  to earn point).

**Visuo-spatial function**
- Ask the patient to copy the intersecting pentagons below.‡    (1)    ___

| **Total Score** (30)    ___ |
|---|

* Prompted answers do not count. However, if the patient cannot recall any of the objects, or just one or two, try prompting with a clue (e.g., "An article of furniture," "A type of coin"). Classically, In Alzheimer's disease, registered objects do not "imprint" into short-term memory.

† Reaching for something with the dominant hand is instinctive, and most people are right-handed. Helpful modification of test: Find out which hand is dominant, then ask the patient to take the paper in the *non-*dominant hand.

‡ In Alzheimer's disease, there often is inconsistency between attempts. If the copy is acceptable but dementia suspected, have patient repeat copy.

**Box 7-5    Geriatric Depression Scale (Short Form) and Very Short Form**

The patient chooses the best answer for how he or she has felt during the past week. Beneath each question, in parentheses, is the yes or no answer suggestive of depression. A total score of greater than 5 suggests depression.

1.* Are you basically satisfied with your life?
    (No = score of 1)

2.  Have you dropped many of your activities and interests?
    (Yes = score of 1)

3.  Do you feel that your life is empty?
    (Yes = score of 1)

4.* Do you often get bored?
    (Yes = score of 1)

5.  Are you in good spirits most of the time?
    (No = score of 1)

6.  Are you afraid something bad is going to happen to you?
    (Yes = score of 1)

7.  Do you feel happy most of the time?
    (No = score of 1)

8.* Do you often feel helpless?
    (Yes = score of 1)

9.* Do you prefer to stay at home, rather than going out and doing new things?
    (Yes = score of 1)

10. Do you feel that you have more problems with memory than most?
    (Yes = score of 1)

11. Do you think it is wonderful to be alive now?
    (No = score of 1)

12.* Do you feel pretty worthless the way you are now?
    (Yes = score of 1)

13. Do you feel full of energy?
    (No = score of 1)

14. Do you feel that your situation is hopeless?
    (Yes =score of 1)

15. Do you think that most people are better off than you?
    (Yes = score of 1)

* Questions 1, 4, 8, 9, and 12 represent components of the five-item (very short) Geriatric Depression Scale. For the five-item scale, a score of greater than 2 suggests depression.

can directly screen for abuse. A considered approach increases the likelihood that screening will be effective. Emphasizing the diagnosis and treatment of the health consequences of abuse, rather than the mistreatment itself, may be less threatening to the victim and abuser. This may allow the physician to retain patient trust and continuity of care during the course of an investigation. If abuse is suspected, the patient and caregiver should be interviewed separately in order to elicit uninhibited disclosure and to identify inconsistencies between the two accounts (21). Confrontation of the suspected abuser should be avoided, and the clinician should appear sympathetic to his or her perceived burden of caregiving. Box 7-4 lists examples of specific questions that may be used to elicit information from the elder about abuse and neglect. General questions should be followed by specific questions designed to identify various forms of elder abuse.

## Management

Once possible elder abuse has been identified, the clinician must act. The victim's safety should remain the paramount concern. Action can occur on several levels: counseling the patient about options, referring the patient to other services (e.g., home health agencies, geriatrician), referring the case to APS, and referring the case to law inforcement. Because states vary in their regulations, clinicians should find out whether or when they are *mandated* to report to APS/law enforcement. Under many states' reporting laws, clinicians are encouraged to report suspected mistreatment even when reporting is voluntary; the patient's informed consent is not required. If a clinician suspects elder abuse but is unsure whether the circumstances justify reporting, he or she may be able to seek guidance from APS, from the risk management department of his or her facility, or from a local medical society.

Although states vary in the time frame in which reports must be filed, clinicians should contact APS (and, depending on local regulations, law enforcement) immediately when the patient appears at imminent risk of severe injury or death, such as escalating physical abuse, credible threats of physical violence, or malicious neglect. For frail, older adults, emergency hospitalization may be the most expedient way to separate victim and abuser.

If the cognitive assessment determines that the patient's decision-making capacity is intact but the patient refuses intervention, the clinician is obligated to refer to APS only if he or she is a mandated reporter. If permitted but not mandated, it is generally preferable to make the referral. The refusal of interventions can then take place at the level of APS, whose skills in counseling may be able to convert an initial refusal into acceptance of services. For the resistant patient, the clinician can frame an APS referral in the following way:

I appreciate that you are reluctant to let the social worker from Adult Protective Services into your home. However, as your physician, I wouldn't be doing my job if I didn't recommend services that I consider necessary to promote your health. If you don't like what they have to offer, you certainly have the right to decline their help, in just the same way you don't have to take a pill I prescribe or take a lab test I order.

In such cases, the physician (and APS, if involved) should educate the patient about the medical consequences of abuse and its tendency to grow in frequency and severity over time. The physician should give the patient the telephone number of APS and counsel the patient to develop a safety plan, such as when to call 911 and installing a "Lifeline" emergency alert system. Often, the patient who refuses interventions for abuse will welcome more frequent monitoring of a specific medical condition, which may secondarily help to curtail the mistreatment. Increased oversight can take the form of more frequent appointments or the engagement of other services, such as home health and adult day health care. A referral to a psychiatrist for the purpose of diagnosing and treating abuse-related affective disorders can also be used to help empower the victim to change his or her living situation.

To minimize the risk of violence, caregivers of demented persons should receive instruction in behavioral management techniques, which may be obtained through the local affiliate of the Alzheimer's Association, its Web site (http://www.alz.org/), or other Web-based and community-based resources. Medication, such as low-dose haloperidol, may ameliorate aggressiveness and threatening behavior in the patient unresponsive to behavioral and environmental approaches, thus decreasing the risk of double-direction violence.

Respite programs, such as adult day health care, can alleviate caregiver burden. Support groups likewise can ease the caregiver's perception of burden and often provide useful coping and management strategies. Because the patient's health depends on the caregiver, the clinician should periodically screen caregivers, especially caregivers of patients with dementia, for depression and burnout, documenting the findings under the patient's "Social History." This should be done away from the patient in a manner that does not arouse anxiety, suspicion, or anger. For example, the caregiver can be briefly interviewed while the nursing assistant is taking the patient's vital signs. If significant emotional (or physical) pathology is identified that may pose a risk for abuse or neglect of the patient, the clinician should encourage the caregiver to seek appropriate professional help and should counsel the caregiver about other long-term care options, such as residential care or nursing home placement. Had these approaches been taken in the case of Mrs. Dennis (Case 7-3), the physical abuse she suffered from her demented husband and her resulting neglect of him might have been prevented.

## Working with Other Services

Home health agencies may be useful in assessing and managing the medical consequences of mistreatment and serving as a "sentinel" for signs of additional abuse. However, the personnel of most agencies have limited experience dealing with elder mistreatment, and the restricted number of visits imposed by Medicare and other insurers limits their involvement.

Busy clinicians may elect to refer complex cases to a geriatrician, if available. Usually working with an interdisciplinary team, the geriatrician may be better able to conduct and coordinate the time-consuming medical, functional, and psychosocial assessments that are integral to understanding the etiology of the mistreatment and its relationship to the patient's health care needs.

## Discussing the Mandate to Report with the Patient or Caregiver

Because the unexpected visit of an APS social worker might anger or alienate the patient or suspected abuser, clinicians should be forthcoming about the fact that a referral will be made to APS. Whenever possible, the law enforcement implications of APS should be de-emphasized, instead portraying APS as an additional resource to help the patient. In Case 7-1, Mrs.

*Let patient and caregiver know when a referral will be made to Adult Protective Services.*

Roberts' niece, who always brought her to the clinic, claimed to visit her daily and help her with her medications. Yet she failed to bring in her blood glucose monitoring record or medication bottles despite frequent requests. Her description of the food she prepared for her demonstrated continued noncompliance with a diabetic diet, despite multiple referrals to the dietician. The physician presented his plan to notify APS in the following manner:

> It must be hard to look after not only your mother and father but also an aunt as sick as Rose. I am therefore going to make a referral to a county social worker and a public health nurse from Adult Protective Services. Their job is to help older people receive the kind of care they need, preferably in their own homes. They also know that caregivers often need support for what they do. Hopefully, they'll come up with some good suggestions after they meet with you, your parents, and your Aunt Rose.

If the patient or caregiver refuses the APS referral, the clinician should explain that he or she is obligated to comply with state regulations that were developed to help seniors who are not receiving the care they need, regardless of the reason. These laws require physicians (in the case of mandated reporting) to notify APS.

# Legal Issues

## Working with Adult Protective Services

Clinicians should have realistic expectations of their local APS. For example, the risk of future abuse is not always routinely assessed by a particular state's APS, and states vary in the criteria they use for providing involuntary protective services. Because the Joint Commission for the Accreditation of Health Care Organizations requires hospitals with emergency departments or outpatient clinics to provide mandatory training about elder mistreatment, APS can use this venue to educate community physicians about their services. APS may be unaccustomed to working closely with the primary care physician in some communities. Physicians therefore should specifically request to be kept informed by APS, especially about whether abuse has been verified and about those interventions that have implications for medical management (e.g., adult day health care).

## Reporting

The first step in managing suspected mistreatment is to report the case to the appropriate protective services agency. Most clinicians do not have the time or training to interview and counsel the victim and alleged abuser, and few can muster the resources offered by most APS agencies.

Although most primary care clinicians are not accustomed to performing an evidentiary examination, it is important that the documentation be as complete as possible, using photographs or diagrams to indicate the location of bruises and injuries. (Photographs require informed consent from the patient or legal proxy.) Accurate, detailed descriptions are essential because physical signs and symptoms recognized by the clinician may resolve before APS, law enforcement, or a forensic examiner can evaluate them. The reporting guidelines in Box 7-6 will help the clinician provide APS with critical information and promote effective collaboration.

Although all 50 states have APS programs, the guidelines for reporting elder mistreatment vary. In all 43 states that have mandatory reporting laws, health care providers are considered mandated reporters. Although suspected physical abuse must be reported in these states, there is inconsistency in the requirement to report other types of abuse. Most states provide reporters with immunity from criminal or civil liability, and the reporting is not considered a legal breach of patient confidentiality. Failure to comply with mandatory reporting generally is considered a misdemeanor. According to California's Welfare and Institutions Code, failure to report abuse that results in death or severe injury is punishable by a fine of up to $5000 and/or 1 year in a county

---

**Box 7-6    Information to Include in a Report to Adult Protective Services**

---

- Urgency of the referral
  - ➤ Likelihood of imminent harm
- History
  - ➤ Description of the suspected abuse
    - ▪ Nature of the abuse (types, frequency, weapons used, etc.)
    - ▪ Medical/psychiatric consequences of the mistreatment and their acuteness or seriousness
    - ▪ List of the patient's chronic illnesses and how they might have been affected
    - ▪ Predicted impact of the abuse on future health
      - ▲ Likelihood of adverse effect
      - ▲ Anticipated time frame (days, weeks, months)
- Pertinent physical findings
  - ➤ If physical abuse, include detailed descriptions of any injuries, using drawings and (if possible) photographs. Forensic photography may be available in some emergency departments.
- Description of patient's functional status and care needs
- Assessed or estimated decision-making capacity of patient
- Suspected abuser's relationship to the patient
- Known or suspected risk factors for abuse (e.g., caregiver stress, substance abuse)
- Other medical and community services being used by patient (e.g., name of home health agency)
- How best to contact you (the physician)

---

jail. It has been argued that a clinician's failure to identify and report cases of obvious abuse and neglect constitute both negligence and medical malpractice (22). Clinicians can obtain reporting guidelines from the social services department of their local hospital, or they can contact their local APS office.

## Summary

Elder mistreatment occurs frequently, may be chronic, and can adversely affect the health and health care of the older patient. Elders with dementia are at particular risk. The intimacy of the physician-patient relationship affords the clinician the opportunity to recognize and report abuse that otherwise might go undetected. Nearly all states require physicians to report suspected physical abuse to the local APS agency, whereas the requirement for reporting other forms of mistreatment varies. The successful management of elder mistreatment requires effective teamwork between the primary care clinician, APS, consultants, and a variety of community agencies. By focusing on the medical conditions caused or aggravated by abuse, physicians can play a critical role in managing elder mistreatment, even when the patient refuses other interventions.

## REFERENCES

1. Vinton L. Working with abused older women from a feminist perspective. J Women Aging. 1999;11:85-100.

2. Wolf SR, Pillemer K. The older battered woman: spouse abuse and parent abuse compared [Abstract]. Gerontologist. 1995;35:306.

3. Lachs MS, Williams C, O'Brien S, et al. Older adults: an 11-year longitudinal study of adult protective service use. Arch Intern Med. 1996;156:449-53.

4. Pillemer K, Finkelhor D. The prevalence of elder abuse: a random sample survey. Gerontologist. 1988;28:51-7.

5. Podnieks E. National survey on abuse of the elderly in Canada. J Elder Abuse Neglect. 1992;4:59-111.

6. National Center on Elder Abuse, Westat I. The National Elder Abuse Incidence Study: Final Report. Administration on Aging, United States Government; 1998.

7. Quinn MJ, Tomita SK. Elder Abuse and Neglect: Causes, Diagnosis, and Intervention Strategies, 2nd ed. New York: Springer Verlag; 1997.

8. Lachs MS, Williams CS, O'Brien S, et al. ED use by older victims of family violence. Ann Emerg Med. 1997;30:448-54.

9. Lachs MS, Williams CS, O'Brien S, et al. The mortality of elder mistreatment. JAMA. 1998;280:428-32.

10. Lachs MS, Williams C, O'Brien S, et al. Risk factors for reported elder abuse and neglect: a nine-year observational cohort study. Gerontologist. 1997;37:469-74.

11. Wolf RS. Major findings from Three Models Projects on elderly abuse. In: Pillemer K, Wolf R, eds. Elder Abuse and Neglect: Conflict in the Family. Dover, MA: Auburn House; 1986.

12. Anetzberger GJ. The Etiology of Elder Abuse by Adult Offspring. Springfield, IL: Charles C Thomas; 1987.

13. Coyne AC, Reichman WE, Berbig LJ. The relationship between dementia and elder abuse. Am J Psychiatry. 1993;150:643-6.

14. Swearer JM, Drachman DA, O'Donnell BF, Mitchell AL. Troublesome and disruptive behaviors in dementia: relationships to diagnosis and disease severity. J Am Geriatr Soc. 1988;36:784-90.

15. Cummings JL, Mega M, Gray K, et al. The Neuropsychiatric Inventory: comprehensive assessment of psychopathology in dementia. Neurology. 1994;44:2308-14.

16. Dinniss S. Violent crime in an elderly demented patient. Int J Geriatr Psychiatry. 1999;14:889-91.

17. Spangenberg KB, Wagner MT, Hendrix S, Bachman DL. Firearm presence in households of patients with Alzheimer's disease and related dementias. J Am Geriatr Soc. 1999;47:1183-6.

18. Folstein MF, Folstein SE, McHugh PR. "Mini-mental state": a practical method for grading the cognitive state of patients for the clinician. J Psychiatr Res. 1975;12:189-98.

19. Wolf-Klein GP, Silverstone FA, Levy AP, Brod MS. Screening for Alzheimer's disease by clock drawing. J Am Geriatr Soc. 1989;37:730-4.

20. Yesavage JA, Brink TL, Rose TL, et al. Development and validation of a geriatric depression screening scale: a preliminary report. J Psychiatr Res. 1982;17:37-49.

21. Lachs MS, Pillemer K. Abuse and neglect of elderly persons. N Engl J Med. 1995;332: 437-43.

22. Moskowitz S. Private enforcement of criminal mandatory reporting laws. J Elder Abuse Neglect. 1998;9:1-22.

# CHAPTER 8

# Pregnancy

MELISA M. HOLMES, MD
LYDIA E. MAYER, MD, MPH

Connections between violence and pregnancy are common and complex. Violence within a relationship may manifest for the first time during pregnancy or may be part of an ongoing problem. A pregnancy may be the direct result of sexual violence. More indirectly, interpersonal violence increases the risk for subsequent unintended pregnancy because past abuse can negatively affect reproductive health behaviors. Research during the past 15 years has described the extent of the problem. It is now recognized that pregnancy offers a unique window of opportunity to identify victimized women. Even if they do not provide routine prenatal care, internists who care for adult women do see pregnant women for a variety of issues, including diagnosis of pregnancy and medical complications of pregnancy.

This chapter reviews the current understanding of the epidemiology and outcomes that are uniquely related to violence that occurs during pregnancy, including the immediate preconception and post-partum periods. Many of the recommendations on screening, acute intervention, and follow-up presented in earlier chapters also apply to violence in pregnant women; therefore, this chapter will address screening and interventions only as they specifically apply to the problem of violence during pregnancy.

## Epidemiology

A recent systematic review of 13 North American studies found that violence during pregnancy has been reported to occur among 1% to 20% of pregnant women, with most studies identifying rates between 4% and 8% (1). This wide variation reflects the problem that data on violence during pregnancy are complicated by the lack of standardized definitions and wide variations in study methodology (2). The available literature suggests that abuse does escalate during pregnancy, although other studies need to confirm these findings. For example, one study found that nearly two-thirds of abused women said that the abuse worsened during pregnancy (3). For some women, the abuse occurs for the first time during a pregnancy, and 60% of abused women experience repetitive episodes throughout the pregnancy.

*Pregnancy may instigate abuse.*

When severe intimate partner violence antedates or occurs during pregnancy, it is likely to continue post-partum (2). Violence may become even more prevalent in the post-partum period than during pregnancy (4). Although differences may exist among certain studies, these variations are most likely attributed to differences in study methods rather than true population differences. For instance, when screening occurs in the third trimester or more than once during the pregnancy, prevalence rates are higher than those found in studies that only screened at the first prenatal visit.

Some populations of pregnant women appear to be at higher risk for abuse than the general obstetrical population (Box 8-1). Among pregnant adolescents, violence is experienced during pregnancy in 20% to 22%, and 32% to 38% report physical or sexual abuse either during the pregnancy or within the past year. Other populations of women at increased risk for violence during pregnancy include women who are divorced or separated, of greater parity, and who report tobacco, alcohol or illicit drug use (5). In pregnant women receiving substance abuse treatment, the vast majority have experienced sexual or physical assault.

Among women experiencing violence during pregnancy, the perpetrator is usually a current or former intimate partner (6). Among adolescents who are pregnant, it is important to recognize that the perpetrator may also be a parent, other family member, or even a female peer. It is critical that providers

---

**Box 8-1    Risk Factors for Violence During Pregnancy and Puerperium**

- Young age
- Divorced or separated
- Substance use
- Higher parity
- History of past abuse
- Male partner concerns regarding paternity
- Male partner feeling threatened by attention given to the baby

recognize that violence occurs as frequently as gestational diabetes and pre-eclampsia, for which screening is routinely done (1,2).

## Violence and Unintended Pregnancy

In addition to addressing violence occurring in pregnancy, it is also important to recognize a causal link between violence (both physical and sexual) and un-intended pregnancy. A population-based study of more than 12,000 mothers of newborns indicates that women with an unintended or mis-timed pregnancy were 4.1 times more likely to have experienced physical violence than women with a planned pregnancy (7). Partner abuse has been linked to unintended pregnancy through several direct and indirect mechanisms. A male abuser may attempt to control his partner by controlling contraceptive options or by having a child with her. Unintended pregnancy can be a direct consequence of sexual assault. A prospective, population-based study in the United States of 4000 women indicates that approximately 30,000 pregnancies per year result directly from rape (8). Indirectly, sexual assault is a cause of unintended pregnancy because it often results in long-term behavioral changes. In the aftermath of sexual assault, for example, victims demonstrate increased risk-taking behaviors, including unsafe sexual practices.

> *Violence is more likely with unintended pregnancy.*

> *Unintended pregnancy can result from sexual assault.*

## Consequences of Violence During Pregnancy

Physical and sexual assault occurring during a pregnancy affect both maternal and fetal well-being. The most severe maternal outcome of intimate partner violence is death due to homicide. Injury is the most common single cause of maternal death, and homicide is the most common injury-related cause of death (9). According to the Bureau of Justice statistics, 28% to 32% of all female murder victims in the United States are murdered by a current or former intimate partner (1,10,11). A multiple-source linked data surveillance analysis of Maryland maternal-associated mortality found

> *Homicide is the most common injury-related cause of maternal death.*

that "enhanced pregnancy mortality surveillance led to the disturbing finding that a pregnant or recently pregnant woman is more likely to be a victim of homicide than to die of any other cause"(12). All evidence consistently found that domestic violence kills more pregnant women than any single medical complication of pregnancy. It should be remembered that this is because of the low risk of death from any single medical complication of pregnancy and the relatively higher risk of death in this age group of women from homicide, not because pregnancy itself increases risk of death from homicide.

Published case reports describe other assault-related complications, including placental abruption, uterine rupture, fetal skeletal fractures, and maternal and fetal death. Neither severity, nor location of maternal injury, nor maternal hemodynamic status predict fetal outcome. Estimated gestational age of the fetus at the time of injury, but not the extent of maternal injury, correlates with the degree of fetal injury (13). More commonly, physical injuries resulting from assault during pregnancy are not severe. The most common sites of physical injury to the pregnant woman involve the head, abdomen, and breasts (6,13). Antenatal hospitalization occurs more frequently among women experiencing domestic violence during pregnancy than among age-matched controls (8,13,14), which correlates with other data showing increased hospitalizations and health care utilization of women experiencing violence. Experiences of abuse appear to affect perinatal health and outcomes, either directly through physical trauma or indirectly through stress mechanisms. However, studies have shown inconsistent associations between violence during pregnancy and specific outcomes. Some studies indicate no significant perinatal morbidity, whereas others reveal higher rates of vaginal bleeding in the first and second trimesters, poor maternal weight gain, anemia, pre-term labor, pre-term rupture of membranes, low birth weight, and an increased risk ratio for caesarian section (9,13,15,16). Pregnancy outcomes may be affected because of other factors associated with experiencing violence during pregnancy: delay in onset of prenatal care, abuse of substances, and experience of depressive symptoms. Although not enough evidence indicates causality, all of these interrelated, abuse-associated complications are recognized risk factors for poor maternal and fetal outcomes.

## Post-Partum Considerations

In addition to the effect of violence on pregnancy, the post-partum period is a critical time for continued surveillance particularly for post-partum depression, escalating violence, and child abuse. Intimate partner violence has been clearly linked with depression and post-traumatic stress disorder in women (17): 53% of the women who had experienced violence during pregnancy met the diagnostic criteria for a major depressive episode during the post-partum period. The added stresses of parenting, financial changes, and sleep deprivation may affect patterns of domestic violence. In a study of 36 physically abused pregnant women, Stewart compared the number of abusive episodes that occurred during the 3 months before conception, the first, second, and third trimesters, and the 3 months following delivery (4). Significantly more abusive episodes occurred in the post-partum period compared to each of the other time frames.

*More abusive episodes occur postpartum than before or during pregnancy.*

Identification of violence during pregnancy can also help identify families at risk for child abuse. Research indicates clear links between domestic violence and child abuse. Abused children are likely to have abused mothers, and abused mothers are likely to have abused children (17). Data from the National Family Violence Survey indicate that marital violence is a statistically significant predictor of physical child abuse.

Finally, the peri-partum and post-partum periods can be physically, emotionally, and financially stressful, thus increasing the risk for tension. During this time period, clinicians should be particularly alert to specific behaviors or concerns that can signal an increased risk for intimate partner violence. A jealous, dominating male partner may feel threatened by the attention given to the infant. The male may be excessively jealous of the baby, resorting to physical or sexual violence as a way of controlling the mother; he may force her to have sex or prevent her from breastfeeding, or he may demonstrate extreme possessiveness and accuse her of having affairs with other men. Male questioning of paternity is felt to be a risk factor for severe violence. The data are limited in this area, but such scenarios should raise suspicion and result in screening, aggressive intervention, and protection for both the woman and the involved children.

## A Unique Screening Opportunity

For health care providers treating pregnant women, a unique opportunity exists for identifying abuse and intervening to effect change. For the pregnant woman, the innate desire to protect the potential life within is often a powerful motivator for change. For both the patient and the health care worker, prenatal care also offers a time frame in which frequent contact, a trusting relationship, and improved access to social service and health care resources exists. These factors enhance

*Prenatal care offers a unique opportunity for abuse intervention.*

the effectiveness of screening and interventions. Furthermore, when domestic violence is suspected or disclosed during pregnancy, transmitting this information confidentially to pediatricians with the patient's consent can help to prevent or detect child abuse. Screening mothers at scheduled well-baby visits in one study detected more domestic violence than had been disclosed during obstetric care (18). When domestic violence is detected in pediatric settings, communication with and referral of the pregnant woman back to her primary care clinician allows the possibility of effective intervention for post-partum abuse and depression. Because the father has a right to the child's pediatric records, it is suggested that the confidentiality issues are carefully discussed before any documentation in the record.

Although routine screening for violence in all pregnant women has been recommended by several professional organizations, research indicates a significant deficit in screening practices (19). A survey conducted among 1339 practicing obstetricians and gynecologists revealed that physicians have a good understanding of the extent of the problem, and the majority have received continuing medical education on the topic (20). Despite appropriate knowledge, however, only 39% of the respondents routinely screen at a first prenatal visit, and screening is most likely to occur when the physician has clinical suspicion of violence. Unfortunately, clinical signs and symptoms are not common, and abused women rarely volunteer information about abuse unless they are directly asked.

General screening techniques have been described in Chapter 2. Screening methods that apply specifically to pregnancy have also been recommended and tested. In general, direct questions that use behaviorally specific phrasing are more effective than legal terms such as "abuse," "domestic violence," and "rape." The Abuse Assessment Screen is a simple, five-question tool that is very useful in pregnancy and can be modified for non-pregnant patients as well. Please refer to Chapter 2 for details on this and other screening methods.

## Interventions

Once screening becomes routine, the health care provider must be prepared to efficiently and effectively assist women with past or ongoing violence (see Chapters 3 and 5). More specific interventions may occasionally be required (Box 8-2). For women who experience physical assault with injury to the gravid abdomen, the obstetrician should assess the severity of the abdominal trauma and initiate a monitoring protocol to assess for placental abruption, other fetal-maternal hemorrhage, and pre-term labor. For the Rh-negative patient with significant abdominal trauma, Rho(D) immune globulin should be given. The hemodynamic changes that normally occur in pregnancy will

---

**Box  8-2    Considerations  and  Interventions  Specific  to  Treating Physical Violence During Pregnancy**

- Physiologic changes in pregnancy may mask large-volume blood loss or alter the physiologic response to internal bleeding; therefore, aggressive evaluation for internal bleeding is necessary.
- Trauma to the gravid abdomen necessitates monitoring protocol to evaluate for
  - Placental abruption
  - Fetal-maternal hemorrhage
  - Preterm labor
  - Uterine rupture
  - Fetal injury
- Pregnant women with Rh-negative blood type and abdominal trauma should receive Rho(D) immune globulin.

---

significantly alter the physiologic response to internal hemorrhage and may even mask massive blood loss. Therefore, it is critical that a pregnant woman with significant trauma be evaluated and managed by a knowledgeable and experienced team, including obstetrical providers.

Because intimate partner violence is usually an indolent, smoldering type of violence, generally there will not be an immediate crisis that needs to be addressed upon disclosure by the patient. In fact, unless the patient is suicidal or wishes to leave the relationship immediately, she could be put at greater danger by trying to make a sudden change: all of the safety implications need to be considered. Instead, once the violence is identified, the clinician should validate the experience as traumatic for the patient, complete a safety assessment, refer to available resources, and continue to offer support (see Chapters 2 and 4). Obstetricians and other health care providers seeing pregnant patients should maintain an active list of available resources, including trauma-specific counseling services, legal advocacy services that focus on family and custody law, and battered women's shelters that will allow women to bring their children. Hospitals can be prepared to manage a domestic violence crisis by establishing a protocol that allows for overnight hospitalization until safe, longer-term shelter can be arranged. Admission under a false name can provide added protection and anonymity.

Only limited data address the outcomes of specific intervention protocols for intimate partner violence. In a quasi-experimental study, a standardized abuse screen was administered over 15 months to all prenatal patients at their routine prenatal intake interview (21). Implementation of this protocol resulted in more pregnant women being assessed and referred for abuse compared to historical controls. In another intervention study, a cohort of abused pregnant women received three education, advocacy, and community referral sessions that focused on safety behaviors (22). After the intervention, there was a significant increase in the adoption of safety behaviors. However, women's use of referral resources was related more to the severity of abuse than to whether the woman had received the intervention. Home visitation by nurses of at-risk families during pregnancy and for the first 2 years postpartum has been found ineffective, improving neither child abuse and neglect nor reproductive control in the cases of severe domestic violence. It may be that severe violence requires significant multifactorial interventions that cannot be accomplished by a few home visits from a nurse.

## Summary

Interpersonal violence occurs in a continuum during pregnancy. Violence may predate a pregnancy and directly or indirectly contribute to the occurrence of unintended pregnancy. It may continue to occur during the pregnancy and result in subtle or devastating complications. It may then carry over into the post-partum period and manifest not only as domestic abuse but also as child abuse. In fact, more abusive episodes tend to occur after the pregnancy than during the pregnancy or before. Therefore, it is critical that health care providers who encounter pregnant women take advantage of the unique opportunity afforded through prenatal care to identify and address the problem of violence during pregnancy.

## REFERENCES

1. Gazmararian JA, Lazorick S, Spitz AM, et al. Prevalence of violence against pregnant women: a review of the literature. JAMA. 1996;275:1915-20.
2. Ballard TJ, Saltzman LE, Gazmararian JA, et al. Violence during pregnancy: measurement issues. Am J Public Health. 1998;88:185-7.
3. Stewart DE, Cecutti A. Physical abuse in pregnancy. Can Med Assoc J. 1993;149:1257-63.
4. Stewart DE. Incidence of postpartum abuse in women with a history of abuse during pregnancy. Can Med Assoc J. 1994;151:1601-4.
5. Berenson AB, Stiglich NJ, Wilkinson GS, Anderson GD. Drug abuse and other risk factors for physical abuse in pregnancy among white non-Hispanic, black, and Hispanic women. Am J Obstet Gynecol. 1991;164:1491-6.
6. McFarlane J, Parker B, Soeken K, Bullock L. Assessing for abuse during pregnancy: severity and frequency of injuries and associated entry into prenatal care. JAMA. 1992;267:3176-8.
7. Gazmararian JA, Adams MM, Saltzman LE, et al. The relationship between pregnancy intendedness and physical violence in mothers of newborns. Obstet Gynecol. 1995;85:1031-8.

8. Holmes MM, Resnick HS, Kilpatrick DG, Best CL. Rape-related pregnancy: estimates and descriptive characteristics from a national sample of women. Am J Obstet Gynecol. 1996;175:320-5.

9. Harper M, Parsons L. Maternal deaths due to homicide and other injuries in North Carolina 1992-1994. Obstet Gynecol. 1997;90:920-3.

10. Tjaden P, Thoennes N. Extent, Nature, and Consequences of Intimate Partner Violence Findings from the National Violence Against Women Survey. Washington, DC: Department of Justice; 2000.

11. Bachman R, Saltzman LE. Violence Against Women: Estimates from the Redesigned Survey. Washington, DC: Department of Justice; 1985:10-8.

12. Horon IL, Chung D. Enhanced surveillance for pregnancy-associated mortality: Maryland, 1993-1998. JAMA. 2001;285:1455-9.

13. Petersen R, Gazmararian JA, Spitz AM, et al. Violence and adverse pregnancy outcomes: a review of the literature and directions for future research. Am J Prev Med. 1997;13:366-3.

14. Council on Scientific Affairs, American Medical Association. Violence against women: relevance for medical practitioners. JAMA. 1992;267:3184-9.

15. Murphy CC, Schei B, Myhr TL, Du Mont J. Abuse: a risk factor for low birth weight? A systemic review and meta-analysis. CMAJ. 2001;164:1567-72.

16. Cokkinides VE, Coker AL, Sanderson M, et al. Physical violence during pregnancy: maternal complications and birth outcomes. Obstet Gynecol. 1999;93:661-6.

17. Campbell JC, Kub J, Rose L. Depression in battered women. J Am Med Womens Assoc. 1996;51:106-10.

18. Siegel RM, Hill TD, Henderson VA, et al. Screening for domestic violence in the community pediatric setting. Pediatrics. 1999;104:874-7.

19. Rodriguez MA, Bauer HM, McLoughlin E, Grumbach K. Screening and intervention for intimate partner abuse: practices and attitudes of primary care physicians. JAMA. 1999;282:468-74.

20. Horan DL, Chapin J, Klein L, et al. Domestic violence screening practices of obstetrician-gynecologists. Obstet Gynecol. 1998;92:785-9.

21. Wiist WH, McFarlane J. The effectiveness of an abuse assessment protocol in public health prenatal clinics. Am J Public Health. 1999;89:1217-21.

22. McFarlane J, Parker B, Soeken K, et al. Safety behaviors of abused women after an intervention during pregnancy. J Obstet Gynecol Neonatal Nurs. 1998;27:64-9.

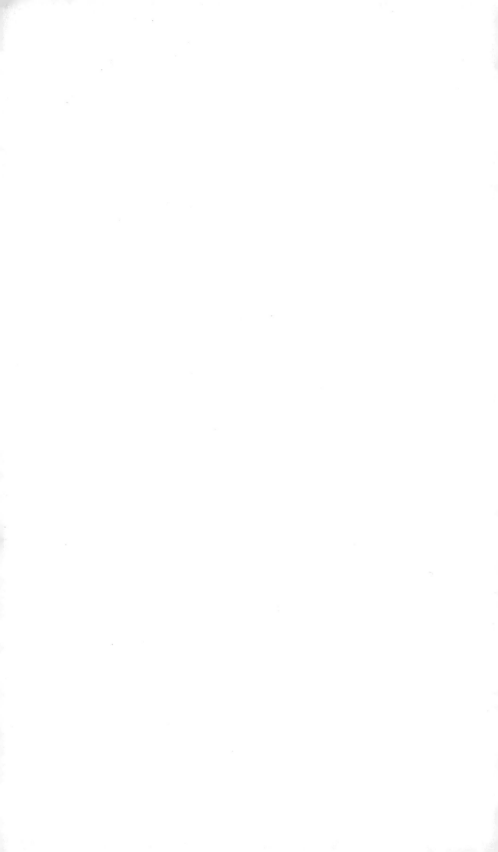

# CHAPTER 9

# Women with Disabilities

MARGARET A. NOSEK, PHD
CAROL A. HOWLAND, MPH

The reaction of the general public, medical professionals, and disability-related service providers to physical and sexual violence against women with
disabilities is often one of shock and disbelief, as if disability could somehow
protect women from violence. Advocates and researchers agree that disability
introduces additional vulnerability for experiencing violence and difficulty in
accessing help. In this chapter, we will define disability and review the epidemiology of disability and prevalence of abuse in women with disabilities.
We will then discuss clinical approaches to abuse in women with disabilities.

## The Disability Experience

The World Health Organization in its most recent classification system, the
ICIDH-2, defines disability as impairment (a significant deviation or loss in
body function or structure) in the context of a health condition. This broad
definition can be further clarified by assessing specific dimensions of the disability's temporality, deviation from the norm, and etiology. Impairments can
be temporary or permanent; progressive, regressive, or static; intermittent or
continuous. The deviation from the norm may be slight or severe and may
fluctuate over time.

The impairment may result from an injury, disease, or congenital condition. Thus, a person with a disability often is not considered ill. Persons with
disabilities have varying degrees of associated activity limitations (difficulties
performing activities in an expected manner) and participation restrictions
(restrictions in the manner or extent of involvement in life situations). The use
of assistive devices or personal assistance may eliminate activity limitations,

**Table 9-1   Demographic Characteristics of Women with Disabilities Compared with Women in the General Population**

| Characteristic | Women with Disabilities* (%) | Women in the General Population (%) |
|---|---|---|
| Married | 40 | 63 |
| Live alone | 35 | 13 |
| High school education or less | 78 | 54 |
| Employed | 14 | 63 |
| Live below poverty level | 23 | 10 |
| Have private health insurance | 55 | 74 |

Data from the 1994–1995 National Health Interview Survey.
* Women with three or more functional limitations. The National Health Interview Survey defines disability similarly to WHO but adds chronic mental disorders.

but the impairment or disability is considered to still exist. Contextual factors associated with having a disability, both environmental and personal, may impose barriers to functioning. Environmental factors include social, attitudinal, and architectural barriers.

According to the 1991-1992 Current Population Reports, 26 million women in the United States have disability-related work limitations, comprising 20% of the population of women as a whole (1). Women with disabilities have demographic characteristics that place them at high risk of social isolation, which has been associated with an increased risk for depression (Table 9-1) (2,3) and other negative health outcomes (4).

## Epidemiology

The prevalence of abuse among women in general is fairly well documented, yet only a few North American studies (5), primarily from Canada, have examined the prevalence among women with disabilities. One national survey compared abuse in 504 women with physical disabilities (most frequently spinal cord injury, cerebral palsy, muscular dystrophy, multiple sclerosis, and joint and connective tissue diseases) and 442 women without disabilities (6). This survey (7) revealed no significant abuse prevalence differences between percentages of women with and without disabilities reporting emotional abuse (52% vs 48%), physical abuse (36% in both groups), or sexual abuse (40% vs 37%). Women with physical disabilities and women with no disabilities were equally likely to have experienced abuse during childhood. The most common perpetrators were intimate partners or members of the family of origin (Fig. 9-1).

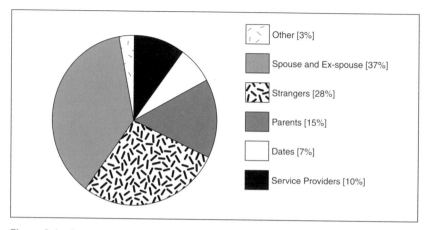

**Figure 9-1**   Perpetrators of violence toward women with disabilities. (Data from Ridington J. Beating the "odds": violence and women with disabilities (Position Paper 2). 1989. Vancouver: Disabled Women's Network.)

However, further analysis revealed that women with disabilities reported significantly longer duration of physical or sexual abuse compared to women without disabilities and that women with disabilities were more likely to experience abuse by health care providers and attendants. Furthermore, women with disabilities were abused by a larger number of perpetrators and were more likely to experience more intense patterns of abuse during their lifetimes than women without disabilities. Other studies have documented abuse in women with intellectual impairments (8) and blindness (9).

*Women with disabilities are more likely to experience intense patterns of abuse than non-disabled women.*

## Risk Factors for Abuse

A small number of studies have investigated why women with disabilities may experience a greater vulnerability to abuse. The cultural devaluation of women and persons with disabilities is a major factor (10). Reduced societal expectations and, paradoxically, overprotection are other significant contributors. Women with disabilities may not experience age-appropriate dating and sexual activity while growing up. They thus have fewer opportunities to learn to establish boundaries around sexual activity and few

*Cultural devaluation of women with disabilities makes them more vulnerable to abuse.*

skills to negotiate a healthy sexual relationship. Furthermore, they frequently believe that no loving person would be attracted to them. In fact, it may be only after reaching adulthood that they have their first sexual encounters, and these encounters may involve little emotional intimacy.

Andrews and Veronen (11) have cited eight reasons for increased vulnerability to victimization among persons with disabilities:

1. Increased dependency on others for long-term care
2. Denial of human rights that results in perceptions of powerlessness
3. Less risk of discovery as perceived by the perpetrator
4. Difficulty in being believed
5. Less education about appropriate and inappropriate sexuality
6. Social isolation and increased risk of manipulation
7. Physical helplessness and vulnerability in public places
8. The push by disability advocates to mainstream and integrate people with disabilities without adequate consideration of each individual's capacity for self-protection.

A qualitative interview study also identified several disability-related vulnerability factors: inability to escape a situation because of architectural inaccessibility; lack of adaptive equipment; social stereotypes of vulnerability; increased risk in institutional settings; increased exposure to medical settings; and dependence on abusive caregivers for daily survival activities such as transferring from bed to wheelchair, eating, using essential orthotic equipment, and taking medications (12). In their analysis of the policy implications of abuse of women with disabilities, Nosek, Howland, and Young (13) cite as additional vulnerability factors the social stereotype that women with disabilities are asexual, passive, unaware, and, therefore, easy prey. The fact that many women with disabilities have been subjected to violence throughout their lives and accept it as normal behavior only contributes to the complexity of abuse issues.

Difficulty locating and retaining persons to provide personal assistance prompts women with disabilities to be more tolerant of abusive assistants. In addition, certain types of disabilities that have associated cognitive impairments, such as traumatic brain injury, mental illness, and mental retardation, may limit the woman's ability to recognize abuse and seek help (6). Furthermore, difficulty financing and obtaining adaptive equipment leaves many women less mobile and unnecessarily dependent on abusers. The woman with a disability may perceive that this is her only living option, that no one else would take care of her, and that abuse is the price she must pay for survival.

Lack of economic independence also adds to the vulnerability of women with disabilities (14,15). However, compared to women without disabilities, and men with disabilities, economic disadvantage is greater for women with disabilities, increasing their susceptibility to entering, and remaining in, abusive relationships. Participation in the labor market is 33% for women with disabilities, dropping to 13% for full-time work, compared with 69% for men with disabilities (16,17). Their employability is also impaired by a lower educational level than for women without disabilities (18). Even college-educated women with disabilities are less successful in obtaining employment than college-educated men with disabilities or college-educated women without disabilities (18). Contrary to societal expectations that women with disabilities are considered asexual and thus exempt from sexual harassment in the workplace, sexual harassment may also lead to job loss, demotion, and interrupted education for women with disabilities (19,20).

## Abuse Specific to Women with Disabilities

Women with disabilities encounter the same types of abuse experienced by women in general. However, women with disabilities also experience abuse that is specifically disability-related (21). As with non-disabled women, disability-related emotional abuse takes the form of emotional abandonment and rejection, threats, belittling, and blaming but may also manifest as threats of physical abandonment, denial of disability, and accusations of faking illness. Disability-related physical abuse may, in addition to physical injury, manifest as physical restraint, confinement, withholding use of orthotic devices or medication, and refusing to provide assistance with essential personal needs such as toileting, hygiene, and eating. Disability-related sexual abuse can occur as expecting sexual activity in return for help, exploiting physical weakness within an isolated environment to force sexual activities.

Certain disability-related settings may create an environment of isolation and diminish the defenses of disabled children and adults by separating them from their mobility devices, restraining them, or isolating them from others who could provide assistance (21). Examples of such settings include special education classrooms or special schools for disabled children, residential facilities, hospitals, clinics, and paratransit vehicles.

## Screening for Abuse

The use of screening tools by health care providers in clinical settings has been found to be effective in detecting abuse that would otherwise go unreported (see Chapter 2) (22). The addition of only two questions to the existing abuse assessment instrument identified 20% of the abuse that would have gone undetected in a clinical sample of 511 women with disabilities (Box 9-1). Women

---

**Box 9-1   Disability-Related Abuse Assessment Tool**

- "Within the last year, has anyone prevented you from using a wheelchair, cane, respirator, or other assistive devices?"
- "Within the last year, has anyone you depend on refused to help you with an important personal need, such as taking your medicine, getting to the bathroom, getting out of bed, bathing, getting dressed, or getting food or drink?"

---

with disabilities have higher than average contact with medical professionals. Because many of the resources women use to seek help with abusive situations are unavailable to women with disabilities, the medical setting may be their only avenue to safety.

There are many barriers to detection of abuse by health care professionals. Physician barriers include insufficient knowledge about abuse (e.g., what to ask and how to ask it), lack of resources, biases and beliefs, and personal experiences. Patients are also unwilling to disclose abuse for numerous reasons, such as fear of retaliation from the abuser and shame. The many barriers to disclosure are discussed in detail in Chapter 2. These barriers apply to disabled women as well as nondisabled women.

For women with disabilities, there may be additional barriers to disclosure. Physicians might not ask about abuse because they may believe that abuse doesn't occur in the population of women with disabilities. The physician may know the assailant and believe he or she is incapable of abuse. He or she may not know what to do if abuse is uncovered or may believe that intervention is the job of other professionals, such as social workers. Or, the physician may know what to do but believe it won't help in the case of a disabled patient.

There are many clues from the medical history that signal abuse. In particular, the physician needs to evaluate whether there is a discrepancy between a description of the incident and the kind of injury suffered. A time delay between injuries and presentation may be purposeful on the part of an abusive caretaker. Before attributing an injury to a disability-related problem (spasticity, falls from the wheelchair), the provider must rule out any intentional acts by a perpetrator. Physicians caring for disabled women must evaluate psychosomatic or recurring physical complaints with a high degree of suspicion of abuse because these may be manifestations of a current or previous abuse history and not just the result of the patient's disability: psychological symptoms can occur in disabled as well as in non-disabled patients.

Clues that will heighten the suspicion of abuse in women with disabilities can be obtained from the physical examination (see Chapter 3 for a detailed description of a physical examination for suspected abuse). In persons who have difficulty communicating because of cognitive impairment, the genital area should be examined for signs of hematomas, bleeding, or the insertion of foreign bodies because such patients may not be able to communicate about or be aware of such injuries.

There are many things a medical professional can do for abused patients with disabilities. These interventions parallel those for non-disabled patients with some special additions. First, in treating disabled women, it is important that clinical staff trained to communicate with persons who have hearing, cognitive, speech, or psychiatric impairments are available. Untrained clinical staff should receive training in recognizing the symptoms of abuse and the characteristics of potential abusers in the case of disabled women. As part of a multi-faceted effort, staff should administer the Abuse Assessment Screen-Disability developed by McFarlane in collaboration with CROWD researchers, which is sensitive to disability-related abuse (23).

## Intervention and Referral to Service Providers

Interventions for non-disabled women include helping with the development of a safety plan and an escape plan in the event of imminent violence and helping the woman escape from the abuser either temporarily to a woman's shelter or permanently to another living arrangement. However, these services (described in more detail in Chapter 4) may not be feasible for a woman with a disability because they may be poorly equipped or unequipped to meet the special needs of disabled persons (e.g., architectural inaccessibility of the shelters) or because the disabled woman depends on the abuser for personal assistance and therefore cannot independently arrange to go to a shelter.

According to a survey conducted in 1998 by the Center for Research on Women with Disabilities (which received responses from 598 battered women's programs), only 35% of these programs offer disability awareness training for their staff, and only 16% have a staff member who is specifically assigned to provide services to women with disabilities. For these reasons, a very small percentage of women with disabilities who are being abused receive services from traditional battered women's programs. For nearly half the programs, less than 1% of the women served had physical disabilities, far less than their proportion in the population.

The National Coalition Against Domestic Violence has issued a manual for battered women's programs on implementing accessibility modifications according to the requirements of the Americans with Disabilities Act. The manual also contains guidelines on how to increase sensitivity and responsiveness among program staff to the needs of abused women with disabilities (24).

*National Domestic Violence Hotline gives information on shelters with accessibility to persons with disabilities.*

The National Domestic Violence Hotline keeps a database of battered women's shelters throughout the country, with indications of their architectural accessibility and availability of interpreter services. The hotline is equipped with telecommunication devices for persons who are deaf, even though it is rarely used. See the Appendix for a list of national and local hotline and resource numbers.

Local abuse intervention programs can collaborate with independent living centers and specialized disability-service providers to enhance services for women with disabilities. A recent survey of 41 independent living centers highlights how this collaboration can successfully address some of the unique barriers encountered by women with disabilities when accessing community abuse programs (25). Independent living centers may help identify women with disabilities experiencing abuse and help these women access appropriate community services. They can also help domestic violence shelters and sexual assault programs improve their accessibility and responsiveness to women with disabilities and have provided personal assistants to women in shelters or who need respite care because of an abusive care provider. Many of the independent living centers in the survey address abuse issues through their individual and group counseling services, and they train abuse intervention program personnel on the unique needs of women with disabilities. In turn, abuse program staff train independent living centers staff on abuse issues.

When a women discloses abuse, the principles of empathy, safety assessment, safety planning, referral to other resources, documentation and plans for follow-up care should be employed. Safety planning should begin by discussing safety risks with the patient. If the caregiver is a paid employee, the patient should look for another caregiver to replace the abusive one. If the caregiver is family member, the patient should be encouraged to pursue outside resources to decrease the dependence on the caregiver. For physically disabled but cognitively intact women, it may be useful to employ a "lifeline," a 24-hour-a-day emergency response system that is activated by pressing a button on a necklace.

As in the case of nondisabled women, clinicians may help directly by brainstorming with women about strategies, but consultation with a provider trained in domestic violence caregiving is also recommended, either in person or by using a local or national hotline. Hotline staff receive extensive training in safety plan development. In some states, medical providers are mandatory reporters for disabled adults. The adult protective services agency in each state can clarify the regulations about a provider's mandatory reporting status, and state-wide domestic violence hotlines may also be able to give this information.

# Summary

Abuse of women with disabilities is a problem of widespread proportions that is only beginning to attract the attention of health care providers, service providers, researchers, and funding agencies. The gaps in our knowledge about abuse and women with disabilities are enormous. For each disability type, different dynamics of abuse come into play. For women with mobility disabilities, limitations in physically escaping violent situations are in sharp contrast to women with hearing impairments, who may be able to escape but face communication barriers in most settings designed to help battered women.

Certain commonalities exist across disability groups, such as economic dependence, social isolation, and the whittling away of self-esteem on the basis of disability as a precursor to abuse. We know very little about what interventions are effective for women with disabilities. Few of the strategies listed in classic safety plans are possible for women who must depend on their abuser to get them out of bed in the morning, dress them, and feed them. Only a handful of programs across the country specifically address the needs of abused women with disabilities.

The assumption has been that abuse falls within the domain of social service providers and should not be addressed by medical professionals, who probably have had no training in how to handle such problems. For women with disabilities, however, medical providers may be their only resource for help. The lack of accessible battered women's programs and the prevailing lack of awareness of the increased vulnerability for abuse that is faced by all women with disabilities limits their ability to benefit from what resources may exist. This barrier-filled landscape places additional responsibility on health care professionals to open the discussion of abuse with their patients who have disabilities, to increase their capacity to recognize and treat the consequences of abuse, and to make appropriate referrals to battered women's programs and other accessible resources for assistance.

## REFERENCES

1. McNeil JM. Americans with Disabilities: 1991-92, Current Population Reports, P70-33. Washington, DC: Bureau of the Census; 1993.
2. Roberts RE, Kaplan GA, Shema SJ, & Strawbridge WJ. Prevalence and correlates of depression in an aging cohort. The Alameda County Study. J Gerontolo Soc Sci. 1997;52B: S252-S258.
3. Pope AM, Tarlov AR, eds. Disability in America: Toward a National Agenda for Prevention. Washington, DC: National Academy Press; 1991.
4. Berkman LF, Syme SL. Social networks, host resistance, and mortality: a nine-year follow-up study of Alameda County residents. Am J Epidemiol. 1979;109:186-204.

5. Sobsey D, Wells D, Lucardie R, Mansell S. eds. Violence and Disability: An Annotated Bibliography. Baltimore, MD: Paul H. Brookes; 1995.

6. Nosek MA, Rintala DH, Young ME, et al. Sexual functioning among women with physical disabilities. Arch Phys Med Rehabil. 1996;77:107-15.

7. Young ME, Nosek MA, Howland C, et al. Prevalence of abuse of women with physical disabilities. Arch Phys Med Rehabil. 1997;78(Suppl 5):S34-S38.

8. Sobsey D, Doe T. Patterns of sexual abuse and assault. Sexuality and Disability. 1991; 9:243-60.

9. Welbourne A, Lipschitz S, Selvin H, Green R. A comparison of the sexual learning experiences of visually impaired and sighted women. J Visual Impairment Blindness. 1983; 77:256-9.

10. Belsky J. Child maltreatment: an ecological integration. Am Psychologist. 1980;35: 320-35.

11. Andrews AB, Veronen LJ. Sexual assault and people with disabilities. J Soc Work Hum Sexuality. 1993;8:137-59.

12. Nosek, M.A. Sexual abuse of women with physical disabilities. In: Krotoski DM, Nosek MA, Turk MA, eds. Women with Physical Disabilities: Achieving and Maintaining Health and Well-Being. Baltimore, MD: Paul H. Brookes; 1996:153-73.

13. Nosek MA, Howland CA, Young ME. Abuse of women with disabilities: policy implications. J Disability Policy Studies. 1997;8:157-76.

14. Farmer A, Tiefenthaler J. Domestic violence: the value of services as signals. American Economic Review. 1996;86:274-9.

15. Schaller J, DeLaGarza D. Issues of gender in vocational testing and counseling. Journal of Job Placement. 1995;11:6-14.

16. Danek MM. The status of women with disabilities revisited. J App Rehabil Counseling. 1992.23:7-13.

17. U.S. Bureau of the Census. Labor force status and other characteristics of persons with a work disability: 1981 to 1988 (Current Population Reports Series P-23, No. 160), 1989. Washington, DC: U.S. Government Printing Office.

18. Fine M, Asch A. eds. Women with Disabilities: Essays in Psychology, Culture, and Politics. Philadelphia: Temple University Press; 1988.

19. Murphy PA. Taking an abuse history in the initial evaluation. NARPPS. 1992;7:187-90.

20. Murphy PA. Making the Connections: Women, Work, and Abuse. Orlando, FL: Paul M. Deutsch Press; 1993.

21. Nosek MA, Foley CC, Hughes RB, Howland CA. Vulnerabilities for abuse among women with disabilities. Sexuality and Disability. 2001;19:177-89.

22. Wiist WH, McFarlane J. The effectiveness of an abuse assessment protocol in a public health prenatal clinic. Am J Public Health. 1999;89:1217-21.

23. McFarlane J, Hughes RB, Nosek MA, et al. Abuse assessment screen-disability (AAS-D): measuring frequency, type, and perpetrator of abuse toward women with physical disabilities. J Womens Health Gend Based Med. 2001;10:861-6.

24. National Coalition Against Domestic Violence. Open Minds Open Doors: Working With Women With Disabilities Resource Manual. Denver, CO: National Coalition Against Domestic Violence; 1996.

25. Swedlund NP, Nosek MA. An exploratory study on the work of independent living centers to address abuse of women with disabilities. J Rehab. 1996;66:57-64.

# CHAPTER 10

# Substance Abuse

JACQUELINE M. GOLDING, PhD
NANCY D. VOGELTANZ, PhD
SHARON C. WILSNACK, PhD
JANE M. LIEBSCHUTZ, MD, MPH

Substance use and interpersonal violence are frequently associated. Substance use in victims of violence can be a reaction to the violence and a risk factor for experiencing further violence. A perpetrator's use of substances can be a marker for risk of more serious injury or increased violence. There are also similarities between substance abuse and interpersonal violence in terms of clinical presentation and treatment approaches. This chapter will focus on substance use in victims of violence, with a particular emphasis on substance abuse and dependence.

## Definitions

*Substance abuse* is the repeated use of mind-altering substances that have adverse effects on work, school, or family, and that exacerbate legal, social, or interpersonal problems. Substance abuse can also be defined as the recurrent use of substances in physically dangerous situations (e.g., driving while intoxicated). Tolerance, withdrawal, and/or compulsive use of the substance is often considered the hallmark of *substance dependence*, a clinical term denoting a more severe and chronic form of substance abuse.

## Epidemiology

### Prevalence of Substance Abuse

In the general population of women, national estimates of the prevalence of active alcohol abuse or dependence range from 4% to 8% (1-3). Lifetime prevalence of alcohol abuse and dependence is 6.4% and 8.2%, respectively, whereas the prevalence for alcohol abuse and dependence over the past 12 months is 1.6% and 3.7%, respectively. For drug abuse and dependence, the lifetime prevalence is 3.5% and 5.9%, respectively, and the prevalence over the past 12 months is 1.3% and 0.9%, respectively.

Substance abuse is also common in women seeking medical care. In one study of a primary care population, the prevalence of active alcohol abuse or alcohol dependence among women was 9%, with a prevalence of 2% for street drug abuse (4). Extracting from studies of male and female hospitalized patients, the prevalence of active alcohol abuse in women is anywhere from 12% in obstetrics/gynecology patients to 43% in orthopedic patients (5,6).

## Association Between Substance Abuse and Violence

Studies typically examine the association between substance abuse and violence against women from two angles: measuring the prevalence of violence in populations of women with substance abuse and measuring substance abuse disorders in women with histories of experiencing violence. In both cases there appears to be a consistent association between the two.

### Exposure to Violence Among Substance Abusers
In studies of women with substance use problems regardless of the type of substance, the prevalence of abuse is astonishingly high (7-10). For example, among women with substance abuse problems, sexual assault ranged from 35% to 73% (Fig. 10-1) (11-14). In samples of women with alcohol problems,

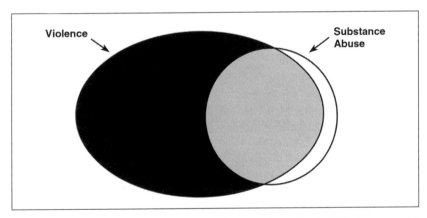

**Figure 10-1**  Overlap between violence and substance abuse. Nearly 90% of women with a history of drug or alcohol abuse have experienced physical or sexual assault. Among women who have been assaulted, the prevalence of alcohol abuse is on average 18.5%.

*Almost all women receiving substance abuse treatment have experienced physical or sexual assault.*

prevalence rates of childhood sexual abuse were 67% to 70% (15). Of women receiving treatment for alcoholism, 87% reported experiencing moderate to severe partner violence (14). Among women seen in drug treatment programs, 60% to 80% had been physically or sexually abused by a male partner (14). Overall, close to 90% of women in alcohol and drug treatment programs have experienced at least one type of physical or sexual assault (7,8,16-19).

### Substance Abuse Among Victims of Violence

In one national survey, 9% of women who had been sexually assaulted at some time in their lives qualified for a lifetime diagnosis of alcohol abuse (20). This rate exceeds the rate of alcohol abuse in the general population (4% to 8%) and the rate for non-assaulted women in the same study (1.5%).

Serious street drug abuse problems also commonly occur in women reporting sexual assault. In Kilpatrick's national study, 3.9% of the women who had been raped developed at least two serious drug abuse problems compared to 0.3% of non-assaulted women in the same study (20). Similarly, in another study, 20% of persons who had been sexually assaulted met criteria for lifetime drug abuse or dependence, compared to 5% of persons who reported no assault (21). A history of rape has also been associated with adverse health behaviors such as sex-for-drugs transactions (22), which further increase the risk for other health problems (e.g., sexually transmitted diseases).

Among women in the general population who report a history of childhood sexual assault, prevalence of alcohol abuse or dependence is remarkably consistent across studies (21% to 22%), as is the abuse of street drugs (14% to 31%) (23-25). Studies of female medical and psychiatric patients also find that alcohol abuse and dependence is highly associated with childhood sexual abuse (26-28). Women reporting childhood sexual assault are more likely than women without such a history to use street drugs (35% vs. 14%; $P < 0.001$) (16,24). Among substance-addicted women, a history of childhood physical abuse is associated with a greater severity of addiction (18).

Date rape commonly occurs in late adolescent and young adult women. This is particularly frequent on college campuses, with 15% to 30% of female students reporting rape by acquaintances, usually fellow students (21,22). The association between sexual assault and alcohol consumption is striking. In one study, approximately half of the college students who were raped reported that they had been drinking alcohol when the assault occurred (29).

Alcohol abuse prevalence is also high among women experiencing intimate partner violence. A meta-analysis of 10 studies found that the average prevalence of alcohol abuse among women battered by intimate partners was 18.5%, with a range of 7% to 44% (30). Women in shelters disclosed a higher prevalence of alcohol abuse than women in other settings (30). Again, these prevalence rates surpass those in general populations; in the four studies that made comparisons to non-abused women, women with a history of intimate partner violence were 5.6 times as likely to abuse alcohol (30). It is thought that the tendency of alcoholic women to have relationships with alcoholic partners may underpin this association (29). However, clinicians should recognize that the alcohol-abusing woman is at increased risk for intimate partner violence, regardless of the causal interpretation.

A meta-analysis of four studies found that street drug abuse among women who had experienced intimate partner violence averaged 9%, with a range of 7% to 25%. Drug abuse was 5.6 times as common among women experiencing intimate partner violence compared with those who did not (30). Among pregnant women, those who misused alcohol or other substances were at higher risk of experiencing intimate partner violence, and violence during pregnancy, which is addressed in Chapter 8, is associated with increased use of alcohol and street drugs during pregnancy (31,32).

## Association Between Violence and Substance Abuse

The question of which is the cause (violence or substance abuse) and which is the effect has been the subject of debate.

### When Substance Abuse Increases the Risk for Experiencing Violence

In some situations, substance abuse may increase the risk for violent victimization because of altered mental state, exposure to potential assailants or societal attitudes about addiction. For example, a national study of college students found that 8% of the women had had unwanted intercourse while impaired from drug or alcohol consumption (22). At one university, 29% of the sexual assaults occurred when the woman could not have consented because she was too incapacitated by alcohol (33). As many as 75% of college men report giving women alcohol or other drugs in an attempt to obtain sex (34). Intoxication may limit a woman's ability to detect (35) or to escape from (34) an assailant. Women who abuse street drugs may sustain more exposure to potential assailants as a result of lifestyles associated with drug use (35). Finally, men's attitudes about women who consume alcohol or other drugs, particularly in dating situations, may increase their propensity to force sex. These attitudes may include seeing such women as "loose" or as more interested in sex (21,22,36). Some men believe that rape is justified if the woman is intoxicated (22). In fact, in one study, female adolescents who had been using drugs or alcohol were only half as likely as their sober counterparts to report that the perpetrator stopped the unwanted sexual activity when requested (37). A double standard exists, at least in college populations, in which women are seen as more responsible for a rape if they were drunk, and men are seen as less responsible (21,38). A similar pattern has been demonstrated for wife abuse (39).

## When Experiencing Violence Increases the Risk for Substance Abuse

Other epidemiological evidence indicates that sexual assault typically precedes the onset of alcohol and drug abuse problems (21,40), suggesting that sexual assault may contribute to the development of substance abuse. One study using a national household sample of 3006 women documented the prevalence of lifetime assaults (physical and sexual) and substance use at baseline and then prospectively measured new assaults and substance use over a 2-year period. At baseline, 11% of the sample had problem substance use and 22% had experienced lifetime assault (14.5% rape and 11% physical assault). Over the next 2 years, 5% of the sample had experienced new assault (1.6% rape and 3.4% physical assault). Analysis revealed that drug use but not alcohol use at baseline was associated with increased risk for new assault, probably because of lifestyle risks associated with drug procurement. A new assault, in turn, was associated with subsequent increase in drug and alcohol use and abuse (35).

## Reciprocal Influences of Substance Abuse and Violent Victimization

We may hypothesize a vicious cycle in which violent victimization and substance abuse each increases the likelihood that the other will occur (35). The combination of the high prevalence of physical and sexual abuse among substance-abusing women and the increased severity of substance abuse among those with victimization histories adds support to this hypothesis (7).

# Post-Traumatic Stress Disorder, Violence, and Substance Abuse

Post-traumatic stress disorder (PTSD) has been examined as a potential mediator of the association between substance abuse and previous experiences of violence in women. A strong epidemiological association links substance abuse disorders with PTSD, with odds ratios ranging from 2.5 to 4.5 (41,42).

Research suggests that women experiencing violence who develop PTSD are at particularly high risk for also developing substance use disorders (43). For example, a national survey found that 20% of women who had been raped and developed PTSD had at least two major substance problems, compared to 4% of women who had been raped but did not have PTSD and 2% of women who had not been raped (20).

Thus, the role of PTSD in the violence-substance abuse association can be seen in at least two ways. First, PTSD represents an adverse psychological response to the trauma, which may be more important than the trauma itself in leading to substance abuse (44). It is widely believed that substance abuse often represents attempts to self-medicate painful feelings about traumatic stress (35), including childhood sexual abuse, rape, and intimate partner violence (15,22,26,45). It has been proposed that substance use may diminish PTSD symptoms such as physiological reactivity to stress, sleep disturbances, behavioral avoidance, emotional distress (44), hyperarousal, and intrusive symptoms (46). Ironically, however, some forms of substance abuse, specifically heavy alcohol use, may worsen PTSD symptoms; for example, sleep disturbances and flashbacks can worsen (44). Also, symptoms of substance use withdrawal can be similar to PTSD symptoms (44). Second, substance use may occur as a way to induce the avoidance that is characteristic of PTSD: dissociation, psychological numbing, or "escape" (46,47).

These conclusions are supported by a study of methadone maintenance clients, which compared substance abuse severity among clients with lifetime trauma, lifetime PTSD, or current PTSD symptoms (7). Current PTSD predicted increased severity of substance abuse. It also predicted other co-morbid psychiatric conditions (depression, anxiety). One resulting hypothesis is that women who have PTSD and are receiving substance abuse treatment may be at increased risk of relapse if the PTSD is not simultaneously addressed.

## Combined Health Risks of Substance Abuse and Violence

The combination of substance abuse and violent victimization is repeatedly associated with worse health indicators and higher rates of health care utilization. As has been pointed out in Chapter 1, studies of women with chronic pain syndromes or somatic symptoms have shown a significant association with histories of physical and sexual abuse, but few of these studies have reported any data on substance use in these subjects (48-56). In one study, women with chronic pelvic pain reported more drug abuse or dependence and more sexual abuse than women in the control group (50). Another study found increased somatic symptoms as well as substance abuse in those with physical or sexual abuse (55). Although neither study specifically examined whether substance abuse mediated the relationship with bodily symptoms and physical and sexual abuse, the consistent findings suggest such a role. Furthermore, chronic pain resulting from abuse-related injuries may impair efforts toward sobriety (14).

Exposure to violence and substance abuse (individually and together) are associated with increased utilization of health care services. For example, one study showed a dose-response relationship between severity of victimization and utilization of outpatient health care but also showed an association between increased utilization and alcohol abuse or other risk-taking behaviors (smoking, overeating, driving without a seatbelt) (57). Another study of women seeking substance abuse treatment found more emergency department visits in the previous 6 months among those with past physical or sexual abuse (75%), despite an already high use among substance abusers without physical or sexual abuse (57%) (10).

*Substance abuse and violent victimization each increase health care utilization.*

## Substance Use Among Perpetrators

Epidemiological data suggest that alcohol abuse and dependence among perpetrators are related to committing violence against women. Several large studies have shown that alcohol abuse has substantial effects on rates of physical abuse of female partners (45,58,59), sexual aggression against dates (60), and rapes in general (59,61). Men screening positive for violent behavior in primary care settings used alcohol more heavily and were more likely to use street drugs than non-violent men (62). The partner's use of drugs was a significant risk factor for more serious injury in a study of intimate partner violence in the emergency department setting (63). However, many batterers who are alcohol or drug abusers exhibit violent behavior when sober (64), and many men who misuse substances do not perpetrate violence against women.

*Most substance-abusing men do not perpetrate violence.*

Conventional wisdom and experimental data indicate that substance use can facilitate or disinhibit aggression, including violence against women (22,38,65). Men who consume alcohol and other psychoactive substances may blame their aggressive behavior on the substance use (21,38), and many may expect others to attribute the aggressive behavior to their intoxication (38).

# Screening

Many of the factors influencing the identification of substance abuse in the clinical setting parallel factors relevant to the identification of a history of interpersonal violence. Like violent victimization, substance abuse can produce social isolation as well as feelings of shame and low self-esteem. Just as women may have difficulty with recognizing certain forms of interpersonal violence, substance abusing women may not realize that they have a problem, particularly with the use of legal substances, such as alcohol or prescription drugs. Furthermore, like some women who have experienced violence, some women with substance use problems may intentionally deny such problems for fear that medical providers will report the information to state child protection agencies. As a result of these factors, medical clinicians may not be aware of the patient's violence exposure or substance abuse.

Because violence and substance use problems affect patients' health, screening for both is an important part of the medical history. Furthermore, if one of the conditions is already known, clinicians must screen for the other condition because of the close relationship between substance use problems and violent victimization. As with the disclosure of violence histories, women with substance use problems will more often answer questions about substance use honestly when asked in a nonjudgmental, confidential, caring manner (45). The key principles of screening include establishing an appropriate setting in which to screen, asking about substance use directly, asking on repeated occasions, and being prepared for follow-up responses. For further information, the reader can refer to Chapter 2 and to other works that directly address substance abuse screening (44,64,66).

In addition to screening for substance use problems in the patient who has experienced violence, asking about the partner's use of substances can help to assess danger risk to the patient. A clinician can ask whether the partner uses alcohol or other drugs, and whether the partner's use of substances plays a role in relationship or episodes of violence.

# Treatment Issues

Treatment of women who have experienced violence is described in detail in Chapters 3 and 5. The reader is referred elsewhere for information about the specific treatment of substance abuse (64,66). Here we address only a few special treatment considerations for patients with histories of violent victimization and substance abuse.

1. It is generally agreed that for the substance abusing patient with violent victimization histories both the substance abuse and the trauma sequelae (e.g., PTSD symptoms) need to be treated, either concurrently or sequentially (44).

2. Providing the patient with information about the fact that many patients turn to substance abuse as a way of self-mediating PTSD symptoms may increase her motivation for modifying exposure to the trauma and substance abuse (44,67).

3. When a patient is being treated for substance abuse, memories of violent victimization or memories that were previously self-medicated by the substance use may resurface (22,46). These memories may lead to depressive episodes and suicidal ideation (22) and may threaten the patient's maintenance of sobriety (25,49). Thus, recognition of these episodes is critical and may help prevent relapse and suicidal attempts.

4. It is important to consider whether to treat the substance abuse or the trauma first, or to treat both concurrently (46). If one or the other condition appears to be more life-threatening, then that is the one to start with.

Because alcohol use suppresses REM sleep, detoxification often causes a REM rebound effect. This may pose particular difficulty for patients with a history of trauma. Specifically, the increased REM sleep may be accompanied by PTSD-related nightmares (44). Thus, alcohol can be discontinued gradually and only after the clinician has prepared the patient for this possibility by providing cognitive-behavioral strategies to manage the potential nightmares (44).

## Physician-Patient Relationship

The physician-patient relationship can play a critical role in the outcome of treatment. The patient may be dually isolated because of the substance abuse and because of her experience of violence. A physician-patient relationship in which the patient feels welcome and cared for and in which she can trust the physician serves as a source of safety. Additionally, a trusting physician-patient relationship probably increases the likelihood that the patient will accept and follow through on referrals. Even when treatment is conducted primarily by mental health and trauma specialists, the medical provider should track the patient's progress, supporting and encouraging her (64). Physicians can counteract the shame and self-blame that are often present by using statements such as, "No matter what, you didn't deserve to be hurt"; "I have seen lots of women like you, who use alcohol [or another drug] to calm bad feelings from [or memories of] having been hurt"; "You are not alone."

## Treatment Programs

Physicians may feel frustrated by the limitations of treatment programs when referring patients with co-occurring trauma and substance abuse. For example, battered women's programs may not have the capacity to house women with active substance abuse problems. Similarly, substance abuse treatment programs may not always address the role of trauma (14). The following material on referral for substance abuse should be considered along with the general principles of making referrals, as outlined in Chapter 4 (e.g., the role of the primary care physician as facilitator, introducing the concept of the referral to the patient).

Despite the seemingly difficult challenges for treating substance abusing and addicted persons, substance abuse treatment does work. For more information on state-of-the-art substance abuse treatment, the reader is referred to the Center for Substance Abuse Treatment, CSAT (www.samhsa.gov/centers/csat/csat.html). In particular, CSAT has developed state-of-the-art practice guidelines for substance abuse and domestic violence and for PTSD and substance abuse. They are available on the CSAT Web site. Finding appropriate referral programs can be facilitated with a substance abuse specialist. Most states and some local governments have publicly funded substance abuse programs that might provide references to such treatment sites. These government programs can be generally located in the government pages in the phone book. Additional options are programs listed under alcohol treatment or drug treatment in the Yellow Pages of the telephone book. The telephone numbers and Web site addresses of Alcoholics Anonymous and Narcotics Anonymous are given in the Appendix.

Substance abuse treatment may include 12-step groups. The social support offered by these groups can contribute importantly to establishing safety during the first phase of treatment (46). For women who have been victimized, a women-only group (such as a women-only Alcoholics Anonymous group, or a Women for Sobriety group) may be preferable (66). Such organizations are particularly important for women who have recently experienced intimate partner violence and who fear that the abuser may be present at meetings that include women and men. The safety of 12-step groups relates to their maintenance of confidentiality and anonymity and to their didactic focus (46). The flexibility of their structure also allows members to decide from moment to moment how intense they wish their experience with the group to be (46). Twelve-step groups can be found in almost any community in the United States and abroad. A contact number for 12-step groups is usually listed in the local phone book and should be called for answers to questions about specific groups.

A cautionary note is prudent because self-help groups can sometimes be exploitative or oppressive (46). In addition, the emphasis on confrontation in Alcoholics Anonymous may be antithetical to the needs of women who feel stigmatized and helpless, both of which are common feelings for women who have also been sexually abused or beaten by partners (66). Likewise, the emphasis on powerlessness, surrender, and humility in Alcoholics Anonymous was meant to reduce the narcissism thought to be common among alcoholic men, which contrasts with the helplessness and low self-esteem that are more common among women who have experienced violence. Thus, it is strongly recommended that women who have experienced violence incorporate from these groups only material that is useful to them individually and discard the rest (46). Physicians may find it helpful in some cases to warn patients about these possibilities when making referrals to Alcoholics Anonymous. Patients who experience Alcoholics Anonymous groups as limited in their helpfulness for these reasons may feel appropriately validated when the physician has discussed these issues. Physicians may also wish to consider offering referrals to alternative self-help organizations. This strategy may be helpful not only in helping patients to locate the most effective self-help setting for their individual needs but also in empowering patients who have been abused to experience self-determination in making choices about their own treatment.

## Summary

Violence against women and associated substance abuse are common health problems and are related to each other in complex ways. The successful management of both requires a thoughtful and coordinated approach by physicians. Physicians can play a key role in coordinating an overall treatment plan, recognizing risks or problems that may jeopardize or delay treatment and modifying the overall treatment plan. When physicians successfully fulfill these roles, the patient's chances of permanent well-being can be optimized.

**REFERENCES**

1. Grant BF, Harford TC, Dawson DA, et al. Epidemiologic Bulletin No. 35. Prevalence of DSM-IV Alcohol Abuse and Dependence: United States, 1992. Alcohol Health and Research World. 1994;18:243-8.

2. Helzer JE, Burnam A, McEvoy LT. Alcohol abuse and dependence. In: Robins LN, Regier DA, eds. Psychiatric Disorders in America: The Epidemiologic Catchment Area Study. New York: Free Press; 1991:81-115.

3. Kessler RC, McGonagle KA, Zhao S, et al. Lifetime and 12-month prevalence of DSM-III-R psychiatric disorders in the United States: results from the National Comorbidity Study. Arch Gen Psychiatry. 1994;51:8-19.

4. Manwell LB, Fleming M, Johnson K, Barry K. Tobacco, alcohol, and drug use in a primary care sample: 90-day prevalence and associated factors. J Addictive Dis. 1998;17:67-81.

5. Bush B, Shaw S, Cleary P, et al. Screening for alcohol abuse using the CAGE questionnaire. Am J Med. 1987;82:231-5.

6. Umbricht-Schneiter A, Santora P, Moore RD. Alcohol abuse: comparison of two methods for assessing its prevalence and associated morbidity in hospitalized patients. Am J Med. 1991;91:110-8.

7. Clark HW, Masson CL, Delucchi KL, et al. Violent traumatic events and drug abuse severity. J Subst Abuse Treat. 2001;20:121-7.

8. Gil-Rivas V, Fiorentine R, Anglin MD, Taylor E. Sexual and physical abuse: do they compromise drug treatment outcomes? J Subst Abuse Treat. 1997;14:351-8.

9. Hien D, Scheier J. Trauma and short-term outcome for women in detoxification. J Subst Abuse Treat. 1996;13:227-31.

10. Liebschutz JM, Mulvey KP, Samet JH. Victimization among substance abusing women: worse health outcomes. Arch Intern Med. 1997;157:1093-7.

11. Dansky BS, Saladin ME, Brady KT, et al. Prevalence of victimization and posttraumatic stress disorder among women with substance use disorders: comparison of telephone and in-person assessment samples. Int J Addict. 1995;30:1079-99.

12. Edwall GE, Hoffman NG, Harrison PA. Psychological correlates of sexual abuse in adolescent girls in chemical dependency treatment. Adolescence. 1989;94:279-88.

13. Deykin EY, Buka SL. Suicidal ideation and attempts among chemically dependent adolescents. Am J Public Health. 1994;84:634-9.

14. Miller BA, Wilsnack SC, Cunradi CB. Family violence and victimization: treatment issues for women with alcohol problems. Alcohol Clin Exp Res. 2000;24:1287-97.

15. Miller BA, Downs WR. Violent victimization among women with alcohol problems. In: Galanter M, ed. Recent Developments in Alcoholism, vol 12. Alcoholism and Women. New York: Plenum; 1995: 81-101.

16. Bennett EM, Kember KJ. Is abuse during childhood a risk factor for developing substance abuse probems as an adult? Dev Behav Pediatr. 1994;15:426-9.

17. Liebschutz JM, Mulvey KP, Samet JH. Victimization among substance abusing women: worse health outcomes. Arch Intern Med. 1997;157:1093-7.

18. Westermeyer J, Wahnamholm K, Thuras P. Effects of childhood physical abuse on course and severity of substance abuse. Am J Addictions. 2001;10:101-10.

19. Young A, Boyd C. Sexual trauma, substance abuse, and treatment success in a sample of African American women who smoke crack cocaine. Substance Abuse. 2000;21:9-19.

20. Kilpatrick D, Edmunds CN, Seymour A. (National Victim Center). Rape in America: A Report to the Nation. 23 April 1992.

21. Beckman LJ, Ackerman KT. Women, alcohol, and sexuality. In: Galanter M, ed. Recent Developments in Alcoholism, volume 12. Alcoholism and Women. New York: Plenum; 1995: 269-85.

22. Koss M, Gidycx C, Wisniewski N. The scope of rape: incidence and prevalence of sexual aggression and victimization in a national sample of higher education students. J Consult Clin Psychol. 1987;55:162.

23. Peters SD. Child sexual abuse and later psychological problems. In: Wyatt GE, Powell GJ, eds. Lasting Effects of Child Sexual Abuse. Newbury Park, CA: Sage Press; 1988: 101-17.

24. Wilsnack SC, Vogeltanz ND, Klassen AD, Harris TR. Childhood sexual abuse and women's substance abuse: national survey findings. J Studies Alcohol. 1997;58:264-71.

25. Stein JA, Golding JM, Siegal JM, et al. Long-term psychological sequelae of child sexual abuse. The Los Angeles Epidmiologic Catchment Area Study. In: Wyatt GE, Powell GJ, eds. Lasting Effects of Child Sexual Abuse. Newbury Park, CA: Sage Press; 1988: 135-54.

26. Salter AC. Transforming Trauma: A Guide to Understanding and Treating Adult Survivors of Child Sexual Abuse. Thousand Oaks, CA: Sage Press; 1995.

27. Wilsnack SC, Wilsnack RW. Drinking and problem drinking in US women: patterns and recent trends. In: Galanter M, ed. Recent Developments in Alcoholism, volume 12. Alcoholism and Women. New York: Plenum; 1995: 30-60.

28. Fleming J, Mullen PE, Sibthorpe B, et al. The relationship between childhood sexual abuse and alcohol abuse in women: a case-control study. Addiction. 1998;93:1787-98.

29. Crowell N, Burgess A. Understanding Violence Against Women. Washingston, DC: National Academy Press; 1996.

30. Golding JM. Intimate partner violence as a risk factor for mental disorders: a meta-analysis. J Fam Violence. 1994;14:99-132.

31. Campbell JC, Poland ML, Waller JB, Ager J. Correlates of battering during pregnancy. Res Nurs Health. 1992;15:219-26.

32. Amaro H, Fried LE, Cabral H, Zuckerman B. Violence during pregnancy and substance use. Am J Public Health. 1990;80:575-9.

33. Meilman PW, Haygood-Jackson D. Data on sexual assault from the first two years of a comprehensive campus prevention program. J Am Coll Health. 1996;44:157-65.

34. Muehlenhard CL, Schrag JL. Nonviolent sexual coercion. In: Parrot A, Bechofer L, eds. Acquaintance Rape: The Hidden Crime. New York: Wiley; 1991, pp. 115-128.

35. Kilpatrick D, Acierno R, Resnick H, Saunders B. A 2-year longitudinal analysis of the relationship between violent assault and substance use in women. J Consult Clin Psychol. 1997;65:834-47.

36. George W, Cue K, Lopez P, et al. Self-reported alcohol expectancies and postdrinking sexual inferences about women. J Appl Soc Psychol. 1995;25:164-86.

37. Rhynard J, Krebs M, Glover J. Sexual assault in dating relationships. J School Health. 1997;67:89-93.

38. Richardson DR, Hammock GS. Alcohol and acquaintance rape. In: Parrot A, Bechofer L, eds. Acquaintance Rape: The Hidden Crime. New York: Wiley; 1991: 83-95.

39. Richardson DC, Campbell JL. Alcohol and wife abuse: the effect of alcohol on attributions of blame for wife abuse. Personality and Social Psychology Bulletin. 1980;6:51-6.

40. Winfield I, George LK, Swartz M, Blazer DG. Sexual assault and psychiatric disorders among a community sample of women. Am J Psychiatry. 1990;147:335-41.

41. Breslau N, Davis GC, Andreski P, Peterson E. Traumatic events and posttraumatic stress disorder in an urban population of young adults. Arch Gen Psychiatry. 1991;48:216-22.

42. Kessler RC, Sonnega A, Bromet E, et al. Posttraumatic stress disorder in the National Comorbidity Survey. Arch Gen Psychiatry. 1995;52:1048-60.

43. Epstein JN, Saunders BE, Kilpatrick D, Resnick H. PTSD as a mediator between childhood rape and alcohol use in adult women. Child Abuse Neglect. 1998;22:223-34.

44. Stewart SH. Alcohol abuse in individuals exposed to trauma: a critical review. Psychol Bulletin. 1996;120:83-112.

45. Galbraith S, Rubinstein G. Alcohol, drugs, and domestic violence: confronting barriers to changing practice and policy. J Am Med Womens Assoc. 1996;51:115-7.

46. Herman J. Trauma and Recovery. New York: Basic Books; 1992.

47. Briere J. Post sexual abuse trauma: data and implications for clinical practice. J Interpersonal Violence. 1987;2:367-79.

48. Drossman DA, Leserman J, Nachman G, et al. Sexual and physical abuse in women with functional or organic gastrointestinal disorders. Ann Intern Med. 1990;113:828-33.

49. Drossman DA, Talley NJ, Leserman J, et al. Sexual and physical abuse and gastrointestinal illness: review and recommendations. Ann Intern Med. 1995;123:782-94.

50. Harrop-Griffiths J, Katon W, Walker E, et al. The association between chronic pelvic pain, psychiatric diagnoses, and childhood sexual abuse. Obstet Gynecol. 1988;71:589-93.

51. Domino JV, Haber JD. Prior physical and sexual abuse in women with chronic headache: clinical correlates. Headache. 1987;27:310-4.

52. Schei B. Psycho-social factors in pelvic pain: a controlled study of women living in physically abusive relationships. Acta Obstet Gynecol Scand. 1990;69:67-71.

53. Rapkin AJ, Kames LD, Darke LL, et al. History of physical and sexual abuse in women with chronic pelvic pain. Obstet Gynecol. 1990;76:92-5.

54. Reiter RC, Shakerin LR, Gambone JC, Milburn AK. Correlation between sexual abuse and somatization in women with somatic and nonsomatic chronic pelvic pain. Am J Obstet Gynecol. 1991;165:104-9.

55. McCauley J, Kern D, Kolodner K, et al. Relation of low-severity violence to women's health. J Gen Inter Med. 1998;13:687-91.

56. Frayne SM, Skinner KM, Sullivan LM, et al. Medical profile of women Veterans Administration outpatients who report a history of sexual assault occurring while in the military. J Womens Health. 1999;8:835-45.

57. Koss MP, Koss PG, Woodruff WJ. Deleterious effects of criminal victimization on women's health and medical utilization. Arch Inter Med. 1991;151:342-7.

58. Kaufman Kantor G, Straus MA. The "drunken bum" theory of wife beating. Soc Prob. 1987;34:213-28.

59. Greenfeld L. Bureau of Justice Statistics, Office of Justice Programs, U.S. Department of Justice. Alcohol and Crime: An Analysis of National Data on the Prevalence of Alcohol Involvement in Crime. Report NCJ-16832; 1998.

60. Koss MP, Gaines JA. The prediction of sexual aggression by alcohol use, athletic participation, and fraternity affiliation. J Interpersonal Violence. 1993;8:94-108.

61. Bachman R. Bureau of Justice Statistics, Office of Justice Programs, U.S. Department of Justice. Violence Against Women: A National Crime Victimization Survey Report. Report NCJ-145325; 1994.

62. Oriel KA, Fleming MF. Screening men for partner violence in a primary care setting: a new strategy for detecting domestic violence. J Fam Pract. 1998;46:493-8.

63. Kyriacou DN, Anglin D, Taliaferro E, et al. Risk factors for injury to women from domestic violence against women. N Engl J Med. 1999;341:1892-8.

64. Burge S, Graham T. Violence and substance abuse. In: Hendricks-Matthews M, ed. Violence Education: Toward a Solution. Kansas City, MO: Society of Teachers of Family Medicine; 1992:155-62.

65. Fromme K, Wendel J. Beliefs about the effects of alcohol on involvement in coercive and consenting sexual activities. J Appl Soc Psychol. 1995;25:2099-117.

66. Volgetanz ND, Wilsnack SC. Alcohol problems in women: risk factors, consequences, and treatment strategies. In: Gallant SJ, Keita G, Royak-Schaler R, eds. Health Care for Women: Psychological, Social, and Behavioral Influences. Washington, DC: American Psychological Association; 1997:75-96.

67. Wajivits LM. Clinicians' views on treating post-traumatic stress disorder and substance abuse disorder. J Subst Abuse Treat. 2002;22:79-85.

# CHAPTER 11

# Immigrants, Refugees, and Survivors of Torture

BEATRICE H. PATSALIDES, PhD

ALEJANDRO MORENO, MD, MPH

JANE M. LIEBSCHUTZ, MD, MPH

The main objective of this chapter is to explore health issues in immigrant women refugees and survivors of torture. The following are reviewed: definitions and the risk factors that make women more susceptible to violence and human rights abuses during uprooting and resettlement; the health effects of violence and human rights abuses on women refugees and survivors of torture; and the clinical approach and treatment considerations for this patient population.

## Definitions and Epidemiology

*Immigrants* are people who live in a country other than their country of origin. They may have chosen to emigrate from their country of origin for economic, educational, or personal reasons. A significant number of immigrants, however, are forced to leave their countries, as in the case of refugees and asylum seekers.

*Refugees* are immigrants who are without adequate protection from persecution based on race, religion, nationality, political opinion, or membership in a particular social group. Both U.S. and international law make a distinction between *refugee* and *asylum seeker*. Refugees enter their host country with the status of refugee, whereas asylum seekers apply for asylum status after entering the host county. Asylum seekers may need medical and/or psychological documentation to support their legal case. The criteria for asylum vary according to the laws of each country but are based on well-founded fear of persecution (1,2).

*Torture survivors* are a subset of refugees and asylum seekers who have been physically or psychologically abused because of their race, religion, nationality, political views, or social associations. Human rights abuses include violations of right to life, liberty, freedom of speech, access to health care, basic public health services, and education. Persecution and torture are just two of the human rights abuses that refugees and asylees may have suffered.

Immigrants and refugees may also be victims of more classic domestic violence relationships, which can be more severe while living in their host country because of increased isolation from the native population, language barriers, cultural differences, and a lack of understanding of the host country's legal system. Fear of deportation from the host country and dependence on a perpetrator of violence for legal residency can further intensify an immigrant woman's helplessness in an abusive relationship.

*Domestic violence among immigrants and refugees can be very severe.*

According to Amnesty International, the number of refugees worldwide has increased to more than 15 million, of which 5% to 35% are survivors of torture (3). In this context, torture includes the deliberate, systematic, or unprovoked infliction of physical or mental suffering by an authority for any reason, including yielding information or confessing a crime. More than 3 million refugees and asylum seekers have resettled in the United States alone during the past 25 years (4). Many refugees and asylum seekers fleeing their homes are not able to reach the safety of a host country and are forced to live in a different region of their country of origin or in refugee camps. Conditions in refugee camps are often substandard, which may exacerbate morbidity, including infectious disease and malnutrition.

Refugees in general have a higher morbidity and mortality compared to other groups of immigrants. Measles, diarrhea, and malnutrition are the leading causes of illness and death (5). Some mental health problems such as posttraumatic stress disorder (PTSD) and depression are also prevalent in this population. For instance, the prevalence of PTSD among survivors of torture can be 70% (6). Surprisingly, significant numbers of refugees and survivors of torture do not develop psychological sequelae. Factors that appear to protect against psychological trauma include mental preparedness, single exposure to traumatic events, support networks, and commitment to a cause, among others (7).

## Women as Refugees and Survivors of Torture

Women and their children comprise more than 75% of the total number of refugees (8), and women are particularly susceptible to violence during uprooting and resettlement. Among the factors that place immigrant women at an increased risk of violence are the breakdown of social protections, discrimination, and social isolation. Depending on the individual immigrant woman, language barriers, poverty, cultural beliefs, and caring for children and elders may also increase vulnerability to violence.

Women refugees endure many forms of violence and torture (Box 11-1), and they are primary targets for sexual violence. Although women are detained and tortured as often as men, they are sexually assaulted approximately twice as often as men (9). Sexual violence is one of the most common forms of torture reported by women refugees. For instance, during the years when a military junta ruled Argentina (March 1976 to December 1983, the "Dirty War"), pregnant women were detained, tortured, and, after delivery of their babies, their newborns were taken away by their perpetrators.

*Refugee women are particularly susceptible to sexual violence.*

Although systematic rape of women was designated as a war crime by the United Nations Commission on Human Rights during the conflict in the Balkans (10,11), only a small percentage of women have admitted to their rape experiences. This may be because of cultural taboos or shame at the individual, family, or community level: in some cultures, for example, rape is considered worse than death.

---

**Box 11-1    Common Types of Torture**

- Asphyxiation: wet, dry, and chemical
- Blunt trauma: whipping, beatings, crushing injuries
- Burns: chemical and thermal (cold and heat)
- Electric shocks
- Extreme physical conditions: forced body positions (prolonged constraint), heat/cold conditions
- Forced human experimentation
- Mental torture: threats, mock execution, solitary confinement, sensory deprivation
- Penetrating injuries: gunshots, stab wounds, slash cuts
- Sexual torture: sexual humiliation, trauma to genitalia, rape
- Suspension
- Traumatic removal of tissue and appendages by avulsion and explosion

Adapted from Moreno A, Grodin MA, Schadt RW, Isasi RM. Caring for Refugees and Survivors of Torture: An Introductory Internet-Based Course. (http://dcc2.bumc.bu.edu/refugees/signs.htm)

# Symptoms and Conditions Found in Women Immigrants, Refugees, and Survivors of Torture

Immigrants, refugees, and survivors of torture can suffer four types of medical problems.

1. Genetic conditions related to the ethnic compositions in the region.

2. Problems associated with political and socioeconomic conditions of a country and its geographical localization (such as intestinal parasites in countries with poor aqueducts and sewage systems).

3. Problems stemming from political and socio-economic conditions of a country that are worsened by the process of uprooting or torture, such as the extensive malnutrition in Somalia after the outbreak of civil war in 1991 (12).

4. Conditions directly related to the process of uprooting and torture. This category can be further divided into mental health (e.g., PTSD, depression) and physical health (e.g., amputations, limb deformities, and head injury).

Although symptoms and specific sequelae in survivors of torture are numerous and beyond the scope of this chapter, the reader may refer to other literature for detailed information (13-15). Combined physical violence and psychological abuse has been shown to cause the greatest number and severity of symptoms in women (16), and permanent physical marks appear to be associated with additional mental health symptoms (17).

## Mental Health Sequelae

Prolonged persecution, detention, and torture may cause (in addition to the well-known symptoms of depression, anxiety, and PTSD) changes in the personality and styles of relating to others that have been described as "complex PTSD" (18) (see Chapter 5 for a detailed discussion of PTSD and complex PTSD). Most torture survivors suffer from a combination of

*Somatic symptoms may represent psychological problems related to torture.*

psychological symptoms that can include disturbed sleep patterns, nightmares, anxiety, depression, memory defects, loss of concentration, dissociative states, and symptoms of hyperarousal alternating with psychic numbing. Prolonged and severe traumatic life circumstances can cause a state of ongoing fear or terror. These symptoms may be further accompanied by changes in the persecution/torture survivor's sense of identity and ability to relate to others (18,19).

Somatization is common among refugees and torture survivors. Somatic symptoms can be a concrete and culturally acceptable way to express psychic pain. The symptoms most frequently take the form of tension headaches, shortness of breath, palpitations, gastrointestinal disturbances, and chronic abdominal, back, or pelvic pain. It must be remembered that these symptoms may represent underlying physical changes related to torture and may not just be a venue to express psychic pain. Of course, psychological and physical trauma are often intertwined, thus complicating the evaluation of symptoms. Conversion disorders, including functional blindness, are found more commonly among female refugees and torture survivors (20,21).

When immigrants or refugees present with non-specific symptoms or are labeled as "somatizers," health care professionals should explore whether these physical and psychological symptoms can be understood within their cultural meaning. A bio-medical model is insufficient to describe culture-related symptoms such as "koro" (*Malaysian:* intense fear that the vagina and nipples will recede into the body and cause death) or "susto" (*Latin American:* an illness attributed to a frightening event that causes the soul to leave the body and results in unhappiness and sickness). Recognizing the subjective meaning of symptoms is thus important to treatment interventions.

## Physical Health Sequelae

Although many of the injuries commonly sustained in acute domestic violence episodes (see Chapter 3) also apply to torture victims, some injuries are particularly important in the context of torture. For example, in some countries in Africa, the Middle East, and the Far East, women are subjected to female genital mutilation (22). According to cultural tradition in these countries, some women and girls may undergo a second and more radical "circumcision" if they are raped. Side effects of the operation include hemorrhage, shock, painful scars, keloid formation, labial adherences, clitoral cysts, chronic urinary infection, and chronic pelvic infections. Later in life, it can cause kidney stones, sterility, sexual dysfunction, depression, and various gynecological and obstetric problems (22). Breast mutilation is also found in parts of Eastern Africa to prevent women from breast feeding.

Fecal incontinence is found among survivors of torture who have suffered sodomy. Damage to the shoulder girdles is associated with certain types of prolonged suspension. Blunt trauma and gunshot wounds can cause a number of deformities and injuries. Amputation and other unusual injuries may result from being tied or restrained by tight ropes or being confined for long periods of time in a small space.

Although torture often results in obvious physical damage, health professionals should remember that physical signs of torture are not the rule. Most physical marks resulting from torture are subtle and require detailed physical examination to detect (17). Not all physical marks in immigrants and refugees represent torture: some may be the results of various cultural practices. For example, the Southeast Asian practice of coining (scraping warm coins on the back) leaves echymoses that may appear to be the result of physical abuse. Asking the patient about what seem to be unusual markings can clarify the circumstances that led to the physical deformities and help the physician determine whether torture or other physical abuse has occurred.

## Evaluation and Interview Considerations

A comprehensive medical and psychological evaluation of immigrants and refugees should include the following: medical and mental health history; current symptoms; physical and psychological functioning; trauma history, including previous psychological trauma and assessment of current safety; and a social history, including life before uprooting and torture and family separation and reunification (7,23,24). In addition, clinicians should update vaccinations and screen for tuberculosis, hepatitis, intestinal parasites, syphilis, anemia, lead poisoning, and HIV, and conduct nutritional and dental assessments (5,7).

Some somatic problems of nonphysical origin may require an awareness of culture-specific syndromes and native language idioms of distress through which symptoms are communicated. Ideally, clinicians should familiarize themselves with cultural materials and basic rules of cross-cultural communication relevant to the countries from which their patients originate. Because it is not realistic that detailed cultural information will always be available in all situations, clinicians should remain sensitive to the possibility that reported symptoms may represent a culture-specific syndrome in a particular patient or patient population. It is always best to ask the patient herself what she thinks is causing the symptoms: she may elucidate an underlying culture-specific syndrome unknown to the clinician. As noted below, interpreters may also be helpful in explaining culture-specific entities.

### Specific Interview Considerations

During the process of resettlement, immigrants and refugees are often interviewed and evaluated by multiple health care providers, as well as legal and allied health professionals. In addition to the specific screening techniques recommended in Chapter 2, there are other interview necessities unique to refugees and survivors of torture (25). The most important of these are for clinicians to overcome language and cultural barriers and to create a safe environment for the patients. Although most American-born women view medical care as a safe, unbiased source of support, refugee women may view medical personnel as potential perpetrators of abuse. This view arises from the fact that in many refugees' countries of origin most health professionals are government employees and may be the people who administer torture or who collaborate in the cover up of government-sponsored or government-administered torture. Health care personnel in the host country who are trying to help these refugees may consequently represent a dangerous figure of authority, thereby triggering a sense of terror in the refugees, despite the good intentions of the host country clinicians. Additionally, patients may fear that providers will report information to the immigration agency of the host country and should be told specifically that the clinician will not give information about them to the INS without their consent.

*Clinicians should assure patients that INS will not receive shared information.*

The interviewer should employ specific tactics to minimize the risk of re-traumatization (Box 11-2). At the beginning of the interview, the clinician should identify himself or herself to the patient, explain the purpose of the interview, and outline the rules and limitations regarding confidentiality, especially if an interpreter is present (26). The clinician should conduct the interview gently and tactfully, avoid rapid questioning (which may resemble an interrogation), and should give a sense of control to the patient by allowing him or her to stop the interview at any time or to decline answering any question he or she finds uncomfortable. Clinicians need to be sensitive and empathetic in their questioning while remaining objective in their clinical assessment and aware of their own potential emotional reactions to the patient's trauma

---

**Box 11-2    Interviewing Considerations**

- Acknowledge that disclosure is difficult
- Do not make the patient wait for long periods
- Educate the patient about symptoms and correct misperceptions
- Arrange examinations rooms to be as unlike cells as possible and provide comfortable climate conditions
- Explain who you are, what your role is, and how the interview will work
- Give patients a sense of control
- Do not hide objects behind screens
- Ask questions gently and tactfully

Adapted from Weinstein H, Dansky L, Iacopino V. Torture and war trauma survivors in primary care practice. West J Med. 1996;165:112-8.

that might distort their perceptions and judgments. Finally, the setting should not engender a feeling of confinement for the patient, particularly in patients who were previously detained by authorities in their country of origin or in their host country (26).

Despite all precautions, psychological and medical assessments may retraumatize the patient, eliciting painful memories and provoking or exacerbating symptoms of PTSD by bringing the traumatic event again into the present. Therefore, it is important for the clinician to express respectful awareness of how difficult disclosure may be and to offer mental health referral and other sources of support as necessary (see Chapter 4) (27).

## Use of Interpreters

Using interpreters with immigrants, refugees, and survivors of torture may hinder or help aspects of history taking, evaluation, and treatment. The interpreter may be a professional interpreter, a relative of the patient, or a fellow national. Clinicians should know the advantages and disadvantages of using each kind of interpreter. Professional interpreters have specific training in technical medical terms and have been trained to protect confidentiality, a feature not found in lay persons who interpret (24,27). Frequently, the professional interpreter has a good understanding of the cultural background of the patient and may be able to explain various cultural concepts specific to the patient's background. Unfortunately, professional interpreters may be expensive and difficult to find. In some instances, professional interpreters know the language but not the culture of a particular patient or patient group (for example, a Puerto Rican interpreter for a Guatemalan patient). If a professional interpreter is unavailable, phone interpreter services are commercially available.

When a professional interpreter is not available, relatives may be needed to interpret for patients. Patients may be reluctant to disclose parts of their trauma history, particularly sexual assault, in order to spare their relatives from unnecessary suffering or to avoid humiliation. Relatives are also more likely to change the patient's history, perhaps because they are too familiar with it or are ashamed of it (24,27). It is also possible that a relative serving as interpreter is a perpetrator of violence, so it may be necessary to avoid asking detailed trauma history questions until an appropriate interpreter is found. Fellow nationals interpreting for a patient may serve as bicultural experts for the clinician, but they must be chosen carefully in consideration of possible conflicts with a refugee's ethnicity, political affiliation, tribal membership, or religion.

Regardless of an interpreter's training, he or she must be sensitized to the task and trained to provide an accurate and a precise translation of the patient's words and an explanation of any nonverbal communications by the patient (Boxes 11-3 and 11-4). He or she must also be made aware of the

---

**Box 11-3    Instructions to Interpreters**

- Avoid drawing attention to yourself
- Correct any mistake as soon as noted, informing the patient and the clinician
- Interpret word by word without summarizing or expanding
- Keep the confidentiality of the patient
- Speak loud and use a clear voice
- Request clarification if a statement was not clear, informing the patient and the clinician that you want to clarify something

Adapted from Moreno A, Grodin MA, Schadt RW, Isasi RM. Caring for Refugees and Survivors of Torture: An Introductory Internet-Based Course. (http://dcc2.bumc.bu.edu/refugees/signs.htm)

---

**Box 11-4    Rules for the Clinician When Using an Interpreter**

- Ask for clarification if the interpreter and the patient have a long discussion and the answer to the questions is a short answer such as a monosyllable
- Avoid long statements or questions
- Use a professional interpreter whenever possible
- Give enough time to the interpreter to translate the question to the patient and to translate the patient's answer
- Stop the interview if confidentiality cannot be ensured
- Keep eye contact with the patient and not the interpreter
- Pay attention to body language and expression while the patient and interpreter are speaking (e.g., do not write in the chart while they are speaking)

Adapted from Moreno A, Grodin MA, Schadt RW, Isasi RM. Caring for Refugees and Survivors of Torture: An Introductory Internet-Based Course. (http://dcc2.bumc.bu.edu/refugees/signs.htm)

---

potentially traumatic content of the interview and given opportunity to debrief with the clinician after the session. Female interpreters have been recognized as essential for the establishment of trust with women refugees and survivors of torture (21,24). Additionally, because of taboos surrounding women's sexuality and feelings of shame and anxiety, women refugees and survivors of torture should be given the choice of also having a female health care provider.

## Treatment

The principles of treatment of survivors of violence outlined in previous chapters apply in the cases of refugees and survivors of torture, but some aspects of treatment, such as physical examination, medication, invasive procedures, and psychiatric evaluation, require more emphasis because of cultural or language barriers common to immigrants and refugees.

The medical clinician must perform an adequate history and physical examination, order diagnostic tests, and treat illness. However, these tasks may be more complicated with refugees and survivors of torture. Patients may not reveal their complete history, permit a full examination, or agree to diagnostic testing. In that case, working with them over time may clarify symptoms or findings. Patients may be skeptical about medications with psychoactive side effects, such as analgesics or tranquilizers, because they may have been drugged as part of their torture. The clinician should take great care to describe side effects of any prescription medication and allow the patients to negotiate the use of medication. Invasive procedures, such as endoscopy, surgery, or colposcopy, may trigger flashbacks of previous physical torture, so the patient needs to be well informed about the details of any invasive procedure and given the option to decline.

Although many immigrants, refugees, and torture survivors need psychiatric services, they may refuse referral because of a stigma associated with psychiatric care. The primary care clinician's clinical sensitivity is of the utmost importance in this situation. Certainly, referrals to social workers, legal counselors, psychotherapists, or psychiatrists should be established according to a hierarchy of needs, addressing the most urgent problems first (see Chapter 4).

*Psychiatric services may be refused because of cultural stigma.*

The patient may require occupational referrals to help get basic needs met, such as safety, legal status, housing, food, and employment. Social workers working for resettlement agencies such as Catholic Charities and the International Rescue Committee can help with housing, employment, and English training. Some of these agencies also provide legal assistance. If an asylum applicant needs a medical-psychological evaluation, the asylum network coordinator at Physicians for Human Rights may help to locate a health professional trained to administer such an evaluation. These agencies can be found in the local phone books or on the Internet.

Documentation of the physical findings and the patient's history is important. If the patient is an asylum applicant, consistent wording of their physical condition and history is necessary for use during court cases. Sometimes patients will request that the trauma history not be recorded in the medical record for fear of a fellow countryman getting the information and hurting others in the country of origin. In those cases, it is helpful to explain to the patient the confidentiality of the medical record. If the patient still does not want the information recorded, it would be appropriate to write, "Trauma

History: kept confidential." The principles of documentation as outlined in Chapter 3 apply here as well. Health professionals should conduct thorough physical examinations, describing the location (with a diagram), size, and characteristics of all lesions (24). Mental health status should also be clearly documented.

## Summary

Immigrant women who are refugees and survivors of torture have experienced a variety of physical and psychological traumas. Psychological sequelae of torture include anxiety, PTSD, and somatization, whereas physical consequences can range from fecal incontinence and head injuries to more immediately apparent injuries such as amputation and mutilation. Although torture can result in obvious injury, it is important for the clinician to remember that most physical marks are subtle and require detailed examination to uncover. For refugee women, violence may occur not only in their native countries but even after immigration because of a breakdown of social protections, discrimination, and social isolation. Furthermore, these women may also experience the more classic domestic violence, which may be more severe because of factors such as lack of understanding of the legal system. Clinicians caring for such patients should be alert to the importance of establishing trust by overcoming language and cultural barriers and by working to create a safe clinical environment for the patient.

## REFERENCES

1. United Nations General Assembly. Declaration on Territorial Asylum Resolution 2312 (XXII) of 14 December 1967. Vol. 2000; 1967.

2. Physicians for Human Rights. Medical testimony on victims of torture: a physicians guide to political asylum cases. 1991.

3. Refugees-Human Rights Have No Borders. New York: Amnesty International; 1997.

4. United States Department of Justice, Immigration and Naturalization Service. 1997 Statistical Yearbook of the INS. Washington, DC: U.S. Government Printing Office; 1999.

5. Ackerman L. Health problems of refugees. J Am Board Fam Pract. 1997;10:337-48.

6. McNally R. Psychopathology of post-traumatic stress disorder: boundaries of the syndrome. In: Basoglu M, ed. Torture and Its Consequences: Current Treatment Approaches. Cambridge: Cambridge University Press; 1992.

7. Piwowarczyk L, Moreno A, Grodin M. Health care of torture survivors. JAMA. 2000;284:539-41.

8. Allotey P. Travelling with "excess baggage": health problems of refugee women in Western Australia. Womens Health. 1998;28:63-81.

9. Allodi F, Stiasny S. Women as torture victims. Can J Psychiatry. 1990;35:144-8.

10. Rape and Abuse of Women in the Territory of the Former Yugoslavia. United Nations Document E/CN.4/1993/L.21. Geneva; 1993.

11. Swiss S, Giller J. Rape as a crime of war: a medical perspective. JAMA. 1993;270:612-5.

12. Howarth J, Healing T, Banatvala N. Health care in disaster and refugee settings. Lancet. 1997;349:14sIII-17sIII.

13. Somnier F, Vesti P, Kastrup M, Genefke I. Psychosocial consequences of torture: current knowledge and evidence. In: Basoglu M, ed. Torture and Its Consequences: Current Treatment Approaches. Cambridge: Cambridge University Press; 1992: 56-68.

14. Skylv G. The physical sequelae of torture. In: Basoglu M, ed. Torture and Its Consequences: Current Treatment Approaches. Cambridge: Cambridge University Press; 1992:35-53.

15. Rasmussen O. Medical aspects of torture. Danish Med Bull. 1990;37:1-88.

16. Fornazzari X, Freire M. Women as victims of torture. Acta Psychiatr Scand. 1990;82: 258-60.

17. Moreno A, Grodin M. The not-so-silent marks of torture. JAMA. 2000;284:538.

18. Herman J. Complex PTSD: a syndrome in survivors of prolonged and repeated trauma. J Trauma Stress. 1992;5:377-91.

19. Bojholm S, Foldspand A, Juhler M, et al. Monitoring the health and rehabilitation of torture survivors. Rehabilitation and Research Center for Torture Survivors; 1992.

20. Arcel TL. Multidisciplinary approach to refugee women and their families. In: Arcel L, Folnegovic-Smalc V, Kozaric-Kovacic D, Marusic A, eds. Psycho-Social Help for War Victims: Women Refugees and Their Families. Copenhagen: International Rehabilitation Council for Torture Victims; 1995:23-62.

21. VanBoemel G, Rozee P. Treatment for psychosomatic blindness among Cambodian refugee women. Women Therapy. 1992;13:239-66.

22. Affairs AMAoS. Female genital mutilation. JAMA. 1995;274:1714-6.

23. Kinzie J. Evaluation and psychotherapy of Indochinese refugee patients. Am J Psychother. 1981;35:251-61.

24. Iacopino V, Ozkalipici O, Schlar C, et al. Manual on the Effective Investigation and Documentation of Torture and Other Cruel, Inhuman or Degrading Treatment or Punishment. The Istanbul Protocol, www.unhchr.ch/html/menu6/2/training.htm.

25. Laws A, Patsalides B. Medical and psychological examination of women seeking asylum: documentation of human rights abuses. J Am Med Womens Assoc. 1997;52:185-7.

26. Weinstein H, Dansky L, Iacopino V. Torture and war trauma survivors in primary care practice. West J Med. 1996;165:112-8.

27. Randall G, Lutz E. Approach to the Patient: Serving Survivors of Torture. American Association for the Advancement of Science; 1991:55-70.

# CHAPTER 12

# Lesbians and Same-Sex Relationships

KIMBERLY J. CLERMONT, MD

A lthough violence against lesbians is in many ways similar to violence against heterosexual women, unique issues pertain to the type of violence experienced by lesbians and their response to it. Lesbians are at risk for not only intimate partner violence but also hate crimes. This chapter will familiarize the clinician with violence issues specific to lesbians and offer strategies for caring for lesbians who have experienced violence.

## Definitions

### Homosexuality and Sexual Identity

What is a lesbian? The terms *lesbian* and *female homosexual* describe a sexual behavior pattern and a sexual identity. *Sexual behavior* is the specific action of a woman engaging in sexual activity with another woman. *Sexual identity* is the woman's sense of emotional-erotic attraction to other women.

Sexual identity and sexual behavior are not interchangeable, although they may overlap within an individual person in the form of sexual orientation. *Sexual orientation* is a collage of physical behavior and sexual attraction and is unique for every individual. Thus, a woman who engages in sexual activity with another woman may or may not self-identify as homosexual or lesbian. A woman who self-identifies as homosexual or lesbian may or may not engage in sexual activity with women. Either group of women may engage in sexual activity with men for a variety of reasons. Experts agree that sexual identity and the awareness of sexuality are formed well before any actual sexual activity occurs (1). The absence or presence of sexual activity does not negate or create sexual identity. In Alfred Kinsey's 1953 investigation of 1749 women, he found that of the 159 (8.6%) women who disclosed any same-sex orientation, many were neither exclusively heterosexual nor homosexual throughout their lives. Kinsey described a range of human sexual expression, from sexual attraction to behavior directed towards the opposite sex (heterosexuality), to both sexes (bisexuality) and the same sex (homosexuality) (Fig. 12-1) (2-4). For this chapter, we will use the term *lesbian* to include women who have sex with women and women with the lesbian sexual identity.

## Homophobia and Heterosexism

*Homophobia,* an unreasonable fear or disdain for homosexuals and/or homosexuality (5), may be expressed by acts such as social avoidance, verbal abuse, and discrimination. Such expressions of homophobia in American culture stigmatize lesbians by implying they are inferior, pathological, and immoral. Homophobia can be communicated through the media, school systems, community organizations, places of worship, and frequently lesbians' families of origin (6). At its most exteme, homophobia is expressed by physical violence, including rape, and even murder.

> *At its most extreme, homophobia is expressed by physical violence, including rape and murder.*

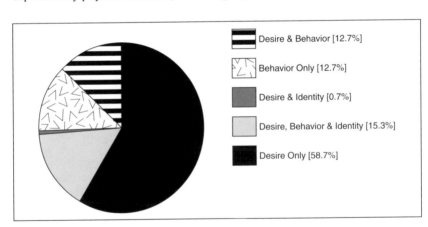

**Figure 12-1**   Sexual orientation. Interrelation of the different dimension of same-sex orientation (current desire, current or past same-sex behavior, current identity as homosexual or bisexual) for 159 women (8.6% of total 1749) who report any adult same-gender orientation. (From Laumann E, Gagnon J, Michael R, Michael S. The Social Organization of Sexuality: Sexual Practices in the United States. Chicago: University of Chicago Press; 1994; with permission.)

*Heterosexism* is the assumption that heterosexuality is the only form of sexual identity and family life (7). Although less stigmatizing than overt homophobia, the assumption of heterosexuality can alienate lesbians in mainstream institutions, including health care settings. A 1995 study using in-depth interviews and focus groups documented the effect of heterosexism in health care and how it adversely affected therapeutic communication and treatment (8). For example, "Are you married?," a question commonly found on intake questionnaires, implies heterosexuality. The corresponding neutral question, "Do you have a significant other, spouse, or partner?" does not assume any particular sexual orientation and is thus more welcoming to homosexuals (9,10).

*Coming out* is the acknowledgement of one's lesbian or gay identity to oneself and to the public (11). Coming out can involve considerable personal risk and pain. Risks may include loss of employment, discharge from the military (12), loss of housing, lost custody of children, direct physical violence (13), stigma, verbal abuse, physical abuse(14), or the loss of the love and support of one's family of origin.There are times that individual lesbians have reported tolerating abusive behavior by others in the hope of avoiding being "outed."

## Epidemiology of Violence Against Homosexuals

### Violence Associated with Hate Crimes

Despite the fact that crime rates are falling nationwide, attacks on lesbians and gays are increasing in number and severity, especially since the identification of AIDS with homosexuality in the mid-1980s (15,16). Gays and lesbians are the fourth highest targeted group for hate crimes (Table 12-1) (17). The 14 national tracking programs of the National Coalition of Anti-Violence Programs (NCAVP), a coalition of organizations serving lesbian, gay, bisexual, transgendered, and HIV-positive persons (LGBTH) who are victims of violence,

**Table 12-1  Hate Crimes Against Target Groups (FBI 2001 statistics)**

| Category | Percent of All Reported 2001 Hate Crimes ($n = 9730$) |
|---|---|
| Race | 45 |
| Ethnicity or national origin | 22 |
| Religion | 19 |
| Sexual orientation | 14 |
| Disability | 0.4 |

documented an overall increase of 2% in bias crimes committed against the LGBTH community nationally in 1999 (Table 12-2). Another study of 1420 homosexual men and 654 homosexual women conducted by the National Gay and Lesbian Task Force found that 19% of respondents reported physical abuse because of their sexual orientation (18).

Historically, a correlation between increased visibility for the lesbian and gay community and increased reports of anti-lesbian and gay incidents exists. For example, anti-lesbian and gay violence is most prevalent during June when communities are celebrating Gay Pride Month. Anti-lesbian and gay incidents are also more frequent in cities and areas of higher lesbian and gay visibility or population. Most attacks occur in areas frequented by lesbian and gay persons (e.g., outside lesbian or gay bars and at Pride marches). Although there are fewer reports of anti-lesbian violence in rural areas, this may be the result of lesbians keeping low profiles and having decreased visibility. Lesbians perceive that rural areas are a higher risk for anti-lesbian violence. Thus in smaller, less lesbian-friendly communities, lesbians frequently adjust their behavior to conceal their sexual identity. Finally, being a lesbian is not a prerequisite for being a victim of anti-lesbian or gay violence, because some victims of such violence identify as heterosexual. Violence may occur because of the attacker's assumptions about sexual identity.

For a number of reasons, the lesbian community perceives that legal and law enforcement professionals often are not sensitive to the issue of anti-lesbian violence. The number of victims refusing to report anti-lesbian and gay incidents to the police increased 21% in 1997. There is a perception that law enforcement professionals can actually perpetrate such crimes. For example, 1997 statistics document an 87% rise in reported anti-LGBTH violence occurring in police precincts and jails. Currently, 49 states and the District of Columbia (DC) have passed some form of hate-crime statute, the exception being Wyoming, and 21 states and DC have hate-crime laws that include crimes based on sexual orientation. Ten states and DC have laws banning discrimination on the basis of sexual orientation (19,20).

## Table 12-2    Hate Crimes Based on Sexual Orientation, 1995–2001

|  | 1995 | 1996 | 1997 | 1998 | 1999 | 2000 | 2001 |
|---|---|---|---|---|---|---|---|
| Total number of hate crime incidents reported | 7947 | 8759 | 8149 | 7755 | 7876 | 8063 | 9730 |
| Hate crimes based on sexual orientation | 1019 | 1016 | 1102 | 1241 | 1339 | 1290 | 1362 |
| Percentage of hate crimes based on sexual orientation | 13 | 12 | 14 | 16 | 17 | 16 | 14 |

Data from National Coalition of Anti-Violence Programs, 2002.

The number of participating agencies reporting hate-crime statistics to the FBI increased from 2771 in 1991 to 11,355 in 1996, representing a 410% increase in reporting of hate crimes by law enforcement agencies under the 1990 Hate-Crimes Statistics Acts. There are 16,000 agencies that regularly report other crime data to the FBI under the Bureau's Uniform Crime Reporting Program (17).

## Same-Sex Intimate Partner Violence

Intimate partner violence in lesbian relationships historically has not been widely acknowledged because of the focus on male perpetration of violence. There are some published studies of the prevalence of same-sex partner violence, although all suffer significant methodological errors. According to these studies, it appears that verbal and physical abuse occurs as frequently in lesbian relationships as it does in heterosexual relationships (21). The National Violence Against Women Survey found that 39% of same-sex cohabiting women experience physical or sexual abuse by a partner at some point in their lives, compared with 20% of opposite-sex cohabitating women (22). Women living with women were still more likely, however, to report men as a perpetrator of intimate partner violence (27% male vs. 11% female perpetrators) (22).

*Intimate partner violence occurs as often in lesbian relationships as in heterosexual relationships.*

Research on heterosexual and lesbian victims of intimate partner violence shows striking similarities with regard to the pattern and perception of intimate partner violence. However, important differences exist between heterosexual and same-sex intimate partner violence (Box 12-1). In addition to the usual forms of physical, verbal, and psychological abuse, the batterer in a lesbian relationship may also threaten to or actually "out" their partner. Lesbians may find it difficult to be believed by health care providers, law enforcement, family, or others. People who express homophobic attitudes may tell lesbian victims they are being battered because they are lesbians (23). Box 12-2 lists some common myths about intimate partner violence in same-sex relationships.

## Sexual Assault

The results from the National Violence Against Women Survey, sponsored by the CDC and National Institute of Justice, revealed that compared to opposite-sex cohabitating women, same-sex cohabitating women were much more likely to have been forcibly raped as a minor (16.5 vs. 8.7%) and as an adult

---

**Box 12-1    How Lesbian Domestic Violence Differs From Heterosexual Domestic Violence**

---

- Absence of family/friend/community support.
- Sexual identity is blamed for the abuse.
- Denial that intimate partner violence exists in lesbians.
- Increased isolation for victims of lesbian domestic violence.
- Fewer appropriate support services.
- Utilizing services may require "coming out."
- The victim is likely to have the same support system as the batterer.
- Domestic violence reinforces the stereotype that the lesbian community is sick or abnormal.
- The survivor may know few or no lesbian persons.
- The batterer can use blackmail to hold the victim in the relationship by threatening to "out" her to the community-at-large.
- The batterer can "pass" (pretend to be heterosexual) and access services and shelters in the heterosexual community.
- The victim may fear losing her children or never seeing them again because courts do not recognize parental rights of a non-biological parent; she may also fear being declared unfit as a biological parent because of sexual orientation.

---

Adapted from Nickel R. Training Materials. Hidden Violence: Domestic Abuse in the Lesbian/Gay/ Transgendered/Bisexual Community.

---

(25.3 vs. 10.3%) (22). About half of the perpetrators were reported to be intimate partners, mostly male partners. Thus, health care providers must have a higher suspicion for history of lifetime sexual assault among their lesbian patients.

## Self-Directed Violence

In the 1994 National Lesbian Health Study, more than 50% of respondents had suicidal ideation and 18% had attempted suicide at some time in their lives (24). Among LGBTH youth, the rates of attempted suicide and suicide ideation are even higher (25). Data from the Youth Risk Behavior Survey concluded that the combined effect of LGB status and high levels of at-school victimization was associated with the highest levels of health risk behavior, including higher levels of substance abuse, suicidality, and sexual risk behavior than heterosexual peers reporting high levels of at-school victimization. LGB youth with low levels of at-school victimization reported levels of health risk comparable to those of heterosexual peers with low at-school victimization (26).

---

**Box 12-2    Myths About Same-Sex Intimate Partner Violence**

- It never happens.
- Women are cat fighting.
- Women are not batterers.
- The level of violence in woman-to-woman abuse is not severe.
- The larger, butch, manly partner is always the batterer.
- Lesbians can leave the relationship easily.
- Children are never an issue.
- One can always recognize a batterer.
- All lesbians are white.
- Same-sex domestic violence only occurs between people of color.
- People in same-sex relationships will automatically disclose their sexual orientation.
- It is easy for lesbians and gay men to get support from the community at large and/or the LGBTH community.
- The reasons lesbians and gay men batter are different than the reasons heterosexual men batter.
- Sadism and masochism is the same thing as domestic violence.
- Lesbians cannot rape each other.

---

## Access to Community Services

Most women's shelters or domestic violence services are focused on heterosexual intimate partner violence. Lesbians may perceive these institutions to be unwelcoming to non-heterosexual women. Also, many sheltering programs have specific rules about barring men, but not women, from the premises. Lesbian-friendly victim services are more plentiful in larger, urban communities and are lacking in smaller, less urban communities.

Going to a medical facility for care related to the abuse entails the risk of disclosure of sexual orientation as the victim fully discloses abuse in a same-sex relationship. The victim may be in a position in which she she needs to choose between getting help or disclosing her sexual orientation to her larger community. To further complicate matters, within the lesbian community the victim and the perpetrator may have the same support network. Such lesbian communities may be reluctant to "choose sides" and may end up giving no assistance at all to either party. Consequently, the victim may feel that she cannot find safety in the largely heterosexual community or in the lesbian community.

*Lesbians are less likely to seek medical care for injuries resulting from intimate partner violence.*

Some resources do exist, however. The 12 member organizations of the NCAVP Domestic Violence Program perform outreach and support for lesbians who have experienced violence. These organizations cover communities that total less than 20% of the nation's total population. Some lesbian communities provide an array of crucial services, including women's centers, women's health services, and hotline services (27). Resources and contact information can be found in the Appendix.

## Provider-Patient Relationship

Establishing trust with a clinician is particularly challenging for many lesbian patients because certain clinician attitudes and beliefs could interfere with clinicians' ability to interact effectively with lesbian patients. This has been substantiated in a number of studies. In a 1987 questionnaire, for example, significant numbers of faculty in a Midwestern nursing school endorsed the belief that lesbianism was a disease (17%), immoral (23%), disgusting (34%), and unnatural (52%) (28). In a 1986 survey of California physicians, 31.4% scored "severely homophobic." This homophobia was directed towards colleagues and potential patients. For example, 31% would deny admission of a highly qualified lesbian or gay applicant to medical school, 40% would stop referring to a colleague found to be lesbian or gay, and 25% would stop using a lesbian or gay surgeon or radiation oncologist. Among obstetric and gynecological physicians, half would not refer to a lesbian or gay pediatrician or psychiatrist. More than 30% of obstetric and gynecological, family practice, and internal medicine providers reported significant hostility towards lesbian and gay patients. Another 40% felt "somewhat uncomfortable" treating lesbian or gay patients (29).

More recently, members of the American Association of Physicians for Human Rights (now known as the Gay and Lesbian Medical Association), an organization of LGBT physicians, medical students, and their supporters, were surveyed. It was found that 52% of the respondents observed professional colleagues denying care or providing reduced or substandard care to LGBTH patients, and 88% heard colleagues make derogatory comments directed towards LGBTH patients. Almost all respondents (98%) felt patients should disclose their sexual orientation to the provider, but 64% believed that patients who did so risked receiving substandard care. Additionally, 17% of survey respondents reported being refused medical privileges, employment, educational opportunities, and referrals from other physicians because of their sexual orientation. One-third of homosexual physicians in practice and 50% of homosexual medical students reported verbal harassment, social ostracism, or insults from medical colleagues (30).

These issues are not unique to the United States. Three Canadian studies—of gay and lesbian physicians in training (31), a national study of general internists and internal medicine residents (32), and a national study of psychiatric and family practice residents and psychiatric faculty (33)—produced similar results of homophobia, feelings of an unsafe environment, and other professional challenges to the gay and lesbian physician.

There are little hard data about lesbian survivors of violence and interactions with health care providers. Based on studies of lesbian health care seeking behavior and anecdotal information, it appears that lesbians are at risk for suboptimal care for violence. Detection is doubly hindered by the lack of interactions with health care providers and general assumptions about heterosexuality among providers. Failure to detect same-sex domestic violence may lead to inappropriate referrals, incomplete use of available resources, and the inability to properly ensure the safety of the lesbian who has experienced same-sex violence.

## Special Considerations

### Adolescents and Young Adults

Developing a fully integrated and positive adult identity is a primary task of adolescents. This task may challenge many lesbian adolescents, who learn from earliest childhood the stigma of a homosexual identity. Such adolescents must frequently negotiate important developmental milestones without the usual emotional support and positive reinforcement or feedback from their families of origin, religious organizations, schools, and peer groups (34). The social and emotional isolation of lesbian adolescents is profound. It is a unique stressor, increasing their vulnerability and risk for a range of medical and mental health problems. Adult lesbian organizations and support groups typically offer little support to lesbian adolescents because they fear the accusation of "recruiting" or exerting "unnatural" influences upon the adolescents. Use of the Internet appears to ease some of the isolation because the lesbian adolescent may be able to come out or explore in a supportive electronic community. However, although the Internet does offer a virtual community of peers, it may also expose the adolescent to sexual predators.

Many gay and lesbian youths report being verbally, physically, or sexually abused and assaulted by family members and peers (35). Data from the National Survey of Midlife Development in the United States (MIDUS) point to adult minority sexual orientation as a risk indicator for history of parental maltreatment during childhood and suggests that gender atypicality may be a causal factor (36). Gay and lesbian youths may additionally find themselves the victims of anti-LGBTH violence. In studies conducted in nine cities and three eastern states, 33% to 50% of lesbian and gay junior and senior high school participants reported being victimized because of their sexual orientation (35). A review of anti-gay violence on college campuses revealed that 55% to 72% of lesbians and gay males sampled reported verbal or physical abuse; 64% of the abusers were peers; and 23% were faculty, staff, and administrators (35). Among lesbian and gay students surveyed at Yale University, more than 42% had been physically abused, and nearly 1 in 5 had been assaulted two or more times because of their sexual orientation (37). The lesbian adolescent or young adult who is a victim of abuse may find it difficult to confront or report abuse within the home or in school for fear of another anti-lesbian reprisal.

Nearly half of all rape victims are adolescents (38). In one study, 50% of lesbians aged 17 to 24 reported rape or sexual assault compared with 27.7% of college women (39). Among college students, 30.6% of lesbians reported being victims of sexual assault compared with 17.8% of heterosexual women (40). Such high rates of lifetime exposure to trauma contribute to the complexity of violence in the lesbian community.

## Lesbians of Color

Sexuality holds different meanings within each cultural and ethnic group. Lesbians of color or of different cultural backgrounds face not only discrimination based on sexual orientation but also racism. Unlike racial stereotypes that may be positively re-framed by the family and ethnic community, negative cultural perceptions of homosexuality are usually reinforced. Within ethnic communities, as in the mainstream community, homophobia is generally high (41). Ethnic lesbians often receive little support from their families of origin and are asked to choose between identities. When seeking support and acceptance from the mainstream lesbian community, they may encounter racism, misunderstanding, devaluation, and other discrimination based on race and ethnicity. Among racial and ethnic minority women, minority sexual orientation seems to be an independent risk factor for increased health risk and lower rates of preventative care (42).

## Transgendered Persons

The term *transgendered* covers a broad range of gender-nonconforming identities and behaviors, including *transsexuals* (people who identify themselves as belonging to the sex opposite their external genital type; they may be preoperative [seeking surgical reassignment], postoperative [having completed surgical reassignment], and nonoperative [living as the opposite sex without surgery]); *transvestites or cross-dressers* (people who wear the clothing of the opposite sex for social or erotic reasons); and *male or female impersonators* (people who perform entertainment acts imitating persons of the opposite sex). Transgendered people may be heterosexual, homosexual, bisexual, or asexual. They have existed throughout history in a variety of cultures (43).

In modern Western society, however, transgendered persons experience more ridicule than homosexual people do. Transgendered people are frequently targeted for verbal and physical abuse. Although the majority are heterosexual, anyone exhibiting gender-atypical behavior is usually considered to be homosexual. Transgendered persons gravitate towards the LGB community because gender norms and roles are more inclusive. Transgendered people face significant discrimination in employment, housing, and access to health care, and they fear abuse, ridicule, refusal of care, and abandonment by physicians and other providers upon the discovery of their atypical gender choices. They sometimes choose to lie about their gender just to obtain emergency treatment. Consequently, transgendered persons usually receive no genital-related health care and no follow-up or continuity of care that requires more in-depth patient disclosure.

## Suggestions to Help Uncover Abuse

There are many ways that providers can improve care for lesbians who have experienced abuse. Most of the suggestions below include specific behaviors intended to make the non-heterosexual patient feel more comfortable, a prerequisite to uncovering abuse and offering appropriate help for abuse.

- Ask gender-neutral questions about intimate partners: "Do you have a spouse or partner?" as opposed to "Are you married?"

- Revise intake forms and documents to be more inclusive by adding "cohabitant," "domestic partnership," or "significant other" to "single, married, divorced, widowed."

- When taking a sexual history, use questions that do not assume exclusive heterosexuality: "Are you sexually active? If so, are you sexually active with men, women, or both?"

- Remind yourself that all women of childbearing age can be pregnant regardless of their sexual orientation.

- Address transgendered patients by the pronoun and/or name of their choice.

- When asking about abuse, do not assume the gender of the perpetrator.

- Interview all women alone when asking about intimate partner violence. Again, do not assume that a female friend of the patient is not the perpetrator.

- As in heterosexual intimate partner violence, an over-attentive same-sex partner may be a red flag for abuse.

- Be aware of community services or shelters that cater to LGBTH clientele. Have this information available when discussing referrals. See the Appendix for resources.

- Maintain confidentiality about abuse and sexual orientation. Despite disclosing her sexual orientation in the patient-provider relationship, a patient may not be comfortable publicly disclosing this in other aspects of her life. Confidentiality includes avoiding unnecessary disclosure to, among others, consultants, family members, co-workers, and employers.

## REFERENCES

1. Savin-Williams R. Gay and lesbian adolescents. In: Bozett FW, Sussman MB, eds. Homosexuality and Family Relations. Binghamton, NY: Harrington Park Press; 1990.

2. Kinsey A, Pomeroy W, Martin C. Sexual Behavior in the Human Male. Philadelphia: WB Saunders; 1948.

3. Kinsey A, Pomeroy W, Martin C, Gebard P. Sexual Behavior of the Human Female Philadelphia: WB Saunders; 1953.

4. Bidwell R. Sexual orientation and gender identity. In: Friedman S, Fisher M, Schonberg S, eds. Comprehensive Adolescent Health Care. St. Louis: Quality Medical Publishing; 1992.

5. Weinberg G. Society and the Healthy Homosexual. New York: St. Martin's Press; 1972.

6. Slater S. The Lesbian Family Cycle. New York: Free Press; 1995.

7. Neison J. Heterosexism: redefining homophobia for the 1990's. J Gay Lesbian Psychology. 1990.

8. Stevens P. Structural and interpersonal impact of heterosexual assumptions on lesbian health care clients. Nurs Res. 1995;44:25-30.

9. Bradford J, Ryan C. The National Lesbian Health Care Survey: Final Report. National Lesbian & Gay Health Foundation; 1988.

10. Smith E, Johnson S, Guenther S. Health care attitudes and experiences during gynecologic care among lesbians and bisexuals. Am J Public Health. 1985;75:1085-7.

11. de Monteflores C, Schulz S. Coming out: similarities and differences for lesbians and gay men. J Soc Issues. 1978;34.

12. Servicemembers Legal Defense Network. The Fourth Annual Report on "Don't Ask, Don't Tell, Don't Pursue." 19 February 1998.

13. Comstock G. Violence Against Lesbians and Gay Men. New York: Columbia University Press; 1991.

14. Savin-Williams R. Verbal and physical abuse as stressors in the lives of lesbians, gay male and bisexual youths: associations with school problems, running away, substance abuse, prostitution and suicide. Special Section: Mental Health of Lesbians and Gay Men. J Counsel Clin Psychol. 1994;62:261-9.

15. Herek G. Hate Crimes: Confronting Violence Against Lesbians and Gay Men. Newbury Park, CA: Sage Publications; 1992.

16. Cooper M. Reports of anti-gay crimes increase by 81%. New York Times. 18 September 1998.

17. FBI Uniform Crime Reports, 2001.

18. Berrill K. Anti-gay violence and victimization in the United States: an overview. J Interpersonal Violence. 1990;5:274-94.

19. Force NGaLT. GLBT Civil Rights Laws in the United States; 1999.

20. Force NGLT. The Right to Privacy in the United States; 1999.

21. Burke L, Follingstad D. Violence in lesbian and gay relationships: theory, prevalence and correlational factors. Clin Psychol Rev. 1999;19:487-512.

22. Tjaden P, Thoennes N, Allison C. Comparing violence over the life span in samples of same-sex and opposite-sex cohabitants. Violence Victims. 1999;14:413-25.

23. Laumann E, Gagnon J, Michael R, Michaels S. The Social Organization of Sexuality: Sexual Practices in the United States. Chicago: University of Chicago Press; 1994.

24. Bradford J, Ryan C, Rothblum E. National Lesbian Health Care Survey: Implications for Mental Health Care. J Consult Clin Psychol. 1994;62:213-20.

25. Muehrer P. Suicide and sexual orientation: a critical summary of recent research and directions for future research. Suicide Life Threatening Behav. 1995;25:72-81.

26. Bontempo DE, D'Augelli AR. Effects of at-school victimization and sexual orientation on lesbian, gay, or bisexual youths' health risk behavior. J Adolesc Health. 2002;30:364-74.

27. Lockard D. The lesbian community: an anthropological approach. J Homosex. 1986;11: 83-95.

28. Randall C. Lesbian phobia among BSN educators: a survey. J Nurse Ed. 1989;28:302.

29. Matthews W, Booth M, Turner J. Physician attitudes towards homosexuality: survey of a California county medical society. West J Med. 1986;144:106.

30. Schatz B, O'Hanlan J. Anti-gay Discrimination in Medicine: Results of a National Survey of Lesbian, Gay & Bisexual Physicians. The Gay & Lesbian Medical Association; 1994.

31. Risdon C, Cook D, Wilms D. Gay and lesbian physicians in training: a qualitative study. Can Med Assoc J. 2000;162:331-4.

32. Cook DJ, Griffith LE, Cohen M, et al. Discrimination and abuse experienced by general internists in Canada. J Gen Intern Med. 1995;10:565-72.

33. Chaimowitz GA. Homophobia among psychiatric residents, family practice residents, and psychiatric faculty. Can J Psychiatry. 1991;36:206-9.

34. Martin A, Hetrick E. The stigmatization of gay and lesbian adolescents. J Homosex. 1988;15:163.

35. Pilkington N, D'Augelli A. Victimization of lesbian, gay and bisexual youth in community settings. J Comm Psychol. 1995;23.

36. Corliss HL, Cochran SD, Mays VM. Reports of parental maltreatment during childhood in a United States population based survey of homosexual, bisexual, and heterosexual adults. Child Abuse Negl. 2002;26:1165-78.

37. Herek G. Documenting prejudice against lesbians and gay men on campus. The Yale Sexual Orientation Study. J Homosex. 1993;25:18.

38. American Association of Pediatrics. Rape and the adolescent. Pediatrics. 1993;92:631.

39. Koss M, Gidyxc C, Wisniewski N. The scope of rape: incidence and prevalence of sexual aggression and victimization in a national sample of higher education students. J Consult Clin Psychol. 1987;55:162.

40. Duncan D. Prevalence of sexual assault victimization among heterosexual and gay/lesbian university students. Psychology. 1990;66:65.

41. Feinberg L. Trans Liberation: Beyond Pink or Blue. Boston: Beacon Press; 1998.

42. Mays VM, Yancey AK, Cochran SD, et al. Heterogeneity of health disparities among African American, Hispanic, and Asian American women: unrecognized influences of sexual orientation. Am J Public Health. 2002;92:632-9.

43. Bullogh V. Transsexualism in history. Arch Sex Behav. 1975;4:561.

# Clinical Vignettes

# VIGNETTE 1

# Boundary Issues in the Management of Patients with Previous Victimization

Marian I. Butterfield, MD, MPH
Susan M. Frayne, MD, MPH

RW is a 40-year-old woman who presents to an internist, Dr. P, as a new patient. RW arrives 30 minutes late for her 4 p.m. appointment. On meeting the physician, RW thanks Dr. P for seeing her at the end of a busy day. She tells Dr. P that she is a hospital administrator and a mother, and asks whether Dr. P has children, how old they are, and if she has a picture of them. Dr. P discloses that she is a mother of two, and she identifies with how challenging it must be for RW to balance her personal and professional life. RW compliments Dr. P on her excellent reputation and inquires if the internist's husband is supportive of her career. Dr. P replies that indeed her husband is supportive, and then redirects RW to describe her current health problem.

RW's chief complaints include fatigue and a swollen lump on her neck. Ever since a family vacation 4 weeks ago, she has been having myalgias and low energy. RW's presentation is also remarkable for tearfulness, insomnia, poor concentration, anxiety, hopelessness, a 10-lb weight loss, and passive suicidality during this same time period. RW denies a history of domestic violence or sexual trauma. The physical examination is remarkable for unilateral cervical adenopathy that is only mildly tender to palpation. Laboratory data reveal a mild normocytic anemia. Dr. P is concerned that RW could have a lymphoma.

To expedite the evaluation, Dr. P pages her otolaryngology colleague for a consult. On hearing of the situation, and personally knowing the individual involved, the otolaryngologist agrees to see RW at 7:30 p.m. for an office consult. A biopsy is performed; throughout the procedure RW cries quietly. RW is told that she will be called when the biopsy results clarify the diagnosis. The following morning RW pages Dr. P to see if the preliminary pathology report is back on the biopsy. She calls the clinic two more times that morning with similar inquiries. Serologic tests and biopsy results confirm a diagnosis of cat scratch disease, which the physician treats with azithromycin.

When RW is being scheduled for follow-up, she requestes a 4:30 p.m. appointment to accommodate her work schedule. RW arrives at 5:00 p.m. for the appointment, just as the clinic staff is locking the office. Dr. P agrees to see her. RW is tearful throughout the clinic visit. Although she says that her neck swelling has resolved, she speaks of how difficult the lymph node biopsy was for her. Her mood symptoms, low energy, and tearfulness have not resolved. Saying that she was not entirely honest in her first visit, RW reveals that she was a victim of incest by her father. Dr. P queries, "When did this happen to you?" and RW gives a detailed description of abuse that occurred after her sixth birthday party. She states that she has never discussed this with anyone. In addition, she says that her father held her neck during their sexual contacts and that the cervical lymph node biopsy procedure felt much the same. RW comments that during her family vacation her daughter had her sixth birthday and that this brought back her own incest memories. Dr. P is empathetic while listening to RW's narrative.

Dr. P realizes that it is 6:15 p.m. and that she is now late in picking up her own daughter, who, like RW's daughter, is 6 years old. Dr. P tells RW that she is running late and explains that her daughter is having behavioral difficulties in school, making her particularly reliant upon consistency in her pick-up time. At this point, RW becomes more unraveled and discusses her intermittent suicidal urges, which have increased since her daughter's birthday. RW states, "I wish I could disappear. I am having urges to drive my car off the road. I won't, but I wish I could." Dr. P suspects major depression and recommends psychiatric consultation to initiate antidepressant therapy. Dr. P has a listing of psychiatrists in the community, but RW is reluctant to accept the referral and pleads with Dr. P to treat her, saying that she has come highly recommended as the "best" in the community. She does not want to see another doctor and tell her story again to someone new, and she fears the stigma of seeing a psychiatrist. RW assures Dr. P that she will take the antidepressant and come regularly for follow-up. Reluctantly, Dr. P agrees to forego a psychiatric consultation.

After carefully assessing suicidal risk and assuring herself that RW is able to contract for safety, Dr. P initiates a sertraline trial. RW agrees to call the office in the morning for a follow-up appointment. RW does not call the following day and cannot be reached by the clinic. That same day a sterling pen set is delivered to Dr. P from RW with a note that reads, "Thanks for your time." Dr. P hears nothing from RW the rest of that week. RW finally calls 5 days later saying that she forgot to call before but wants to schedule follow-up with Dr. P. She requests a clinic appointment that Friday afternoon because of work conflicts. Although the internist does not usually see patients on Friday afternoons, she reluctantly agrees because of concerns about RW and the need to solidify a follow-up plan.

## Discussion

Several clinical questions are raised by this vignette:

- What are the boundaries of the patient-provider relationship?
- What is a boundary violation?
- How can a clinician know when a boundary violation has occurred?
- What harm is done to the patient, the provider, and the patient-provider relationship when a boundary violation occurs ?
- What should the clinician do when the patient or the clinician him/herself violates a boundary?

### Overview of Boundaries in Patient Care

This case illustrates several common ways boundary issues can arise when working with survivors of trauma. Readers may have felt uneasy as RW asked questions about Dr. P's children and sent an expensive gift or as Dr. P extended herself to accommodate RW's schedule and additionally agreed to forego a psychiatric consultation. At the same time, readers may be unsure whether any of these represented true boundary violations. The patient-provider relationship is a complex human interaction in which the clinician must balance caring and empathy on the one hand with professional distance and respect on the other. Physicians must understand and maintain professional boundaries to decrease the risk of unintentionally harming their patients.

### Definitions

What, then, are boundaries? "Boundaries define the expected and accepted psychological and social distance between physicians and their patients" (1). Although "clinicians tend to feel that they understand the concept of boundaries instinctively" (2), it is actually difficult to clearly define the perimeter of these boundaries (1). Many patient actions (such as seeking a prolonged visit, asking personal questions of the physician, and gift giving) and physician actions (such as self-disclosure or providing care outside the physician's scope of practice) constitute *potential* boundary violations. They become *actual* boundary violations when the psychological and social distance between patient and provider are narrowed in such a way that the patient is harmed. Sexual boundary violations are clearly prohibited: the AMA Council on Ethical and Judicial affairs states, "Sexual contact or romantic relationships concurrent with the physician-patient relationship are unethical" (3).

Many types of boundary crossing are more ambiguous, however: there is generally a lack of objective rules for what constitutes a definite boundary violation. For example, agreeing to see a patient after normal business hours may be appropriate in some cases but may constitute a boundary violation in others. Although there is a need for considerable clinical discretion in deciding what the psychological and social distance should be with a particular patient, the patient's needs, rather than the clinician's, must come first.

## Why Boundary Violations Occur

Boundary crossings are especially common in interactions between patients with a history of childhood trauma and their health care providers and pose a particular risk of harm to patients with a trauma history. An individual's ability to establish healthy interpersonal boundaries is shaped, in large part, by early life experiences. Adults with a childhood history of physical or sexual victimization have not had healthy boundaries modeled. Pathological patterns of interpersonal interaction (including pathological feelings of attachment to and dependency upon the perpetrator [4]) are thus learned and reinforced. These behaviors can persist into adulthood.

Pathological behaviors may become amplified in the setting of a medical encounter (5). This is because the patient-provider interaction can mirror certain aspects of the child-perpetrator interaction. In both situations, there is a substantial power differential and the expectation of a fiduciary relationship. In both situations the relationship is intimate, involving the sharing of secrets as well as forms of physical contact not acceptable in ordinary social relationships. Thus, the patient can experience the physician-patient relationship as a re-enactment of earlier boundary violations.

In response to the strong feelings engendered by the clinical encounter, the patient may turn to coping mechanisms she learned as a child. Such coping mechanisms may have been adaptive in childhood but prove maladaptive in the context of an adult relationship. Indeed, these behaviors may alienate the physician and result in a situation opposite to that which the patient intended. The similarities between the childhood victimization experience and the clinical encounter can lead to strong transference reactions in the patient. The patient unconsciously "transfers" the characteristics of another person from his or her past onto the clinician.

Clinicians, too, can have blurry boundaries and be initiators of boundary crossings. The literature on physician boundary crossings (including sexual boundary violations) suggests that the clinician may be at particular risk of initiating a boundary violation at difficult times in his or her personal life, such as when going through divorce or financial difficulties (6). Dr. P was coping with her daughter's behavioral difficulties, and the strain may have decreased her ability to carefully monitor her boundaries. Thus, a variety of personal vulnerabilities shape the physician's behaviors. Every clinician has a distinct way of responding emotionally to others, and every clinician is at risk of boundary violations, especially during challenging times in his or her life.

Such "countertransference" reactions on the physician's part are particularly likely to occur in interactions with a patient who has a trauma history. Physicians often have particularly strong countertransference reactions to neediness and idealization. Having entered the profession with a desire to help people, physicians may feel drawn by the patient's need, and easily lured into a heroic role. This happened to Dr P: seeing RW after hours and accepting responsibility for her psychiatric care. However, there is hazard in this. As soon as the provider fails to live up to this unrealistic idealization (which is inevitable), the patient may quickly devalue the provider. RW's childhood experiences also explain her distressed reaction to learning that Dr. P needed to terminate the interview to go pick up her own daughter. This raised abandonment issues for RW that arose from role confusion in her family of origin.

## Common Boundary Crossings

Several classes of boundary crossing are common in interactions between patients with a trauma history and their providers (2,7,8). Boundaries often crossed by patients include:

- *Time*—Patients may seek large amounts of the provider's time or may ask to be seen outside of the clinician's normal hours.

- *Place*—Patients may catch the provider in the hallway, at the grocery store, or at a social event, asking the clinician to address a health concern outside of the office.

- *Interpersonal distance*—Patients may seek closeness with the physician. They may ask questions about the clinician's personal life and offer gifts, money, or services to the clinician. They may engage in overtly seductive behaviors or disclose too much of the details of the trauma history to the clinician. Conversely, patients may distance themselves from the clinician. Such "approach and avoidance" (9) can be understood as a coping mechanism, a desire for relationships (approach) juxtaposed against a fear of judgement or betrayal (avoidance). In RW's case, avoidance was illustrated by her failure to follow-up despite assuring Dr. P that she would. Her failure to keep an important scheduled appointment reflected her attempts to control her distance from Dr. P and to modulate her own affect.

- *Clinical role*—The patient may urge the clinician to give her special treatments or to engage in nonstandard approaches to care. For example, she may ask the clinician to provide a treatment (e.g., psychotherapy, opioid analgesics, herbal remedies) that the clinician is not trained to administer or does not feel is indicated for the condition. RW asked Dr. P to prescribe an antidepressant, and Dr. P complied, even though she felt RW needed expert psychiatric consultation.

## Consequences of Boundary Crossings

Medical objectivity is lost when boundaries are compromised. This can interfere with a clinician's decision-making, leading to lower quality medical care. For the patient, psychological consequences of boundary crossings can include feelings of anxiety and distrust. Excessive clinician self-disclosure may cause the patient to experience the strain of role reversal (where the patient becomes caregiver to the physician). In RW's case, boundary violations led her to panic at the end of her second visit and to flee from treatment for 5 days at a very high-risk time (i.e., when she was feeling suicidal).

Boundary crossings can also take a toll on the physician. They can lead to conflicts with family (the physician spends time away from home), less self-care and sleep (the physician gets over-extended and over-involved in patient care), guilt about accepting an expensive gift, and worries about what is wanted by the patient in return. The physician who is cajoled into providing care outside his or her area of expertise is at risk of decision-making errors and even malpractice allegations. In more extreme boundary violations, such as a sexual relationship with a patient, the physician jeopardizes personal relationships, professional status, and his or her license to practice medicine.

The physician-patient relationship also suffers problems from boundary violations. For example, the physician who engages in self-disclosure uses time that could have been used for clinically relevant communication between patient and provider. The slippery slope of boundary crossings can start out small but progress to exploitative and harmful boundary violations.

## How Physicians Can Respond to Boundary Crossings

How can the clinician avoid crossing a boundary, particularly in response to a patient boundary crossing? In psychotherapy, the patient with a trauma history may learn new boundary-related skills. However, in the medical setting, the onus is on the clinician, not the patient, to address boundaries in a professional manner that will be safe and therapeutic for the patient.

- *Be aware of the patient's transference.* "Is she idealizing me?" "Is she seeing me as a rescuer?" "Is she seeing me as a parent?" "Is she seeing me as an assailant?" Recognizing the patient's transference and coping behaviors will decrease the likelihood that the physician will have a countertransference reaction in response.

- *Be aware of countertransference.* It is useful for a physician to step back and consider whether he or she is having a countertransference reaction. "Do I experience particularly strong feelings in the care of this patient (e.g., pride in how well the relationship is going, frustration with the patient's behaviors, anxiety in relation to the patient's care, sexual attraction)?" Such feelings can be clues that a countertransference reaction may be occurring. These reactions may be even stronger if the physician has a personal trauma history.

- *Look for clues that suggest boundary crossings are occurring.* It can be illuminating for a physician to ask himself or herself, "Am I doing things for this patient that I would not do for other patients?" "Am I being clear about my own use of time?" If the clinician has crossed a boundary (e.g., through self-revelation), he or she should examine the motivation: "Whose need [the patient's or mine] was this crossing serving?" Recognizing the boundary crossing increases the likelihood that that physician will be able to rectify an inappropriate situation.

- *Set limits.* By thoughtfully setting limits, the physician protects the patient from harmful boundary crossings. For example, "I appreciate your interest in my family situation, but this is your clinic time, so let's work together to keep the focus on you and your health." "Because you arrived at 3:10 today, we just have 10 minutes for our visit, so let me know what you want to focus on during this time. If we find that we need more time, we can schedule an additional visit." "Thank you for complimenting my reputation. There are many excellent physicians in this community besides me. I will do my best to take care of you, as I do for every patient, but no one is perfect. Please let me know when I do not meet your expectations."

- *Use approaches that communicate the professional nature of the relationship.* Simple measures such as the use of last names and the use of chaperones for sensitive examinations can help to maintain clarity about the professional nature of the relationship.

- *Consult with a colleague if a boundary crossing has occurred.* It is helpful to get the perspective of a clinician who is not himself or herself entangled in the doctor-patient relationship.

- *Help the patient not to disclose more than she is ready to disclose.* As this text emphasizes throughout, screening for a history of violence exposure, validating feelings about traumatic experiences, and facilitating mental health referral are essential tasks for medical providers. However, the screening process, too, must be bounded. A patient with poor boundaries may impulsively relate an extremely detailed account of the trauma to the provider, only to feel ashamed, violated, and overwhelmed after the visit. Attempt to recognize how much disclosure represents a healthy opportunity to tell her story and be validated, without becoming invasive or voyeuristic. In general, medical providers will be able to provide better care if they know basic, relevant facts about the trauma history. However, they generally do not need to know details of what happened during the assault. Detailed processing of the assault is ideally reserved for trauma-focussed psychotherapy. In addition to helping the patient not say so much that she later regrets the disclosure, it is helpful to ask the patient at the end of the visit how she is feeling about the disclosure. For example, "Many of my patients have had traumatic experiences. Sometimes when they first tell me about those experiences, they go home afterwards and feel worried that they should not have told me. I want to assure you that the information you have provided is confidential, and also that it will be helpful for me to be able to provide good medical care for you in the future."

- *Be particularly vigilant about maintaining boundaries during the physical examination and procedures.* It is important to seek permission before touching the patient. The presence of a chaperone can increase the patient's feeling of safety, particularly during examination of areas such as the breasts, pelvis, and rectum.

- *Resist the temptation to go beyond scope of practice.* The patient does not have a right to expect the physician to administer a treatment that is not indicated or is outside the physician's scope of practice. When in doubt, the adage "Follow standard procedure" can be helpful.

Despite such precautions, all clinicians will inevitably cross boundaries with their patients, because of the ambiguity inherent in recognizing boundaries. The goal is to minimize the frequency and severity of boundary violations. To have effective boundaries with patients, clinicians must be aware of limits and able to state them clearly. To model them in professional work can be particularly therapeutic for those who have had their boundaries exploited during childhood.

## REFERENCES

1. Linklater D, MacDougall S. Boundary issues. What do they mean for family physicians? Can Fam Physician. 1993;39:2569-73.
2. Gutheil TG, Gabbard GO. Misuses and misunderstandings of boundary theory in clinical and regulatory settings. Am J Psychiatry. 1998;155:409-14.
3. Council on Ethical and Judicial Affairs, American Medical Association. Sexual misconduct in the practice of medicine. JAMA. 1991;266:2741-5.
4. Herman J. Trauma and Recovery. New York: Basic Books; 1992.
5. Butterfield MI, Panzer PG, Forneris CA. Victimization of women and its impact on assessment and treatment in the psychiatric emergency setting. Psychiatr Clin North Am. 1999;22:875-96.
6. Vaillant GE, Sobowale NC, McArthur C. Some psychologic vulnerabilities of physicians. N Engl J Med. 1972;287:372-5.
7. Farber NJ, Novack DH, O'Brien MK. Love, boundaries, and the patient-physician relationship. Arch Intern Med. 1997;157:2291-4.
8. Gabbard GO, Nadelson C. Professional boundaries in the physician-patient relationship. JAMA. 1995;273:1445-9.
9. Roth S, Lebowitz L. The experience of sexual trauma. J Trauma Stress. 1988;1:79-107.

# VIGNETTE 2

# Dissociation

Arlene D. Bradley, MD

DB is a 37-year-old white female with a history of chronic post-traumatic stress disorder and dissociation with frequent suicidal attempts and gestures. Her psychotherapist has referred her to an internist, Dr. J, for cervical cancer screening.

After having obtained DB's permission, the therapist contacts Dr. J and explains that DB, who has not had a Pap smear in 15 years, is anxious because her female partner has been diagnosed recently with cervical cancer. The therapist expresses his concern that, because of a history of early childhood sexual and physical interpersonal violence, DB could have an adverse reaction to the pelvic examination (e.g., anxiety, panic, dissociation, even subsequent self-mutilation). The psychotherapist advises Dr. J that DB has been able to avert panic attacks and dissociative episodes in the past by using the "square breathing" technique (inhalation and exhalation of equal duration that is counted by the provider and patient).

DB arrives for her medical appointment on time but appears nervous. She occasionally appears to not really hear some of the initial questions posed by the nurse. When Dr. J enters the room, DB is sitting in a chair, fully clothed, with a blank stare and her body posture statue-like. Dr. J says, "Hello. My name is Dr. J." DB's entire body jerks in a startled response and her eyes quickly focus on the provider with a panicked look. Dr. J asks, "Is it OK if we talk for a few minutes?" DB nods quietly. "How would you like me to address you?" asks Dr. J. DB says, "You can call me 'Deb.'" The provider then lets DB know that she has spoken with her therapist. DB appears relieved and mentions that she last saw a medical provider 15 years ago. Dr. J, reviewing her chart, notes a scheduled visit 1 year ago for a routine Pap smear. The progress note states, "Patient refuses exam." Dr. J is confused about these discrepancies and asks DB about the visit last year. She assures Dr. J that it has been 15 years since her last examination. Dr. J decides not to pursue the issue.

DB relays her fears about cervical cancer. When asked why she has not had a recent cervical cancer examination, DB explains that previous examinations have been painful. She has been afraid of them ever since her first vaginal examination, which was performed at age 12 when her mother accused her of "playing around." DB then admits hesitantly that her father frequently "did things" to her throughout her childhood. Dr. J makes an empathetic response and reassures DB that details are not needed because she is addressing these issues with her psychotherapist.

Throughout the interview, Dr. J notes multiple 3 to 5 second episodes in which DB develops a blank stare, associated with her entire body being slightly stiff and immobile. DB then becomes responsive again and says nothing about these spells.

Dr. J says, "I agree that you should be checked. A physical exam and Pap smear seem reasonable. Is it OK if we do this exam today?"

"Yes, I guess so."

"I'd like to tell you how I do this exam. First, I usually have an assistant in the room for your comfort and to help me. Next, before I do anything, I will tell you exactly what I'm going to do and ask if it's OK to keep going. If you feel uncomfortable at any time, I will stop. At any time. Is all this OK with you?"

"Yes."

"Your therapist also told me that square breathing sometimes helps when you're feeling anxious. Maybe we could use that if you feel really anxious during this exam?"

"That's a good idea."

DB changes into a gown. When she is ready, the nurse comes in to set up materials for the pelvic examination. After obtaining permission, Dr. J auscultates DB's lungs and heart while talking in a low-pitched, soothing voice, explaining what she is listening for and the results of her examination. Dr. J then asks permission again to perform a breast exam. DB again gives permission. Immediately before performing the examination, while DB's chest is still draped, Dr. J explains the entire procedure in detail. At the completion of the breast examination, Dr. J asks, "Are you ready for the Pap and pelvic exam?" DB assents.

During the gynecological examination, Dr. J describes what she is going to do before she does it (examples: "I'm going to start by looking at the outside"; "I will touch and examine the outside"; "Here's the speculum; you'll feel some pressure as I get your cervix in view"). In addition, just before each step, the provider asks, "How are you doing? Should I keep going or stop?" The drape is kept low so that Dr. J can watch DB's face and body movements. As the speculum is opened and DB's cervix is fully visualized, DB's body suddenly becomes very still and she stares upwards at the ceiling.

"Deb? Are you OK?" Dr. J firmly asks, stopping all movement related to the examination.

There is no response.

"Deb? Deb! Let's count together and practice that square breathing. Ready? Let's go."

Still no response.

"Breathe in, two, three, four. Breathe out, two, three, four."

DB starts breathing, according to the directions. After 15 seconds, she also begins counting with Dr. J.

"Breathe in, two, three, four. Breathe out, two, three four," the two echo together.

Dr. J tells DB that she looked as though she had "spaced out" for a bit. DB says, "I'm OK. Let's finish the exam." The rest of the examination is unremarkable. When dressed again, DB tells Dr. J, "That was a good exam. It didn't hurt a bit. I'm so glad you told me what was happening."

Since that examination, DB has seen Dr. J three more times for cervical cancer screening. No dissociative episodes or panic attacks have occurred during cervical cancer screening examinations.

## Discussion

This vignette addresses two important questions:

- How might dissociative disorders present clinically?
- What should a provider do when a patient dissociates during a medical procedure?

## Definitions

Dissociative disorders, officially recognized as a category of psychiatric diagnoses in 1980, are defined as "disruption in the usually integrated functions of consciousness, memory, identity, or perception of the environment" (1). Dissociation often presents in the medical setting, especially during physical examination or medical procedures. However, many primary care providers have never been trained to recognize and manage dissociative episodes. The causes of dissociation and its manifestations are discussed in detail in Chapter 5.

## Clinical Presentation

Many aspects of the medical experience can serve as triggers for a woman with a proclivity to dissociate, particularly if they elicit memories of the original trauma. A breast examination or pelvic examination could be such a stressful, triggering event. DB clearly displays this. Sensory reminders of previous trauma (e.g. touch, smells) or behavioral cues from another person (whose interpersonal style reminds her of the perpetrator's style) can also trigger dissociation.

Dissociative phenomena occur across a clinical spectrum. The mildest form (which can be non-pathological) is "spacing out." The patient would experience this as a memory gap or as time for which she cannot account (e.g., not having heard someone ask her a question, or, in DB's case, not remembering her visit from a year ago). To the provider, the patient may appear to be staring or have a glazed look, possibly with body stiffening. In this vignette, Dr. J noted DB's postural stiffening and staring, signaling dissociative change. Notably, this dissociation (appearance of "spacing out") was triggered by a stressful situation (pelvic examination) and was reversible (by helping her to feel safer). Such transitory dissociation suggests the patient is in acute distress, usually secondary to a strong emotion like fear or anger. Other physical cues that may suggest a patient is dissociating include blinking, eye rolling, changes in body posture, trance-like behavior, and changes in behavior.

Other phenomena across the spectrum of dissociation include *déjà vu* phenomena, depersonalization (out-of-body experiences and other distortions of the sense of one's body), derealization (distortions in visual perception, such as seeing things as if they are in a tunnel or seeing things in black and white), and identity disturbance (fragmentation of the sense of the self). Instances of "pseudoseizure" have been associated with dissociative events (2).

The most extreme example of dissociation is dissociative identity disorder (previously referred to as multiple personality disorder), in which a person experiences herself as another person or people. Often, a person is unaware of what she did or said while experiencing herself as this other person (alter personality states). The different alter personality states sometimes have different names, speech patterns (accent, rhythm, vocabulary), emotional range (one persona may be hostile and aggressive, while another may be timid and child-like), nonverbal communication style (body stance, use of gestures), etc. In other instances, the changes betweeen alter personality states may be much more subtle.

Establishing a diagnosis of a dissociative disorder can be complex; diagnostic assessment by a mental health expert is normally indicated. However, medical providers should strongly consider the diagnosis in a patient who is exhibiting some of the symptoms described above, particularly if the patient has a trauma history.

## Clinical Approach

The major goal in managing dissociation is to help the patient feel safer and in better control. If objective findings suggest that a patient may be dissociating (e.g., if she suddenly becomes rigid with staring), the provider should immediately check in with her, as Dr. J did (e.g., "Are you OK?"). After recognizing that a patient may be experiencing a dissociative episode, the triggering event should be identified and stopped, if possible. Dr. J did this when she stopped moving the speculum: she was prepared to remove the speculum completely if necessary. The next step is to focus on concrete, simple tasks that are free of abstract connotations. This helps resolve dissociation and relegate control back to the patient.

Several methods can help accomplish this: counting aloud with the patient (as Dr. J and DB did), asking simple math questions, discussing the color or temperature of the room, or asking the patient to focus on her breathing. Calling the patient's name may also help to ground her although, if her assailant used to call her by name, this may not facilitate resolution of the dissociative episode. The clinician should make every effort to remain aware of the patient's emotional state throughout the examination.

Although a clinician's intuitive response might be to reach out to an acutely distressed patient, touching a patient during a dissociative episode is not recommended. Touch can be a sensory reminder of previous trauma. This, in turn, can lead to a flooding of memories and risks alienation within the provider-patient relationship, or even misinterpretation of physician behavior and allegations of physician misconduct.

When a patient has recovered full cognitive function and has regained control, the clinician should objectively relay exactly what he or she saw and help normalize the event. For example, the clinician might say, "Many people have events like this happen when they are experiencing a stressful situation." Dr. J in this vignette relayed what she saw, a "spaced out" state. Medical providers should avoid exploring what a dissociative episode means to the individual; this should be left to mental health experts. Psychiatric evaluation is recommended for all patients experiencing dissociative phenomena. Careful framing of this suggestion is imperative so the patient does not misunderstand the provider's intentions (e.g., believing the provider thinks she is "crazy"). See Chapter 4 for further recommendations about referral to mental health.

Specific strategies can be used to prevent dissociative episodes from occurring in the first place, or at least to decrease their frequency and severity. First, the clinician should determine whether the patient is at high risk for dissociation. Women with a history of trauma (especially childhood sexual trauma) are at increased risk, so screening all women for trauma is important (see Chapter 2). (When a patient does disclose a history of trauma, the clinician should avoid eliciting details because an incapacitating flood of memories can themselves trigger dissociation.) Trauma survivors with a previous history of dissociation are at particularly high risk of recurrent dissociation. The clinician can screen for this (e.g., "Are there periods of time that you cannot account for?" or "Have you ever found yourself somewhere and did not know where you were or how you got there?"). Second, the clinician should take steps to decrease anxiety-provoking aspects of the medical encounter, which are likely to trigger dissociative episodes. The clinician should discuss beforehand potentially anxiety-provoking aspects of the health care experience and ask permission before performing a physical examination. Other approaches to minimizing patient discomfort during medical procedures are discussed in Chapter 5.

A heightened awareness of dissociative phenomena can facilitate identification and improve clinical management. Steps taken to decrease patient anxiety can help prevent dissociation. A provider can help resolve a dissociative episode by facilitating a return of control to the patient and helping the patient feel safer, in some cases through simple tasks like counting or "square breathing." Although medical clinicians can help women acutely during dissociative episodes, these patients should be referred to mental health professionals for more treatment.

## REFERENCES

1. Diagnostic and Statistical Manual of Mental Disorders, 4th ed. Washington, DC: American Psychiatric Association; 1994.
2. Harden CL. Pseudoseizures and dissociative disorders: a common mechanism involving traumatic experiences. Seizure. 1997;6:151-5.

# VIGNETTE 3

# Child Abuse, Incest, and Somatization

### Diane S. Morse, MD, MPH

KG is a 38-year-old woman presenting to her internist as a new patient with a variety of physical symptoms: diarrhea, abdominal pain, sore throat, headaches, muscle aches, painful menses, difficulty concentrating, and palpitations. The physician, Dr. S, initially feels overwhelmed by the patient's rapid-fire sequence of complaints and suspects somatization disorder. He elects to listen to her complaints, waiting for an opportunity to pursue psychosocial leads. Eventually, one occurs:

KG: This morning, I had diarrhea again. Sometimes I think I'm going crazy.

Dr. S: What do you mean by "going crazy"?

KG: My symptoms are driving me crazy.

Dr. S: It can be very stressful to feel as sick as you do. Sometimes when you have a lot of symptoms, it's hard to figure out why you have them. There can be more than one cause. Does it seem as if stress has an effect on any of your symptoms?

KG: Kind of . . .

Dr. S: Can you be more specific?

KG: Being around my family this weekend. On Monday I had a stomach ache.

Dr. S: I ask all my patients about family and personal issues to help take better care of them, if that's all right with you.

KG: OK.

Dr. S: How were things in your family when you were growing up?

KG: Well, we're not the closest family.

Dr. S: In this day and age, I ask all my patients about violence in the family.

KG: Actually, there was quite a bit of violence in my family, but why do you ask about that?

Dr. S: I ask all my patients these questions to help understand them better and help me better understand their needs. I'm sorry to hear that you've had some really tough experiences. You said your symptoms were worse after seeing your family, so I wonder if these experiences could be affecting you in some way now. Have you ever talked about them with anyone?

Dr. S and KG continue their discussion in a collaborative fashion and agree that she'll sign the forms to have her records sent for his review before initiating any new treatment and that she'll consider going to a therapist. He also screens her for domestic violence, which she denies currently but admits to experiencing in the past. Her records indicate a history of multiple surgeries and invasive procedures for various pain disorders. Extensive work-ups have been unrevealing. Dr. S continues to suspect somatization disorder, complicated by a history of childhood abuse, and a history of domestic violence.

Two weeks later, Dr. S asks the patient how things have been going since her last visit:

KG: Actually, I've been feeling kind of worse. I've been having palpitations and stomach aches. Also, I've been having some terrible dreams, nightmares, in fact.

Dr. S: That sounds scary.

KG: Yes, it has been. When you asked me about my family, it made me remember things I hadn't thought about in a long time. I just don't know if I can deal with it.

Dr. S: I hope we can figure out a way to help you with all this. Have you thought about the therapist idea?

KG: Yes, I think I should see one. But what about all my physical symptoms? I'm worried there may be something wrong with me.

Dr. S: When I reviewed your records, I couldn't find any test that hasn't been done for these symptoms. That makes me think that although you have substantial pain and other physical symptoms, and we don't know the exact cause, it isn't dangerous to you right now. It is well known that when people have experienced trauma in the past, their bodies often go through physical changes that can last for many years, leading to chronic symptoms. For example, some people develop high levels of adrenaline on a chronic basis, which can cause symptoms like palpitations. Other people experience a sensitivity to physical sensations. It is possible that these types of changes could be at least part of what is going on with you. There are some approaches that might help you feel somewhat better.

KG: What are they?

Dr. S: There are many strategies that can help patients with these types of symptoms. We can try them one at a time to see which ones help you feel somewhat better. As we go along, we will continue to monitor your symptoms and readjust our course if needed.

Dr. S and KG elect to start with an SSRI that has analgesic properties and may help with the post-traumatic stress symptoms that KG is experiencing. Dr. S asks her if she wants to share her thoughts and feelings, but she says she'd rather discuss it with a female therapist. He asks if she is suicidal, which she denies. Dr. S calls a local battered woman's shelter to get the names of some therapists who have expertise treating women who have experienced violence and makes the referral. When KG starts therapy, Dr. S asks her to sign an agreement allowing the therapist and Dr. S to discuss her case openly and KG agrees.

Dr. S schedules KG for a visit every 2 weeks for the first three visits, gradually increasing the time between visits to 1 month. He asks her to refrain from seeing other physicians without discussing it with him first. They devise a system where she can "check out" symptoms with him, do limited work-ups as needed, and avoid invasive interventions.

The therapist shares with Dr. S the severe nature of KG's history of childhood physical and sexual abuse (her parents have also had chronic physical symptoms). KG tells Dr. S that she tried to tell her pediatrician and wasn't believed. This helps him understand her better, including the meaning of the symptoms that are reminiscent of those she had experienced during the period of abuse in her childhood.

## Discussion

Several clinical questions are raised by this vignette:

- What is the nature of the association between somatization disorder and a history of childhood abuse?
- How do childhood experiences of abuse influence adult patterns of health care utilization?
- How do childhood experiences of abuse influence interpersonal interactions in adulthood, including patient-provider interactions?
- What can a clinician do to help?

## Somatization Disorder and Childhood Abuse

There is a known association between childhood physical and sexual abuse and later somatization disorder (1-4). Somatization and somatoform disorders are also seen in victims of domestic violence (5). The mechanisms for these associations remain unclear, but a variety of theories have been postulated (6-12). One possibility is that the victim identifies with the abuser(s), who may have multiple symptoms. For example, KG had parents with chronic physical symptoms. Like KG, a woman may continue to experience the distressing sensations she felt during the abuse (such as pain in an injured area) long after the physical precipitant is resolved, without conscious awareness that the physical symptom is related to the abuse. She may also experience symptoms that symbolize the meaning of her experience. For example, she may experience pain as the "punishment" she feels she deserves for having had sexual relations with her father.

Childhood abuse can lead to chronic psychiatric conditions such as anxiety, depression, and post-traumatic stress disorder, each of which has a known constellation of associated physical symptoms. Family or cultural styles may also contribute to the way in which physical symptoms are interpreted and disclosed. Poor self-care (including smoking and/or substance abuse) is also seen in women with a victimization history and may lead to chronic illness and pain. Having been taught in childhood to repress emotional pain, women may confuse emotional pain, expressing it instead as physical pain. Physical symptoms may also reflect chronic physiological derangements caused by the abuse.

## Health Care Utilization in Women with History of Childhood Abuse

In women with a history of childhood abuse, excessive health care utilization can begin at an early age for a variety of reasons. As children, they may articulate dilemmas to professionals they view as safe through physical symptoms, which symbolize the abuse (11). Given the opportunity of private empathetic dialogue, children may reveal abuse to a professional and may be seeking an emotional respite from the abuse through the nurturing they receive from nurses or physicians. There may even be a physical respite from sexual or physical trauma during a hospitalization (1-4,6,13). Patterns of increased health care utilization can continue into adulthood. Although clinicians may regard the frequent telephone calls and urgent care visits as difficult, it is helpful to recognize that such over-utilization represents help-seeking behaviors learned in childhood.

A woman with a history of childhood abuse learns to hide from both reality and feelings through adaptations that may include dissociation and somatization

(6,13-15). KG's experiences taught her that disclosing the abuse only made things worse, which lead to feelings of hopelessness about her ability to effect a change (16). The lack of validation and protection that the survivor of child abuse experiences leads to an inability to trust her own feelings, which can be compounded by her interactions with physicians. For example, although a woman knows she has symptoms, work-ups reveal no pathology and she may be told explicitly or implicitly that "it's all in your head." This tends to be a counterproductive experience.

## Clinical Approach

Medical providers caring for women with somatization disorder and a history of childhood physical or sexual abuse can help their patients if they follow some basic strategies:

- Schedule frequent visits at a regular interval, setting appropriate boundaries on visit duration and unscheduled contacts (6). Recognize that heavy utilization of the health care system reflects adaptive behaviors learned in childhood.

- Understand that it may be very difficult for the patient to develop a trusting relationship; establishing a trusting relationship takes time and empathy.

- Acknowledge the reality of the patient's symptoms, even if there is no clear physiological basis (6-8,10,13). Given the lack of certainty that exists in medical diagnosis, the clinician should express a sense of humility when discussing the possible etiology of a patient's symptoms. One way to frame the symptoms is in terms of "a sensitivity to bodily sensations." It is important to remember that the suffering is real, regardless of its mechanism.

- Limit diagnostic and therapeutic interventions to avoid iatrogenic complications, but remain alert to the fact that patients with somatization disorder do also develop organically based illnesses.

- Consider mental health referral (11,17). Referral to mental health providers to treat the somatization disorder itself is typically not helpful ("My doctor thinks my pain is all in my head"). A mental health referral designed to treat a physical symptom is likely to alienate the patient. However, mental health referral may be more acceptable and useful if it is framed in terms of stress reduction (especially because life stressors can exacerbate physical symptoms) and helping her cope with her chronic suffering. A mental health professional knowledgeable about trauma and its sequelae is likely to have a particularly therapeutic approach.

- Screen and treat appropriately for domestic violence, which, like a history of childhood abuse, is often associated with somatoform disorders (5).

## REFERENCES

1. Springs FE, Friedrich WN. Health risk behaviors and medical sequelae of childhood sexual abuse. Mayo Clin Proc. 1992;67:527-32.
2. McCauley J, Kern DE, Kolodner K, et al. Clinical characteristics of women with a history of childhood abuse: unhealed wounds. JAMA. 1997;277:1362-8.
3. Drossman DA, Leserman J, Nachman G, et al. Sexual and physical abuse in women with functional or organic gastrointestinal disorders. Ann Intern Med. 1990;113:828-33.
4. Walker EA, Katon WJ, Hansom J, et al. Medical and psychiatric symptoms in women with childhood sexual abuse. Psychomatic Med. 1992;54:658-64.
5. McCauley JM, Kern DE, Kolodner K, et al. The battering syndrome: prevalence and clinical characteristics of domestic violence in primary care internal medicine practices. Ann Intern Med. 1995;123:737-46.
6. Morse DS, Suchman AL, Frankel RM. The meaning of symptoms in 10 women with somatization disorder and a history of childhood abuse. Arch Fam Med. 1997;6:468-76.
7. Lipowski ZJ. Somatization: the concept and its clinical application. Am J Psychiatry. 1988;145:1358-68.
8. Quill TE, Lipkin M Jr, Greenland P. The medicalization of normal variants: the case of mitral valve prolapse. J Gen Intern Med. 1988;3:267-76.
9. Engel GL. Psychogenic pain and the pain-prone patient. Am J Med. 1959;6:899-918.
10. Kaplan C, Lipkin M Jr., Gordon, GH. Somatization in primary care: patients with unexplained and vexing medical complaints. J Gen Intern Med. 1988;3:177-90.
11. Griffith JL, Griffith ME. The Body Speaks: Therapeutic Dialogues for Mind-Body Problems. New York: Basic Books; 1994.
12. Van der Kolk, BA. The psychobiology of posttraumatic stress disorder. J Clin Psychiatry. 1997; 58:16-24.
13. Drossman DA, Talley NJ, Leserman J, et al. Sexual and physical abuse and gastrointestinal illness: review and recommendations. Ann Int Med. 1995;123:782-94.
14. Beutler LE, Williams RE, Zetzer HA. Efficacy of treatment for victims of child sexual abuse. Sexual Abuse of Children. 1994;4:156-75.
15. Epstein JN, Saunders BE, Kirkpatrick DG. Predicting PTSD in women with a history of childhood rape. J Trauma Stress. 1997;10:573-88.
16. Alpert EJ. Violence in intimate relationships and the practicing internist: new "disease" or new agenda? Ann Intern Med. 1995;123:774-81.
17. McDaniel S, Campbell TL, Seaburn DB. Integrating the mind-body split: a biopsychosocial approach to somatic fixation. In: Family-Oriented Primary Care: A Manual for Medical Providers. New York: Springer-Verlag; 1990:248-62.

# VIGNETTE 4

# Domestic Violence in an American Indian Tribe

Mona Polacca, MSW, LICSW

BT is a 28-year-old female member of the Pima Indian tribe whose husband is a Vietnam veteran. BT is brought to the Indian Health Service hospital by a tribal member. She has numerous bruises on her face and a sprained ankle. The tribal member reports that BT was found walking on the road. When the doctor, who is not American Indian, questions her about her injuries, BT says her husband trapped her at home and beat her. She escaped when he fell asleep intoxicated. While running through a field to get to the road, she twisted her ankle. BT tells the doctor that there is no telephone at home and the nearest neighbor is 5 miles away. The doctor says, "I'm sorry that your husband hurt you" and asks her if this has happened before. She tells him this usually happens on weekends, after her husband drinks. "The beatings are getting worse," she says.

BT tells the doctor that her grandfather approached her husband after a recent beating. He asked her husband, "Why do you beat my granddaughter? You should never beat your wife. She is your partner; you don't beat your partner. The way it used to be, the first time you beat your wife the family would get together and have a talk with you. The second time you beat her we would do something to you. The third time you beat her, you would be banished from the village. We didn't raise her so you could beat her." The husband responded, "That's old stuff. Besides, you made your women walk five steps behind you. What's up with that?" The grandfather said, "We walk in front of our women to protect them."

The doctor is new to the Indian Health Service and recognizes that he has a limited knowledge of Native American culture and the unique domestic violence management issues, if any, that exist in this population. To address this limitation, with the patient's permission he asks a social worker who is herself American Indian to see BT as well and consult with him about management issues.

The social worker conducts a safety evaluation and learns that BT does not feel safe going home for fear her husband might hurt her again. The social worker notes that there are no domestic violence shelters or support groups on the patient's reservation. However, the social worker knows of some programs at a neighboring reservation that accept women from a variety of tribes. The social worker also discusses with BT the possibility of bringing a trusted family member to the next visit, and BT expresses an interest in this.

The social worker also asks BT if she has ever used American Indian traditional healing methods. BT indicates that she participated in a women's sweat lodge ceremony and in talking circles but hasn't felt up to going in recent months because of the shame caused by the abuse. The social worker supports BT in her intention to seek comfort in the future from these sources.

BT tells the doctor that she does not want any authorities to know about the beatings. She does not want to report her husband to the police. The doctor feels uncomfortable, wanting to respect the patient's wishes but at the same time recognizing the he has a legal responsibility in the Pima tribe where he is practicing to report the domestic violence to the police. The social worker provides additional supportive counseling to the patient to address her feelings of fear and betrayal regarding the mandatory reporting issue. BT has called the police in the past but says that "the tribal police came and took a report, but they did not do anything." The social worker acknowledges BT's feelings and helps her to recognize that police sensitivity and response has improved in recent years and that the reporting requirements for health care providers are new. With the social worker's help, BT comes to understand the reasons for reporting and agrees to report the beatings to the police.

## Discussion

This vignette addresses three important questions:

- What aspects of tribal life and American Indian culture increase or decrease the risk of domestic violence for American Indian women?
- What resources are available to American Indian women who are experiencing domestic violence?
- What unique legal issues arise for clinicians caring for American Indian women who have experienced domestic violence?

## Epidemiology and Risk Factors for Violence Among American Indians

This case raises issues relevant to the care of women of American Indian and Alaska Native descent. It also illustrates general considerations that apply in the care of women from diverse cultural backgrounds and women who live in rural areas. For the purposes of this chapter, we will use the term *American Indian* to encompass both American Indians and Alaskan Natives.

The epidemiology of partner violence among American Indians is not well studied. Preliminary data suggest that American Indian women living on Indian reservations experience high levels of domestic violence (1-3), and various tribes have identified domestic violence as a common issue in their populations (4). Despite the focus of American Indian tribes upon this issue, it has been difficult to estimate accurately the scope of the problem because abuse is frequently not reported.

Certain distinct factors may put American Indian women at a particularly high risk for violence. Because most tribal communities are rural, these women tend to be geographically and socially isolated. Resources for abused women are concentrated in larger population areas, which may be difficult to access because of a paucity of transportation or even telephone services. A related problem in rural areas is an absence of the anonymity that exists in larger urban areas. For women of any ethnic background, residence in a closely knit, isolated community increases the risks associated with disclosure of violence to family, friends or health care providers, particularly risks of confidentiality violations.

Substance abuse by the perpetrator is a risk factor for violence and serious injury (see Chapter 10) (5). The rates of alcoholism are high in some American Indian tribes (6) and in American Indian military veterans (7). Given the high prevalence of post-traumatic stress disorder (PTSD) among Vietnam veterans (8), BT's husband may well have PTSD, a known risk factor for violent behavior. If he is without access to treatment, he may be especially likely to be abusive.

It has been recently argued that problems common in modern American Indian society (including domestic violence, child abuse, and substance abuse) have their roots in American Indians' long history of victimization by colonists and post-colonists (8a). According to this argument, historical oppression becomes internalized by the Native American man, who projects his anger upon his partner. Other ethnic and cultural groups, such as African Americans, may also experience such internalized oppression. However, although these factors might be acknowledged in the course of discussions with patients, they cannot be used to excuse or discount violent actions of any individual.

## Cultural Issues

For any ethnic group, a number of specific cultural issues may arise in the care of a woman who has experienced violence (9). For example, although mainstream American society often perceives Indians as a homogeneous group with the same appearance, customs and language, the reality is much different. Tribes vary greatly in history, culture, economy, location, size and government (10). Similar heterogeneity accompanies people from Asia, Latin America, the Middle East, and Africa. These differences make it imperative for clinicians to avoid assumptions about a patient's culture. General principles of caring for patients from diverse cultural backgrounds are presented in Chapter 11.

The following example illustrates heterogeneity in two tribal groups living in close proximity in the southwestern United States, the Pima and the Navajo Nation. The Pima have an intact culture and actively participate in special ceremonies. However, the geographic proximity to Phoenix, Arizona has led to increased levels of acculturation into mainstream American culture, as well as access to the resources of a large city (including domestic violence shelters). The Pima tribe also has more financial resources than some other tribes: proximity to a metropolis has led to an economic boom in recent years, fueled by income and jobs generated by the tribe's casinos and shopping mall. In contrast, the Navajo Nation is the largest tribal reservation in the country (in population and geographically) and is located in the high desert of the Four Corners area of the states of Arizona, New Mexico, Utah, and Colorado. The tribe is more rural: access to telephones and electricity, for example, is limited, which potentially increases the isolation of a victim of violence. Tribal members must travel great distances to reach medical care, shelters, and law enforcement agents. Employment opportunities and economic resources are scarcer than in the Pima tribe. There is strong adherence to traditional cultural practices; indeed, a substantial number of Navajos do not speak English. This may make it more difficult for them to seek help from English-speaking medical providers. The strong cultural orientation may also provide them with additional sources of support and comfort.

Cultural heterogeneity is further complicated because of the intergenerational variation seen in the constantly evolving customs within a single ethnic group. Most families from ethnic groups will vary along a continuum, from those who retain and are only comfortable with traditional ways to those who are completely assimilated into mainstream American culture. Acculturation tends to be greater in younger members of American Indian tribes, and such differences can contribute to intergenerational conflict, as reflected in the case presented. BT's grandfather attempted to use traditional methods to convince BT's husband to change his behavior, but BT's husband rebuffed this effort. BT's husband may have become assimilated into mainstream American culture during his tour of duty in Vietnam and may now feel less confined by the traditional tribal behavioral codes. It should be noted that some younger Indians who have been assimilated into mainstream American culture are now returning to traditional cultural practices.

In a situation of domestic violence, the tribe or extended family can provide a positive or negative influence on the victim and the perpetrator. Close-knit extended families can be very loyal to each other, as in the American Indian community. This can work in the victim's favor, if family members support her, as BT's grandfather did. The tribe may even ban the perpetrator from returning to the community. However, small, closely interconnected communities often function as the main support for both victim and perpetrator and may therefore hesitate to intervene in the problem. Family loyalty can also work directly against the victim: the perpetrator's family may be loyal to him and turn against the victim; this can be particularly serious when tribal officials are related to the perpetrator. If the husband and wife are from two different tribes or communities that have been traditional enemies for generations, the domestic violence conflict can trigger previous animosities. This may escalate the domestic violence or marginalize it.

A unique aspect of providing care for American Indians is the variability in their societal governance, a variability that can have legal ramifications relevant to the care of domestic violence victims. Some American Indians live on sovereign tribal reservations (11), and they have their own tribal police who will respond to reports of domestic violence and remove one or both partners from the home, depending upon their assessment of the situation (e.g., bruises on one partner) and statements of witnesses. Other American Indians live in tribes that fall under Public Law 280; for these tribes, the state in which they are located has legal jurisdiction over the tribe. In this case, state police would respond to domestic violence reports. Still other American Indians do not live on a tribal reservation (e.g., urban Indians). They typically utilize health care facilities and law enforcement systems within the mainstream community.

In addition to the variance in geographic, familial, and governance structures, all cultures and societies have unique beliefs and superstitions. American Indian tribes, for example, believe that if someone speaks of death, that person will bring death to someone close to him or her: clinicians must take this belief into account when counseling American Indian patients about the potential lethality of a domestic assault or when screening for suicidal ideation.

## Legal Issues

Laws mandating physicians to report intimate partner violence do not exist uniformly in the United States and are considered controversial for a variety of reasons. First, there is a fear that such laws will discourage women from seeking health care to help for abuse. Second, there is a worry that the police response will be ineffectual and might even threaten the victim's safety if the perpetrator finds out. Few studies have examined the effect of mandatory reporting, so much of the controversy is based on anecdotal evidence and expert opinion.

Law and order codes of several Indian tribes include mandatory reporting of domestic violence. When mandatory reporting requirements do exist, the health care provider should notify the patient that he or she is a mandated reporter *before* screening for domestic violence. The patient should be advised of the risks (e.g., potential for escalation of the abuse when the perpetrator learns of the disclosure) and benefits (e.g., potential to get shelter or other help) associated with deciding to disclose that she is experiencing violence. In this vignette, the physician and social worker worked together to acknowledge the legal mandate to report as well as BT's feelings about it. This contributed to the success of the intervention. They also conducted a safety evaluation to make sure that BT would have a safe living arrangement during this high-risk period.

## What Medical Providers Can Do

Medical professionals can take concrete steps to ensure they provide culturally competent care to women from different backgrounds who have experienced domestic violence. One very useful step is for a clinician to recognize that he or she might not understand all the cultural issues relevant to the management of domestic violence in a particular patient. The clinician can then obtain a cultural translator to facilitate the communication, who would ideally be a clinician (nurse, social worker, nursing assistant) or trained language interpreter. In the case of BT, the provider enlisted the help of a social worker from the same tribe in order to learn what might be useful to the patient. By asking permission to refer to the social worker, he conveyed a sense of respect to the patient and also helped establish continuity between the social worker and himself. Rather than having to research all of the specifics of BT's culture, he instead engaged an ally to facilitate the encounter.

## Resources for American Indian Women

In an effort to make domestic violence resources and shelters available to American Indian women, a number of tribes are establishing STOP Violence Against Indian Women projects, funded by the United States Office of Justice. These projects integrate Indian values and customs with mainstream program ideas. For example, such projects emphasize inclusion of the family in intervention. Tribal programs also typically use mediators who have personal knowledge of the families involved. In the case study, BT would have been encouraged to draw upon her talking circle and sweatlodge ceremonies as sources of support.

In a typical talking circle, a woman tells her story in a safe, nonconfrontational, nonjudgemental group environment. A facilitator reviews the ground rules at the outset, such as an emphasis upon mutual respect, sharing, and listening. The ceremony involves the use of symbolic items (candle, eagle feather, and sage or cedar) as part of traditional Native American teachings. Classically, no one questions what a woman says in the talking circle: what she says is her own story and is accepted as her own truth. The use of traditional symbols and practices may make this a more effective form of group support than techniques developed by non-Indians.

A sweatlodge ceremony can be used as a healing ceremony for domestic violence, in which case it would include women only. The women would enter a heated structure and perform prayers and rituals, the goal being for the participants to gain spiritual, physical, and emotional purification through prayer and ritual in the presence of others. Individual tribes may have other ceremonies specific to their tribe. For example, the Navajo Nation has a "peacemaker court," which utilizes traditional Native American mediation techniques when working with the perpetrator and the victim of violence.

When there is a cultural or ethnic group that is predominant in a clinical practice, clinicians should take steps to increase their cultural competence regarding the customs, language, and traditional health care practices of the populations they care for. This can include talking with patients themselves or with medical colleagues from the same cultural group, attending lectures, watching documentaries or movies that accurately depict the culture, reading textbooks (a good reference for information on the medical care of Native Americans is *Primary Care of Native American Patients: Diagnosis, Therapy, and Epidemiology* [1]), and browsing the Internet. When encountering a patient from an unfamiliar ethnic group or tribe, it is especially important to ask the patient about cultural practices that affect her perception of a domestic violence problem.

Clinicians must make sure that recommendations are realistic and sensitive to the patient's situation. For example, safety planning often includes a recommendation for the woman to open her own bank account, which will

## Mandatory Reporting Requirements Among Indian Tribes

American Indians receive their health care in different ways, which complicates the issues involved in mandated reporting. Some receive their health care from the mainstream American health care delivery system and some from clinicians hired by the reservation. Those living in tribal reservations often receive care from the Indian Health Service. The Indian Health Service is an agency of the United States Department of Health and Human Services, responsible for providing health services to tribes on reservations and in urban Native American and Alaska Native clinics. Special legal considerations apply to physicians caring for American Indian domestic violence victims in the Indian Health Service setting.

Because most Indian Health Service hospitals and clinics are located within the boundaries of a tribal reservation, legal jurisdiction is under the tribe (unless the tribe is covered by Public Law 280, in which case jurisdiction is under the state). Therefore, it is important for clinicians working within the Indian Health Service system to be knowledgeable of tribal mandatory reporting requirements. At present, the law and order codes of several tribes require health care providers to report domestic violence to police (Valencia-Weber G, Zuni CP. Domestic violence and tribal protection of indigenous women in the United States. St. John's Law Review. 1995;69:124). It is important for clinicians practicing in an Indian Health Service setting to become familiar with the function and operation of tribal agencies and with the legal mandates governing their policies. Most Indian Health Service hospitals and clinics have established domestic violence prevention and intervention policies and procedures. However, the Indian Health Service itself does not currently have a domestic violence policy.

be useful in a future attempt to escape from her home. However, because many American Indian women lack access to a regular inflow of money, this may be unrealistic. Likewise, giving the patient a domestic violence hotline number may be useless, and insensitive, if she does not have access to a telephone.

Similar to the need for a cultural translator, clinicians often need to identify a resource that is a conduit to other resources. Depending on the setting, this can include a social worker, local domestic violence advocate, or a national or local hotline. In addition, many ethnic and cultural groups have domestic violence resources specific to that group. In the case of American Indian women, information can be obtained from Mending the Sacred Hoop, STOP Violence Against Indian Women Technical Assistance Project (telephone, 888-305-1650) (see Chapter 4 for information on referral). State domestic violence coalitions (see Appendix for telephone numbers) often have information about culturally specific resources.

# REFERENCES

1. Chrestman K, Polacca M, Koss MP. Domestic violence. In: Galloway JM, Goldberg BW, Alpert JS, eds. Primary Care of Native American Patients: Diagnosis, Therapy, and Epidemiology. Burlington, MA: Heinemann; 1999.

2. Skupien MB, & Hamby, S.L. Domestic Violence on the San Carlos Apache Indian Reservation: Rates, Associated Psychological Symptomology, and Cultural Considerations. Tenth Annual Indian Health Service Research Conference. Albuquerque, NM; 1998.

3. Bachman R. Death and Violence on the Reservation: Homicide, Family Violence, and Suicide in American Indian Populations. New York: Auburn House; 1992.

4. Office of Planning and Legislation. Indian Health Service, U.S. Department of Health and Human Services. Final Report: A Case Study of Family Violence in Four Native American Communities. Contract 282-90-0035; 1994.

5. Kyriacou DN, Anglin D, Taliaferro E, et al. Risk factors for injury to women from domestic violence against women. N Engl J Med. 1999;341:1892-8.

6. Leung PK, Kinzie JD, Boehnlein JK, Shore JH. A prospective study of the natural course of alcoholism in a Native American village. J Stud Alcohol. 1993;54:733-8.

7. Walker RD, Howard MO, Anderson B, Lambert MD. Substance dependent American Indian veterans: a national evaluation. Public Health Rep. 1994;109:235-42.

8. Kulka R, Schlenger W, Fairbank J, et al. Trauma and the Vietnam War Generation; Report of Findings from the National Vietnam Veterans Readjustment Study. New York: Brunner/Mazel; 1990.

8a. Duran E, Duran B. Native American Post-Colonial Psychology. Albany: State University of New York Press; 1995.

9. Chester B, Robin RW, Koss MP, et al. Grandmother dishonored: violence against women by male partners in American Indian communities. Violence Victims. 1994;9:3.

10. U.S. Congress Office of Technological Assessment. Indian Health Care. OTA-H-290. Washington, DC: U.S. Government Printing Office; 1990.

11. Valencia-Weber G, Zuni C. Domestic violence and tribal protection of indigenous women in the United States. In: Carillo J, ed. Readings in American Indian Law. Philadelphia: Temple University Press; 1998:264-75.

# VIGNETTE 5

# Sexual Trauma in the Military Workplace

Maureen Murdoch, MD, MPH
Arlene D. Bradley, MD

JD, a 31-year-old female veteran, is referred to an internist, Dr. S, for on-going problems with alcohol use, possible depression, and anxiety. She is seeking Veterans Administration (VA) disability benefits for service-related post-traumatic stress disorder (PTSD). JD has adamantly refused to see a mental health specialist, insisting that "It won't help." On presentation, JD gives Dr. S a copy of her "Request for Benefits," a narrative describing her experiences while in the military and an integral part of her VA disability benefits claim. JD requests a Letter of Support for her VA claims file. Skimming the narrative, Dr. S learns the following information.

At the time of her third year of duty with the Air Force, JD was 21 years old. Because of consistently stellar work performance, she had been given a prestigious posting to gain further training in her specialty, which was fire protection. JD found herself the only woman in a work group of 11 men. The men at her new posting had worked together for a long time, and they made it clear they did not believe women could be capable fire protection specialists. When she first reported to duty, several of them made offensive, sexist comments. Later, her ranking officer, a staff sergeant, asked her for a date. When she refused, the sexual harassment escalated to include lewd comments when she walked by co-workers, fondling from her co-workers, and sexually explicit drawings and notes left on her desk.

The harassment continued for several months, during which time JD tried various strategies for coping with and changing her co-workers' aggressive behavior, all without success. For example, she tried working harder to gain their acceptance and also avoided the men as much as possible. Then, one night after a work-related celebration that JD attended, she was raped by the staff sergeant. The sergeant threatened to ruin her career if she ever reported the assault. In addition to being intimidated by him, JD was also reluctant to report the rape because she felt that she had to some extent brought it upon herself, by "stupidly" allowing herself to be alone with the sergeant (he had told her that he needed to speak with her privately) when she could tell that he had been drinking.

Three days after the rape, she presented to the health clinic with headaches. She requested testing for pregnancy, sexually transmitted diseases, and HIV but did not explain why she wanted them. Her tests returned negative and she was given ibuprofen for her headaches.

Over the next few months, JD became increasingly withdrawn and broke all contact with friends and family. Her concentration deteriorated, and her work ratings declined precipitously. She also began having heart palpitations. She again presented to the clinic where she was diagnosed as having panic attacks. JD began drinking heavily to help her to sleep and began to neglect her personal hygiene. At work she was cited for dishevelment. Finally, when a concerned friend confronted her, she told her friend what had happened. Her friend urged JD to report the case.

The lawyer at Criminal Investigation Command was supportive, but he warned JD that the sergeant would probably say the sex had been consensual. Furthermore, there was no physical evidence to prove a rape had occurred, and the fact that she had delayed reporting the assault would probably be exploited by the defense as well. In addition, he warned, if her assailant prevailed in court on the consensual sex defense, she would be liable for prosecution under the fraternization codes of the Uniformed Code of Military Justice. In absence of a court finding in her favor, rightly or wrongly, the fact that she had made what appeared to be an unsubstantiated rape charge against an officer would probably be construed as a permanent black mark on her own record, effectively ending all chances of advancement.

At her military hearing (similar to a grand jury hearing in civilian court) the judge ruled there was insufficient evidence of a sexual assault to refer to court-martial. JD declined to extend her tour of duty when it expired a month later.

Dr. S decides to open the interview with an empathetic remark: "I just read your Request for Benefits, and it looks as if you had a very difficult time during your last year in the service." JD nods and becomes tearful. Dr. S continues, "No one deserves to be treated that way." Dr. S then asks, "What can I do to help you feel better today?" JD goes on to explain that she has never felt well since leaving the service. Her family, aware of the rape, told her it was her fault for joining the service. She has been having nightmares of the rape with increasing regularity and can no longer sleep well. When she sees men with a short, stocky appearance, she develops palpitations (the staff sergeant is short and stocky). She has been drinking more, though she defensively adds that it "isn't a problem." She no longer sees her friends and hasn't worked for a year and a half. "Look," JD says, "The lady who's been helping me with my disability claim sent me here. All I want is a Letter of Support for my claim. I just want my benefits so I can afford to live."

## Discussion

Several clinical questions are raised by this vignette:

- What are the interpersonal dynamics facilitating sexual trauma in the workplace?
- In what ways is sexual trauma unique when it occurs in a military environment?
- What is the clinical presentation (physical and emotional symptoms) of women who have experienced sexual harassment?
- What clinical issues can arise when the woman's decision to pursue legal action forces her to relive the sexual trauma?
- What services are available to help women address such adverse working conditions?

### Sexual Trauma in the Military Workplace

Approximately 2% of women seen in primary care settings have served in the United States Armed Forces, and there are currently more than 2 million female veterans living in the United States. Although this is a fictitious account, JD's case was created from a composite of actual histories, and it illustrates a number of features often seen in instances of *work-related sexual trauma,* a term that includes both sexual harassment and assault (1). As in the civilian sector, JD's age, gender, low rank, outsider status, and employment in a "gender-discordant" occupation all increased the likelihood that she would be a victim of sexual harassment (2-4). Up to 58% of female veterans have experienced some type of physical or sexual abuse while in the military (2). However, in the military workplace, sexual trauma is more common than combat exposure (2-10) and more common than domestic violence that spills over from the home into the workplace.

A number of features unique to military service can compound the damage that occurs after sexual trauma. For example, frequent mobilization of service men and women interferes with the building of strong social networks, and traumatized women often find themselves isolated from friends and family at a time when they most need support (10). Access to spiritual care or to mental health support may be limited, absent, or of poor quality, depending on where the victim is posted (10). Military peers may pressure victims to keep quiet about their experiences to maintain the appearance of a smooth-running unit, and women who do "disrupt" the unit by reporting sexual trauma may be ostracized. War-zone sexual assaults may be particularly traumatizing in that victims are harmed not by the "identified enemy" but by colleagues sworn to upholding their safety and the safety of all Americans (10).

According to anecdotal experience at several VA Medical Centers, one of the single greatest regrets many sexual assault victims report is having told military authorities about the crime. Women who experience sexual trauma in the workplace, whether in the military or civilian setting, often feel they have little redress. They may feel trapped, fearing that if they report the trauma to a supervisor they will be retaliated against or fired. In the 1995 Armed Forces Sexual Harassment Survey, 69% of women who filed a sexual harassment report said that they were not taken seriously, were pressured to drop their complaint, saw no action taken in response to their complaint, or experienced retaliatory hostility from co-workers and supervisors in their work unit (11). Approximately 59% of women filing rape charges said the same (11).

Again, because of features specific to the armed forces, such concerns may be magnified among military women relative to women in the civilian sector. For example, when a crime occurs between two employees, the military is simultaneously responsible for treatment of the victim and for the adjudication of the assailant (10). The victim's medical records are not confidential and may be used against her (10,12). Concerns for the community's safety, maintenance of military readiness, and upholding the integrity of the fact-finding process may outweigh victim's therapeutic needs (10,12). Women who do not feel mentally well enough to pursue prosecution or who fear the career consequences of pursuing prosecution may nonetheless be required to do so. Although successful prosecution can bring to victims a sense of validation and closure, just slightly more than half of all courts-martial for sexual assault adjudicate for the plaintiff (12).

Perhaps one of the most potent barriers to filing rape charges in the military is the ban against fraternization across ranks (12,13). Under these laws, a rape victim who cannot prove her case in court is at risk of being charged with fraternization with the assailant. Consequently, instead of her assailant, it may be she who ends up the target of a court-martial. Married victims or victims raped by married men may find themselves facing not only charges of fraternization but also those of adultery (12).

An additional feature of military service that may compound the effects of sexual trauma is the homecoming experience. Women veterans commonly report being stigmatized as either "lesbians" or "whores" when they return from active duty (6). Such stereotyping may be especially pronounced in women who experienced sexual assaults while in the service (6). Furthermore, these judgmental attitudes and the lack of social support increase the risk of PTSD after sexual assault (5,6). In JD's case, the judgmental attitudes of her family may have contributed to her poor post-service adjustment. Primary care physicians should be aware of the negative attitudes to which their women veteran patients may have been exposed, and, if possible, counter them. Routinely asking women about their veteran status and thanking them for their service may be a useful validating and re-affirming action, as may be directly asking female veterans if they have encountered negative stereotypes and assuring them that such beliefs are not endorsed.

## Clinical Implications

Medical providers need to be aware of the spectrum of physical problems (e.g., chronic pain, irritable bowel syndrome, gynecological symptoms, sexual dysfunction) and emotional distress (e.g., depression, PTSD, anxiety) that can persist for years after a sexual trauma. However, providers should also be aware that female veterans with a history of sexual trauma in the military may have more unexplained physical symptoms than civilian women with sexual trauma histories (14,15). Since 1999, all VA providers are required to screen veterans for military sexual trauma. Non-VA providers should also consider screening women veterans for such histories. When screening is positive, referral to a mental health specialist may be appropriate. Veterans with histories of sexual trauma in the service are eligible for free mental health counseling and related services through the Department of Veterans Affairs. It is not necessary for veterans to "prove" they were sexually traumatized to receive these services. For the nearest VA Medical Center, providers may consult the phone book or the Department of Veterans Affairs Web site (www.va.gov). For non-veterans or female veterans experiencing current workplace sexual trauma, providers can also point women toward workplace-specific programs and toward the local Equal Employment Opportunity Commission, which can counsel women about options for addressing current adverse working conditions.

In addition to counseling services, veterans who develop psychiatric or physical illness as a direct result of military sexual trauma may be eligible for disability compensation through the Department of Veterans Affairs (16). Unlike the free mental services offered to any veteran who reports a military sexual trauma, veterans seeking disability benefits because of illness related to military sexual trauma must provide a reasonably credible basis for their claim.

Although these benefits are useful in stabilizing veterans' health and economic status, the process of obtaining such benefits can be extremely stressful (17). As in criminal proceedings, victims must recount their traumatic experiences to multiple people, all of whom serve in a forensic capacity. For many veterans, VA compensation offers external validation of their heroism, their service to their country, or, as in the case of JD, their disablement while in the service. VA disability benefits may therefore offer therapeutic value to veterans above and beyond any cash award (18).

Unfortunately, by the same token, failure to receive benefits may be psychiatrically devastating to veterans. Physicians should proactively educate their patients that failure to receive benefits does not necessarily mean that the VA believes they are lying about their experiences. Because of the stresses associated with applying for VA disability benefits, the applicant should ideally already be in a stable, therapeutic relationship with a mental health provider before starting the application process. Women who are not in a therapeutic relationship should be encouraged to develop one. Because physical symptoms also tend to flare during these stressful times, primary care physicians should also offer more frequent visits.

A similar strategy can be employed for civilian women considering legal redress for workplace sexual trauma. As with female veterans, therapists and physicians should explore with civilian women the potential risks and benefits to emotional well-being that are associated with filing a claim. Should a patient decide to pursue legal actions, a care provider should be aware that the process can take up to 2 years and sometimes longer, and it is common for women's mental and physical health to deteriorate during this time (19). More frequent medical visits should be offered, and women should be encouraged to develop a stable, therapeutic relationship with a mental health provider before filing their claims.

## Resources for Patients

Up-to-date information about VA-sponsored treatment options for sexually traumatized veterans can be accessed through the VA Intranet (vaww.sites.Irn. va.gov/wvhp) or through the Internet (www.va.gov/womenvet or www.va.gov). In general, these resources allow victims the option of remaining anonymous. Active duty victims of sexual trauma might also be able to take advantage of chaplaincy services, mental health services, and Equal Opportunity Advisers at their local post or base. Most local services will honor victims' requests to remain anonymous. However, when the harassment is especially egregious or represents an ongoing risk to others, confidentiality requests may not be honored.

## Resources for Patients

Armed Services Supported Hotlines
- Army Hotline: 1-800-752-9747
- Naval Equal Opportunity Adviceline: 1-800-253-0931 (use also for Marine Corps personnel)
- Air Force Equal Opportunity Line: 1-800-468-6661
- Coast Guard Women's Policy and EO Line: 1-800-242-9513
- Department of Defense Hotline: 1-800-424-9098
- Civilian EEO Hotline: 1-800-533-1414

### National Hotline

- Rape Abuse and Incest National Network (RAINN): 1-800-656-HOPE

### Armed Services Supported Web Sites

- www.chinfo.navy.mil
- www.bupers.navy.mil
- www.hqmc.usmc.mil/manpower/mpe/mpe.nst
- www.aetc.af.mil/sh_policy.html

### National Web Sites

- www.MilitaryWoman.org (highly recommended)
- www.feminist.org/911/1_support.html

## Follow-Up

At the end of the visit, Dr. S informs JD that she will mail a statement of disability to her at the end of the week and asks JD if she would like a referral to a mental health specialist, which JD declines. Dr. S then explains that the disability process can be very stressful and that although JD will be seeing mental health specialists as part of her claims process, none will be seeing her within the context of a therapeutic relationship. Dr. S gives JD educational information about PTSD and tells her to call the office if she changes her mind about a referral. Dr. S considers initiating therapy with sertraline but is concerned that SSRI-class medications may initially worsen JD's insomnia and anxiety. Instead, Dr. S suggests treatment with clonidine at 0.1 mg bid to reduce some of JD's intrusive recollection and avoidant symptoms (19). Knowing that female veterans represent an exceptionally mobile demographic group (moving, on average, across state lines every 5 years [20]), Dr. S asks if JD is planning to move any time soon. JD answers, "I just moved, and I'm not sure how long I'll be here." Dr. S asks JD to come back in 2 weeks to assess her response to the clonidine and makes a note to address JD's alcohol consumption at that time.

# REFERENCES

1. Department of Veterans Affairs: Women Veterans Health Programs. Counseling and Treatment for Sexual Trauma. VA Pamphlet 10-114; 1994.
2. Coyle B, Wolan D, Van Horn A. The prevalence of physical and sexual abuse in women veterans seeking care at a Veterans Affairs Medical Center. Military Med. 1996;161:588-93.
3. Culbertson A, Rosenfeld P, Newell C. Sexual harassment in the active-duty Navy. Findings from the 1991 Navy-wide survey. San Diego: Navy Personnel Research and Development Center. TR-94-2;1993.
4. Rosen L, Durand D, Bliese P, et al. Cohesion and readiness in gender-integrated combat service support units: the impact of acceptance of women and gender ratio. Armed Forces Society. 1996;22:537-53.
5. Fontana A, Spoonster Schwartz L, Rosenheck R. Posttraumatic stress disorder among female Vietnam veterans: a causal model of etiology. Am J Pub Health. 1997;87:169-75.
6. Fontana A, Rosenheck R. Duty-related and sexual stress in the etiology of PTSD among women veterans who seek treatment. Psychiatr Serv. 1998; 49:658-62.
7. Wolfe J, Schnurr P, Brown P, Furey J. Posttraumatic stress disorder and war-zone exposure as correlates of perceived health in female Vietnam War veterans. J Consult Clin Psychol. 1994;62:1235-40.
8. Wolfe J, Brown P, Kelley J. Reassessing war stress: exposure and the Persian Gulf War. J Soc Issues. 1993;49:15-31.
9. Baker D, Boat B, Grinvalsky H, Geracioti TJ. Interpersonal trauma and animal-related experiences in female and male military veterans: implications for program development. Military Med. 1998; 163:20-5.
10. Furey J. Women Veterans Issues. C&P Training Operations Teleconference. 17 Dec 1996.
11. Bastian L, Lancaster A, Reyst H. Department of Defense 1995 Sexual Harassment Survey (Report 96-014). Arlington, VA: Defense Manpower Data Center; 1996.
12. Ritchie E. Reactions to rape: a military forensic psychiatrist's perspective. Military Med. 1998;163:505-9.
13. Manual for Courts-Martial. 1995 ed. Washington, DC: Government Printing Office; 1995.
14. Golding J. Sexual assault history and physical health in randomly selected Los Angeles women. Health Psychol. 1994;13:130-8.
15. Frayne S, Skinner K, Sullivan L, et al. Medical profile of women VA outpatients who report a history of sexual assault occurring while in the military. J Womens Health and Gender Based Med. 1999;8:835-45.
16. Department of Veterans Affairs. Manual M21-1. Adjudication Procedures—Compensation and Pension, Dependency and Indemnity Compensation, Accrued Amounts, Burial Allowance, and Special Benefits;1995.
17. Eldridge G. Contextual issues in the assessment of post-traumatic stress disorder. J Trauma Stress. 1991;4:7-23.
18. Department of Veterans Affairs Employee Education System. The National Center for PTSD. Part IV: Effectively Working with Trauma Survivors in a Primary Care Setting. Veterans Health Initiative: Post-Traumatic Stress Disorder: Implications for Primary Care. Washington, DC: Dept. of Veterans Affairs; 2002:114-8.
19. Wexler D. Therapeutic jurisprudence in clinical practice. Am J Psychiatry. 1996;153:453-5.
20. Cowper D, Manheim L, Dienstfrey S, et al. Final Report: Migration Patterns of US Veterans. Chicago: VA HSR&D, IIR#95-065, 1998.

# VIGNETTE 6

## A Patient Who Is a Batterer

Rebecca A. Griffith, MD

JG is a 42-year-old man who has been Dr. Johnson's patient for the past 3 years. She has been treating him for hypertension and hyperlipidemia. Today he presents for a routine follow-up visit. Upon entering the examining room, Dr. Johnson notices that JG has a bandage on his right hand. When she asks what happened, JG is evasive, answering "I hurt it." Worried about a missed injury, Dr. Johnson asks, "How did you hurt it?" and the patient reveals that he was injured during a fight with his wife. The doctor then probes further by asking, "What happened during the fight?" and discovers that the injury occurred when he hit the doorjamb after his wife ducked to escape his attempted blow to her. He was evaluated for the injury in the emergency department and told that there were no fractures of his hand, just minor abrasions and contusions. He says that his hand is improving and that over-the-counter analgesics have been beneficial.

Dr. Johnson remains concerned about the incident. She asks a series of questions. "Do you often fight with your wife?" "What happens?" "Has either of you been hurt before?" "How do you usually deal with your anger?" She learns that his fights with his wife often result in pushing, shoving, and throwing of objects. This is the first time that JG has tried to punch his wife, and neither has required medical treatment for injuries before this incident. JG states that his wife initiated the argument by asking him too many questions about where he had gone after work (he had been at a local bar with some friends and was drinking). The fights seem to occur more frequently when he has been drinking, but JG denies daily drinking and says that he never has more than three or four beers at a time. He denies drug use.

Questioning JG about his childhood reveals that he witnessed his mother often being hit by his father. His father also hit or spanked him "whenever I did something wrong, which was all the time." Recently, JG lost his job at a local warehouse and has been doing odd jobs to make money. He has been having difficulty sleeping for the past 4 weeks, has no energy, feels worthless, and doesn't know what to do with his life. He denies suicidal ideation. He says that things are "just bad right now" because he is unemployed. He thinks his wife is "too sensitive" and becomes aggravated easily. She has suggested that they go for marriage counseling, but JG feels that counseling is completely unnecessary. Dr. Johnson, as his primary care provider, would like to help him but doesn't know where to begin.

## Discussion

Three questions arise from this vignette:

- What is the primary care provider's role in identifying and addressing the perpetration of intimate partner violence?
- What treatment options are available for perpetrators of intimate partner violence?
- Are available treatments effective?

### Characteristics of Batterers

Most domestic violence research has focused on identifying and treating the victims of domestic violence. Studies of perpetrators have primarily been limited to men who have come to the attention of the criminal justice system for domestic violence crimes. Thus, the prevalence of batterers in the primary care setting is unknown, but undoubtedly many perpetrators pass through the health care system undetected.

A number of theories attempt to explain battering behavior, but none offers a complete explanation. Nevertheless, research has recently identified several characteristics associated with the perpetration of violence (these and other risk factors are discussed in detail in Chapter 1) (1,2).

Risk factors include

1. Family history of violence
2. Alcohol or substance abuse
3. Unemployment
4. Antisocial personality
5. Insecurity or low self-esteem
6. Poor impulse control
7. Relationship conflict or separation
8. Poor communication skills
9. Young age

The attempt to categorize the personality or characteristics of a typical batterer is particularly complex. Many batterers do not have any of these risk factors. Despite the compilation of extensive data on the personalities, behavior, and socialization of many batterers, no distinct profile has emerged and most interventions utilize a generalized approach to treatment. Therefore, it is essential that primary care physicians explicitly screen for perpetration of violence.

## Identification of Abuse

Most abusers are in denial and minimize the severity of their behavior: they may not consider their behavior to be abusive. Typically, they do not volunteer a history of abuse, so the identification of violence requires that the physician watch for red flags that suggest the possibility that a patient is a batterer: substance abuse, psychiatric or personality disorders, and history of experiencing or witnessing victimization as a child. Specific interviewing skills are also necessary. Although optimal approaches to screening have not been studied, providers should be attuned to code words, such as "fighting," "lost my [his/her] temper," "self-defense," and "anger" (3). The provider should then follow up indirect references to violence with more direct questions without being accusatory. Such follow-up may include questions about what happens during fights, whether either party gets injured, and how the patient deals with anger control.

The physician should also look for physical signs of violence such as cuts, scratches, bruises, and fractures. In the case presented in this chapter, Dr. Johnson appropriately recognizes that JG's injury could be a sign of violence, investigates the cause of his injury, and discovers that JG is a perpetrator of intimate partner violence. She elicits the history by starting with nonjudgmental, open-ended questions ("How did you hurt it?" "What happened during the fight?") and then progresses to more specific questions about JG's patterns of fighting and responses to anger.

The revelation that a patient may be a batterer can be difficult for a provider, and many may avoid the issue altogether. To combat the negative feelings that may arise when it is revealed that a patient is a perpetrator of violence, it is important to remember that the overall goal is to stop violence. Identification is the first step. By maintaining a professional relationship with the abuser, the provider has an increased opportunity to initiate treatment before the batterer is forced into treatment by the court system, which is currently the most common circumstance under which batterers enter treatment.

## Treatment Options

Successful treatment options primarily include group therapy models, but programs vary widely. Most effective programs use a combination of educational and psychotherapeutic techniques. Some studies evaluating psychoeducational group therapy have indicated that, by the partner's account, two thirds of participants are non-violent after 18 months of therapy. These studies further indicate that there is a significant reduction in violence perpetration in the majority of treated men even after a 10-year follow-up period (4).

A common treatment approach is to help batterers identify what abusive behavior and inequality of power actually are and then to teach them how to participate in their relationships in a nonviolent, equality-based manner. This approach is used by the Domestic Abuse Intervention Project in Duluth, Minnesota and is known as "The Duluth Model" (5). Anger management therapy can also be used, but critics feel that it does not always address the power/control issue that often is an element in the abusive relationship. Alternatively, compassion-based therapy de-emphasizes the gender aspect of domestic violence and focuses on the unmanageble feelings experienced by perpetrators that ultimately manifest themselves through violent acts (5). This therapy is also used to treat same-sex partner abuse, in which the theory of the patriarchal aspect of society does not have as clear a role in the perpetration of violence.

Another program that has shown benefits in treating batterers is the Emerge intervention, a program founded in 1977 with the express purpose of treating abusive men. Eighty-five percent of men who participate in Emerge enter through the criminal justice system, and the recidivism rate is decreased in abusers who complete the program (6). Emerge intervention is based on the idea that partner violence is a learned behavior. The goal of the intervention is for abusers to identify and take responsibility for their behavior through insight therapy and specific counseling regarding attitudes that contribute to the perpetration of violence (3,6). Simultaneous treatment of the perpetrator's substance abuse or psychiatric conditions is recommended.

Many mental health professionals consider the initiation of couples or family counseling to be a threat to the victim and do not recommend it until the perpetrator has been treated (4). Therefore, primary care providers should not attempt to intervene by counseling the couple in a joint primary care visit because there may be unintended negative consequences for the victim: paradoxically, such counseling may lead to the escalation of intimate partner violence because the perpetrator may retaliate against the victim for disclosures made during the session. Primary care providers can, however, play a pivotal role in the *identification* of battering and can intervene with the perpetrator by referring him to treatment programs, much as they do with the victim of violence. Research has shown that treatment of perpetrators of domestic violence does lead to a decrease in abusive behavior.

## Making a Referral

Referrals to mental health professionals who are specifically trained in domestic violence batterer treatment may help a perpetrator who is willing to pursue such help. Primary care physicians should learn about the counseling options available in their area. Many domestic violence hotlines provide referrals for treatment of perpetrators as well as victims (see Appendix). Physicians should also become aware of whether the state in which they practice has certification standards for batterer treatment programs and refer only to those programs that are certified. Marriage counselors, for example, are not necessarily qualified to handle domestic violence cases, and a therapist who is not specifically trained in this area may do more harm than good.

Although making referrals is a worthwhile intervention because treatment programs can be effective, batterers may resist referral. As with other behavioral counseling techniques, the provider needs to assess the patient's willingness to change before initiating intervention. JG's low motivation to change is fairly typical of batterers, for example. He offers the usual rationalizations and explanations in an effort to deny responsibility for his behavior by blaming his wife for starting the fights. In such cases, it may be helpful to illustrate for the batterer an association between the violence and its effects on the health and well-being of the patient himself and his family.

## Legal Issues

The legal issues surrounding the identification of a perpetrator of domestic violence are not clearly defined. States have adopted individual laws regarding domestic violence issues and reporting. Most states have mandated reporting requirements for suspected child abuse or elder abuse, and some have mandated reporting for domestic violence as well. Physicians should be aware of the requirements of their state. It is also important to consider confidentiality issues: a physician who is told about a batterer's intention to kill or harm a partner may have a duty to warn (called the *Tarasoff requirement*) (4). As with any legal issues, the provider should also consider consultation with an attorney to discuss these complex confidentiality issues.

Dr. Johnson correctly makes the connection between JG's bruised hand and his violent behavior, identifies JG as a perpetrator of violence, and speaks with him about the fights he has with his wife. Her next step is to discuss with JG the fact that both he and his wife appear to be unhappy with the present status of their relationship and to suggest to him that he may benefit from counseling and antidepressants for his history of childhood victimization and depression. Dr. Johnson can further suggest that JG consider treatment for alcohol abuse and enrollment in a batterer treatment program, which may help him take responsibility for his behavior and learn how to change it, for the benefit of himself, his marriage, and his wife. By framing these suggestions in terms of JG's personal benefit, Dr. Johnson may be able to penetrate the barrier established by JG's denial of his violent behavior and thus achieve a benefit not only for her patient but also for his wife.

## REFERENCES

1. Crowell N, Burgess A. Understanding Violence Against Women. Washington DC: National Academy Press; 1996.
2. Kaufman Kantor G, Jasinski J. Dynamics and risk factors in partner violence. In Jasinski J, Williams L, eds. Partner Violence: A Comprehensive Review of 20 Years of Research. Thousand Oaks, CA: Sage Press; 1998:1-43.
3. Adams D. Guidelines for doctors on identifying and helping their patients who batter. JAMA. 1996;51:123-6.
4. Mintz HA, Cornett FW. When your patient is a batterer. Postgrad Med. 1997;101:219-28.
5. Palmer K. Treating the batterer: help for men who hurt. Minnesota Med. 1997;80:14-9.
6. Bullock K. Treatment programs for batterers. Can Fam Phys. 1997;43:307-11.

# VIGNETTE 7

# Teaching the Care of Survivors of Violence

Jeffrey R. Jaeger, MD
Nadja G. Peter, MD

Dr. Jackson, a second-year internal medicine resident, presents a patient case to his preceptor, Dr. Lee, during his primary care clinic. The patient is a 28-year old woman whom he is seeing for her first primary care visit. She has a history of asthma and is admitted for serious flares two or three times per year. She has been treated with albuterol inhalers as needed but has not refilled her prescription in months. A review of systems is notable for headaches for the past 6 years. The headaches present daily and last several hours. The patient denies any aura but does note photophobia. She reports some ongoing nasal congestion, as well as chest pain, heartburn, and vaginal itching. She has been married for 8 years and has two young children. She is a stay-at-home mom and does not smoke, drink, or use illicit drugs. She is sexually active with her husband only and uses oral contraceptive pills for contraception. Her examination is unremarkable except that she is overweight and has wheezing on her lung examination.

When asked what he would like to do about the patient's asthma, Dr. Jackson states he would like to restart her albuterol, start an inhaled steroid, and add cromolyn before exercise. He also wants to check a glucose and some other baseline labs. When Dr. Lee asks what he thinks is causing the headaches, Dr. Jackson replies that it is possible that they are migraines but agrees that the time course and location are atypical. He lists chronic sinusitis, rebound headaches from acetaminophen, and tension as other possibilities.

Regarding the patient's tension, Dr. Lee asks Dr. Jackson whether there any stressors in her life. Dr. Jackson replies that because the patient is a stay-at-home mom with two kids, there is a lot of stress. Dr. Lee then asks him how her relationship with her husband is. Dr. Jackson replies he did not ask her because he feels as if he is prying into her private business and that he feels it is his job to take care of her medical problems not her marital relations. Dr. Lee replies that it is important because her headaches could be related to her mood or to marital problems.

Dr. Lee then asks Dr. Jackson how he would ask the patient about possible abuse. Dr. Jackson replies that he would ask the patient if she were a victim of domestic violence. Dr. Lee points out that many patients in abusive relationships don't view themselves as victims and believe that domestic violence happens to other people. Dr. Lee suggests that Dr. Jackson go back and ask the patient in non-judgmental language whether she is currently in a relationship with her husband or anyone else in which she is being hurt or threatened. Dr. Jackson is uncomfortable with this but is willing to practice asking the question with Dr. Lee. After he practices with her, he returns to talk further with the patient.

After the patient has left, the resident reports to Dr. Lee that the patient denied any abuse and current depression. He was surprised to find that his patient had required hospitalization for depression in the past but that she has been off her fluoxetine for years and reports doing well. He has started her on fluticasone and cromolyn, asked her to stop her daily acetaminophen, and scheduled a follow-up for 2 weeks later. However, the patient misses her next two appointments.

Two months later the patient comes in urgently because she has chest tightness and wheezing. She has been out of her inhalers for 2 weeks. Dr. Jackson seems frustrated by the patient's lack of adherence to the treatment plan. After two nebulizer treatments, he talks to the patient about her non-compliance. Dr. Lee reminds Dr. Jackson to consider factors that might be related to non-compliance, including side-effects, financial problems, and psychological stressors, including emotional or physical abuse.

Dr. Jackson returns to speak to Dr. Lee after some time. He tells Dr. Lee that the patient reports a long history of physical, emotional, and verbal abuse. The patient was too embarrassed to talk about the abuse the first time she visited but knew that because Dr. Jackson had asked her about it before, she could bring it up when she felt comfortable. Dr. Jackson is shocked by the details of her story and visibly upset. He tells Dr. Lee that the patient said her husband only hits her when he drinks and that at other times he is supportive and kind. The husband has not hurt the children, but he hides the patient's medications when he is angry. The patient is very sad and frustrated. She and her husband were both abused as children.

Dr. Jackson and Dr. Lee go back into the room together to see the patient. Dr. Jackson introduces Dr. Lee to the patient and explains her role. After completing an examination, Dr. Lee references the previous conversation about the patient's history of abuse. She tells the patient that no one deserves to be hurt and expresses concern about her safety and well-being. The patient assures Dr. Lee that her situation is stable and that she feels safe to return home. She also reassures Dr. Lee that the children have not witnessed or experienced violence. Dr. Lee offers her the opportunity to talk to a social worker and gives her the names of local mental health workers who have experience treating victims of violence. The patient declines the referral but is willing to take a card with the numbers of local hotlines. Follow-up is scheduled for 2 weeks later.

Two weeks later, the patient is late but does arrive for the appointment. Dr. Jackson reports that the patient has not taken any concrete steps to change her situation but is taking her medication as prescribed and her asthma is under good control. The patient tells Dr. Jackson that her husband would become suspicious if she were to go to the psychologist Dr. Lee recommended but that because her husband does let her come to the clinic she would like to return in a week to meet with just the social worker.

## Discussion

Three questions arise from this vignette:

- What are the core elements of caring for victims of violence that all trainees should learn?
- How can teachers balance the sometimes conflicting needs of patients and trainees?
- What are some examples of teaching techniques that can be used to increase trainees' knowledge and skills in the management of women who have experienced violence?

Screening for and care of victims of violence are critically important to the effective practice of primary care. In most medical education settings, however, issues such as family violence are marginalized, and trainees may complete all of medical school and residency without any exposure to the principles of caring for victims of family violence. When family violence does arise in the course of caring for a patient, the trainee may feel ill-prepared to handle this complicated "social" issue.

A patient such as the one described above presents an excellent opportunity for trainee education. The attending physician plays several complementary roles as clinic supervisor, including teaching and demonstration of core skills, overseeing the care of the patient, and promoting insight and introspection on the part of the trainee. Care of survivors of violence in the clinic setting also allows for the optimal use of several key principles of successful teaching, such as role playing, modeling, and providing feedback to learners.

# Core Skills

The attending can use a case such as the one above to guarantee that the core elements of caring for the victim of violence are taught to the trainee. These include screening, counseling, safety assessment, appropriate referral, and follow-up (1-3). The attending should encourage the trainee to use non-judgmental language and direct questions when screening all patients (1). Questions should not be asked in the presence of other persons, especially family members. As in the case above, the attending should point out warning signs that should alert the trainee to the necessity of asking certain questions in a different way or waiting for a future visit to raise the issue of violence again. Once a patient has disclosed abuse, a safety assessment should be conducted, as the attending physician did in this case (2).

It is important to have resources available at the clinic site because a resident's screening efforts could be negatively affected if a patient discloses violence and the resident cannot offer her help. For example, training programs should give residents and other trainees cards with important phone numbers for patients experiencing violence. Frequently, local or state domestic violence organizations have wallet sized cards available either for free or for a nominal fee. Additionally, practitioners teaching residents and students should identify institutional resources for victims of violence (1,2,4-6). As in the case above, a resident should be taught to encourage patients who have disclosed violence to agree to a follow-up appointment soon after the visit in which the disclosure took place (7). Such measures, along with proper training, will relieve the pressure on the resident to solve every problem during a patient's initial visit and convey to the patient that the medical team considers violence to be an important issue requiring attention and care.

## Duty of the Attending to the Patient

Ultimately, the attending is the individual responsible for the care of the patient. This must be balanced with the resident's need to learn the skills of managing wellness and disease and the patient's desire to bond with her primary care provider.

Safety assessment is a critical part of caring for victims of violence. Until the attending is comfortable enough with a trainee's skills to be sure of his or her thoroughness, the attending should perform this critical assessment with the resident, even if this means doing the asssement twice. This provides verification of the patient's history and an opportunity for the attending to model history-taking for the trainee, a tactic that has been cited as an effective teaching method in the ambulatory setting (8). Depending on the expertise of the resident and the degree of suspicion of violence, the attending physician may choose to get involved immediately, during the initial screening of the patient. However, the attending should do everything possible to reinforce the notion that the resident-patient relationship is the primary relationship in the room. The attending can do this by referring to the resident as the patient's doctor and by having the resident or trainee sit across from the patient during the evaluation.

Issues of doctor-patient confidentiality often arise in the resident clinic setting. Patients who have experienced domestic violence may not answer screening questions candidly if they are not sure of the confidentiality of their answers. However, the patient of a trainee is often already aware that other more experienced physicians play some role in her medical management. The resident should make sure that the patient knows about this arrangement at the beginning of the resident-patient relationship (8). The patient should be informed of the limits of confidentiality and the necessity of involving the attending. The resident should reassure the patient: "Situations like the one you describe sound very difficult. I want to support you to become safe, but I can't do it alone. These kind of situations require a team approach, and I want to involve someone who has more experience helping women like yourself." When it is clear that her disclosure will result in additional participants getting involved to help her, the patient may better tolerate the necessary breach of confidentiality.

The attending can use the patient's disclosure to expose the resident to the important role that representatives of other disciplines play in the care of patients. Residents (like many physicians) often feel that they should be able to handle every situation by themselves. Debunking this myth is an important part of teaching of primary care to trainees and best serves the needs of the patient. In this case, the care of the resident's patient will, by necessity, include a more experienced physician (the attending) but may also include social workers, victim advocates, and even law enforcement if the situation dictates and the patient desires (4,7,10).

## Promoting Insight and Introspection

Dr. Jackson was reluctant to delve into social issues because he felt that his job was to treat medical problems rather than marital conflicts. This notion, that the medical problems are somehow distinct from the social milieu, is instilled into physicians early in their training (4,11). In first-year physical diagnosis courses, students are taught to first document the history of present illness, then, after a review of symptoms and family history, to get to the social history. This approach is reinforced throughout medical school and residency, by which time the social history is usually just a detailing of alcohol and drug addictions. Such simplification and separation does not serve trainees or patients well. A case such as the one described offers the teacher an excellent opportunity to point out that the patient's environment, her acute illness, and her ability to achieve and maintain wellness are inextricably linked. Here, the patient's asthma will not improve if her husband continues to withhold her medications and her headaches will be more effectively relieved by eliminating the stressors in her home situation than by prescribing a pill. One of the greatest challenges of primary care teachers is to help trainees to recognize the effect social environment has on illness.

Asking questions about abuse, sexual orientation, or poverty is initially difficult and uncomfortable Residents must, however, be taught that asking questions is not optional but as crucial to the practice of good medicine as physical examination skills (4). In the case above, the patient's disclosure provided critical insight about why she was failing to follow through with her treatment. No laboratory test or physical examination indication would have detected this barrier to care, and the resident should be congratulated for his excellent "doctoring." Asking questions compassionately and confidently will promote patient trust. In the case, the patient felt more comfortable disclosing abuse at her second visit because she knew that the resident was aware of the dynamics of domestic violence.

The disclosure, however, also made the resident visibly upset. Had the attending stopped there, the resident might not have ever viewed this scenario as a positive learning experience. There are techniques, including encouraging reflection and giving feedback, that the attending can use to help the resident channel his or her discomfort into the development of empathy and even activism. Physicians rarely examine in any formal fashion how their own feelings might either improve or hinder clinical practice. An important but rarely acknowledged role of the preceptor is to provide a safe environment in which such personal and emotional issues can be discussed (4). As our trainees ask the questions and listen to the answers, educators must make sure to get them to reflect on their feelings about the issues that arise. The attending in this chapter's case might have asked the resident what he was feeling after the second visit. A resident caring for such a patient might express frustration with the situation and perhaps even anger at the patient for not leaving her abusive husband. By helping the resident to verbalize and identify these very natural emotions, the attending can identify barriers (e.g., knowledge deficits, attitudes) that might exist to the resident's providing similar care to future patients.

One way this can be done is by reframing success in caring for victims of violence. The attending in the above case can point out that although the difficult screening and disclosure process did not result in an end to the violence, the patient is feeling better, has followed up as instructed, and is taking more control of her care. Seeing these developments as successes, and her verbal responses as effective "treatment," may make the resident more likely to screen and treat his next patient. The preceptor might even use this opportunity to encourage the resident to investigate available resources for family violence victims by phone or site visits (12).

Positive feedback is crucial to reinforcing skillful care of patients involved in abusive relationships. Feedback should be provided to the resident at or close to the time of the interaction and should be based on direct observation of the resident and the patient (13). It can be provided through a role-play scenario, with the attending acting as a patient. This strategy is also an effective means of allowing residents to try risky or uncomfortable patient care strategies without the fear of embarrassment or doing harm, which might stand in the way of providing effective care for patients (7,14). The role-play should be quite short, approximately 1 to 2 minutes in length. The instructor can demonstrate the correct behavior before asking the resident to perform. Feedback should be limited to behaviors that are remediable and should deal with decisions and actions ("I'm interested in why you didn't ask that patient about her relationship") rather than assumed intentions ("It seems you don't consider domestic violence important") (13). In addition to pointing out the behaviors that need improvement, the attending should reinforce positive behavior. In the case above, the attending should highlight what a critically important job the resident did in "setting the stage" at the first visit for the disclosure that occurred on the second visit.

It may take repeated attempts over a long time for medical providers to adopt new behaviors during training and throughout their careers. In bringing a trainee from the point at which he or she says "That is not my problem" to the time when he or she routinely screens and cares for all patients experiencing violence, a teacher has done the trainee and patients a great service.

## REFERENCES

1. Brandt E. Curricular principles for health professions education about family violence. Acad Med. 1997;72:S51-8.
2. Ambuel B, Hamberger L, Lahti J. Partner violence: a systematic approach to identification and intervention in outpatient health care. WMJ. 1996;95:292-7.

3. Short L, Johnson D, Osattin A. Recommended components of health care provider training programs on intimate partner violence. Am J Prev Med. 1998;14:283-8.

4. Warshaw C. Intimate partner abuse: developing a framework for change in medical education. Acad Med. 1997;72(1 Suppl):S26-37.

5. Kripke E, Steele G, O'Brien M, Novack D. Domestic violence training program for residents. J General Intern Med. 1998;13:839-41.

6. Osattin A, Short L. (Centers for Disease Control and Prevention and National Center for Injury Prevention and Control). Intimate Partner Violence and Sexual Assault: A Guide to Training Materials and Programs for Health Care Providers; 1998.

7. Weiss L, Coons H, Kripke E, O'Brien M. Integrating a domestic violence education program into a medical school curriculum: challenges and strategies. Teaching and Learning Medicine. 2000;12:133-40.

8. Heidenreich C, Lye P, Simpson D, et al. The search for effective and efficient ambulatory teaching methods through the literature. Pediatrics. 2000;105:231-7.

9. Hyman A. Domestic violence: legal issues for health care practitioners and institutions. J Am Med Womens Assoc. 1996;51:101-5.

10. Petersdorf R, Turner K. Are we educating a medical professional who cares? Am J Dis Child. 1992;146:1338-41.

11. Warshaw C. Limitations of the medical model in the care of battered women. Gender and Society. 1989;3:506-17.

12. Ende J. Feedback in clinical medical education. JAMA. 1983;250:777-81.

13. Phelps B. Helping medical students help survivors of domestic violence. JAMA. 2000; 283:1199.

# Appendix

# Resources

JEANNE CAWSE
JULIETA HOLMAN
RASHNA IRANI, MD
ERIC SLEEPER

Each of the 50 States has (though the names may differ) a Coalition Against Domestic Violence that provides educational materials as well as legal and shelter referrals for domestic violence and sexual assault. In addition, most states have a telephone hotline that can quickly refer callers to the nearest shelter or program. States that do not have their own hotline use the National Domestic Violence Hotline.

This Appendix of resources for domestic violence and related topics comprises four tables:

Some terms and abbreviations in Tables 1 and 2 require a brief explanation. "Referrals" signifies that the organization does not have specific programs for survivors of same-sex intimate partner violence but can provide appropriate referrals. Some organizations (denoted by *) do not offer either services or referrals directly intended for these survivors, but most programs do welcome *any* victim of domestic violence, regardless of sexual orientation. Organizations with bilingual staff members have the appropriate second language(s) listed. Other programs can call upon translators or refer to multilingual resources ("translator"). Programs with neither bilingual staff nor access to translators are indicated by an em dash (—). "TDD" indicates the availability of a telecommunications device for the deaf.

**APPENDIX Table 1   Domestic Violence Resources State-By-State**

| State | Organization | Contact Information | Hours | Lesbian, Gay, Bisexual, Transgendered, Homosexual Services | Foreign Languages |
|---|---|---|---|---|---|
| | **National Domestic Violence Hotline** | **1-800-799-SAFE (7233)** 1-800-787-3224 (TDD) | 24/7 | Referrals, crisis counseling | Spanish, translators |
| **Alabama** | Alabama Coalition Against Domestic Violence | (334) 832-4842 www.acadv.org | M-F 8-5 (CST) | * | Spanish |
| | Statewide Hotline | 1-800-650-6522 | 24/7 | * | — |
| **Alaska** | Alaska Network on Domestic Violence | (907) 586-3650 www.andvsa.org | M-F 9-5 (AKST) | * | Translators |
| | AWAIC (Abused Women's Aid in Crisis) | (907) 272-0100 (accepts collect calls) TTY: (907) 274-6882 Admin: (907) 274-6882 Fax: (907) 279-7244 www.awaic.org | 24/7 | * | Spanish |
| **Arizona** | Arizona Coalition Against Domestic Violence | (602) 279-2900 www.azacadv.org | M-F 8-5 (MST) | Referrals | — |
| | Statewide Hotline | 1-800-782-6400 hotline | 24/7 | * | — |
| **Arkansas** | Arkansas Coalition Against Domestic Violence | (501) 812-0571 acadv@acadv.org www.law-enforcement.org/cji/acadv | M-F 8-5 (CST) | Referrals | — |
| | Women and Children First | (501) 376-3219 (accepts collect calls) 1-800-332-4443 (in-state only) wcf@aristotle.net | 24/7 | * | — |

| State | Organization | Contact | Hours | Services | Translators |
|---|---|---|---|---|---|
| **California** | California Alliance Against Domestic Violence | (916) 444-7163 www.caadv.org | M-F 8-5 (PST) | Referrals, published resources | Translators |
| | WEAVE (Women Escaping A Violent Environment) | (916) 920-2952 hotline (916) 448-2321 admin. www.weaveinc.org | 24/7 | Lesbian survivors support group, referrals | Spanish |
| *Southern California* | YWCA | 1-888-305-7233 (in-state only) (619) 239-0355 | 24/7 | * | Spanish |
| **Colorado** | Colorado Coalition Against Domestic Violence | (303) 831-9632 www.ccadv.org | M-F 8-5 (MST) | * | — |
| | T-E-S-S-A (Trust, Education, Safety, Support, Action) | (719) 633-3819 | 24/7 | Referrals, published resources | Spanish |
| **Connecticut** | Connecticut Coalition Against Domestic Violence | (860) 282-7899 | M-F 9-5 (EST) | Referrals | — |
| | Statewide Hotline | 1-888-774-2900 | 24/7 | * | Spanish |
| **Delaware** | Delaware Coalition Against Domestic Violence | (302) 658-2958 www.dcadv.org | M-F 9-5 (EST) | * | Translators |
| | Domestic Violence Hotline | (302) 762-6110 (collect calls in-state only) Admin: (302) 762-6111 www.childinc.com | 24/7 | * | Spanish |
| | Abriendo Puertas Bilingual Hotline | (302) 745-9874 | 24/7 | Referrals | Spanish |
| | Families in Transition | (302) 422-8058 | 24/7 | * | Translators |

*(Cont'd.)*

**APPENDIX Table 1    Domestic Violence Resources State-By-State (continued)**

| State | Organization | Contact Information | Hours | Lesbian, Gay, Bisexual, Transgendered, Homosexual Services | Foreign Languages |
|---|---|---|---|---|---|
| **District of Columbia** | District of Columbia Coalition Against Domestic Violence | (202) 299-1181 | M-F 9-5 (EST) | Referrals | Spanish, French, Urdu |
| | SOS Center | (202) 783-3003 | M-Th 9-8 F 9-5 | Referrals, group for lesbian survivors, counseling | — |
| | My Sister's Place Shelter and Hotline | (202) 529-5991 www.mysistersplace.org | 24/7 | Referrals | Spanish, Vietnamese |
| | House of Ruth | (202) 347-2777 www.houseofruth.org | 24/7 | Referrals | Spanish |
| **Florida** | Florida Coalition Against Domestic Violence | (850) 425-2749 tcarr-fcadv@worldnet.att.net | M-F 9-5 (EST) | Referrals | Translators |
| | Statewide Hotline | 1-800-500-1119 (in-state calls only) | 24/7 | Referrals | Translators |
| **Georgia** | Georgia Coalition on Family Violence | (404) 209-0280 gacoalition@mindspring.com | M-F 9-5 (EST) | * | — |
| | Statewide hotline | 1-800-33-HAVEN | 24/7 | Referrals | Translators |
| | Liberty House | (229) 439-7065 Admin: (229) 439-7094 | 24/7 | * | Spanish |
| | Project Safe | (706) 543-3331 (accepts collect calls) Admin: (706) 549-0922 www.project-save.org pjctsafe@bellsouth.net | 24/7 | Referrals, information | Spanish |

| State | Organization | Contact | Hours | Services | Language |
|---|---|---|---|---|---|
| **Hawaii** | Hawaii State Coalition Against Domestic Violence | (808) 486-5072 hscadv@pixi.com | M-F 8-4 (HST) | * | — |
| | Honolulu Shelter Hotline | (808) 841-0822 (in-state only) | 24/7 | * | — |
| **Idaho** | Idaho Coalition Against Sexual and Domestic Violence | (208) 384-0419 domvo@micron.net | M-F 8:30-6 (MST) | Referrals, educational material | — |
| | Statewide hotline | 1-800-669-3176 | 24/7 | Referrals | Spanish |
| **Illinois** | Illinois Coalition Against Domestic Violence | (217) 789-2830 www.ilcadv.org | M-F 9-5 (CST) | Referrals | — |
| | DOVE | (217) 423-2238 (217) 428-6559 (TTY) | 24/7 | Group for same-sex violence, referrals | — |
| | A Friend's Place | 1-800-603-HELP www.afriendsplace.org afriendsplace@worldnet.att.net | 24/7 | Referrals | Spanish |
| | Mercer County Family Crisis Center | (309) 582-7233 (accepts collect calls) www.mcfcc.com | 24/7 | * | — |
| | Oasis Women's Center | (618) 465-1978 | 24/7 | Referrals | — |
| | Sarah's Inn | (708) 386-4225 sarahsinn@sarahsinn.org www.communityresources.net/sarahsinn.html | 24/7 | Group for Lesbian survivors, referrals | Spanish |
| **Indiana** | Indiana Coalition Against Domestic Violence | (317) 917-3685 www.violenceresources.org | M-F 8-5 (CST) | * | Translators |
| | Statewide Hotline | 1-800-332-7325 | 24/7 | * | Spanish |

*(Cont'd.)*

**APPENDIX Table 1  Domestic Violence Resources State-By-State (continued)**

| State | Organization | Contact Information | Hours | Lesbian, Gay, Bisexual, Transgendered, Homosexual Services | Foreign Languages |
|-------|-------------|---------------------|-------|-----------------------------------------------------------|-------------------|
| Indiana | Albion Fellows Bacon Center | 1-800-339-7752<br>(812) 422-5622<br>Admin: (812) 422-9372<br>www.albionfellowsbacon.org | 24/7 | * | Spanish |
| Iowa | Iowa Coalition Against Domestic Violence | (515) 244-8028<br>www.icadv.org | M-F<br>8-4 (CST) | Referrals | Spanish |
| | Statewide Hotline | 1-800-942-0333 | 24/7 | Referrals | Spanish |
| | Children and Families of Iowa Family Violence Center | (515) 243-6147<br>1-800-942-0333 (in-state only)<br>www.cfiowa.org/fvc | 24/7 | * | Spanish, translators, TTD |
| Kansas | Kansas Coalition Against Sexual and Domestic Violence | (785) 232-9784<br>kcsdv@cineworks.com | M-F<br>8:30-4:30 (CST) | Referrals | Translators |
| Kentucky | Kentucky Domestic Violence Association | (502) 695-2444<br>www.kdva.org | M-F<br>8:30-4:30 (EST) | Referrals | Translators |
| | Center for Women and Families | (502) 581-7222<br>(877) 803-7577<br>www.thecenteronline.org | 24/7 | * | Translators |
| Louisiana | Louisiana Coalition Against Domestic Violence | (225) 752-1296<br>www.lcadv.org | M-F<br>8:30-4:30 (CST) | Referrals | Spanish |

| State | Organization | Contact | Hours | Services | Languages |
|---|---|---|---|---|---|
| | Statewide hotline | 1-888-411-1333 (in-state only) | 24/7 | Referrals | — |
| | YWCA Battered Women's Program | (504) 486-0377 (accepts collect calls) | 24/7 | Referrals | Spanish |
| **Maine** | Maine Coalition to End Domestic Violence | (207) 941-1194 www.mcedv.org | M-F 9:30-4 (EST) | * | — |
| **Maryland** | Maryland Network Against Domestic Violence | (301) 352-4574 www.mnadv.org | M-F 9-5 (EST) | Referrals | — |
| | Statewide Hotline | 1-800-634-3577 | 24/7 | * | Spanish |
| | Montgomery County Crisis Center | (240) 777-4000 | 24/7 | Referrals | Translators |
| | Maryland Abused Persons Program | (240) 777-4210 | M-W 9-9 Th, F 9-5 | * | Spanish, French |
| **Massachusetts** | Casa Myrna Vásquez | 1-800-992-2600 www.casamyrna.org | 24/7 | * | Spanish, translators |
| | Massachusetts Hotline for Battered Women | 1-800-992-2600 | 24/7 | Shelter, groups, hotline | Haitian Creole, Spanish |
| | Safelink Domestic Violence | (877) 785-2020 | 24/7 | Referrals | Spanish, translators |
| | New Beginnings | (413) 562-5739 (accepts collect calls) 1-800-479-6245 | 24/7 | Groups for same-sex survivors | Spanish |
| **Michigan** | Michigan Coalition Against Domestic and Sexual Violence | (517) 347-7000 www.mcadsv.org | M-F 8:30-5:00 (EST) | * | — |

*(Cont'd.)*

**APPENDIX Table 1    Domestic Violence Resources State-By-State (continued)**

| State | Organization | Contact Information | Hours | Lesbian, Gay, Bisexual, Transgendered, Homosexual Services | Foreign Languages |
|---|---|---|---|---|---|
| **Minnesota** | Minnesota Coalition for Battered Women | (651) 646-6177 mcbw@pclink.com | M-F 8-4:30 (CST) | Referrals | — |
| | Statewide Hotline | 1-800-289-6177 | 24/7 | * | Spanish |
| **Mississippi** | Mississippi Coalition Against Domestic Violence | (601) 981-9196 mcadv@misner.com | M-F 8:30-4 (CST) | * | Spanish |
| | Statewide hotline (in-state calls only) | 1-800-273-9012 | 24/7 | * | — |
| **Missouri** | Missouri Coalition Against Domestic Violence | (573) 634-4161 http://mova.missouri.org/ members/mcadv.htm | M-F 8:30-4:30 (CST) | Information groups | Referrals |
| **Montana** | Montana Coalition Against Domestic and Sexual Violence | (406) 443-7794 mcadv@mt.net | M-F 8-5 (MST) | * | — |
| | YWCA – Pathways Hotline | 1-800-483-7858 | 24/7 | * | Spanish, translators |
| **Nebraska** | Nebraska Domestic Violence and Sexual Assault Coalition | (402) 476-6256 ndvsac@mailcity.com | M-F 9-5 (CST) | * | Spanish |
| | Statewide hotline (in-state calls only) | 1-800-876-6238 | 24/7 | * | — |
| | Rape & Spouse Abuse Crisis Center | Crisis line: (402) 475-7273 Office line: (402) 476-2110 www.rsacc.org | 24/7 | Groups, information | Spanish |

| State | Organization | Contact | Hours | Information | Language |
|---|---|---|---|---|---|
| **Nevada** | Nevada Network Against Domestic Violence | (775) 828-1115 nnadv@powernet.net | M-F 9-5 (PST) | Information | Spanish |
| | Temporary Assistance for Domestic Crisis – Safe Net | 1-800-500-1556 | 24/7 | * | Spanish |
| **New Hampshire** | New Hampshire Coalition Against Domestic and Sexual Violence | (603) 224-8893 www.mv.com/ipusers/nhcadsv | M-F 8:30-4 (EST) | Referrals | Translators |
| | Women's Crisis Center | (603) 352-3782 1-800-852-3311 | 24/7 | * | Spanish, translators |
| | New Hampshire Help Line | 1-800-277-5570 (in-state calls) www.nhhelpline.org | 24/7 | * | Translators |
| **New Jersey** | New Jersey Coalition for Battered Women | (609) 584-8107 www.njcbw.org | M-F 9-5 (EST) | Yes | Spanish, Polish, Haitian Creole |
| | Statewide hotline | 1-800-572-7233 (in-state only) | 24/7 | * | — |
| **New Mexico** | New Mexico Coalition Against Domestic Violence | (505) 246-9240 www.nmcadv.org | M-F 8-5 (MST) | * | Spanish |
| | Statewide hotline | 1-800-773-3645 | 24/7 | * | — |
| **New York** | New York State Coalition Against Domestic Violence | (518) 432-4864 NYSCADV@aol.com | M-F 9-5 (EST) | Referrals | Translators |
| | Statewide hotline | 1-800-942-6906 (in-state only) | 24/7 | Referrals | Translators |
| | Statewide Spanish hotline | 1-800-942-6908 | 24/7 | Referrals | Spanish |
| **North Carolina** | North Carolina Coalition Against Domestic Violence | (919) 956-9124 www.nccadv.org | M-F 8-5 (EST) | Lesbian caucus | Spanish |

*(Cont'd.)*

**APPENDIX Table 1    Domestic Violence Resources State-By-State (continued)**

| State | Organization | Contact Information | Hours | Lesbian, Gay, Bisexual, Transgendered, Homosexual Services | Foreign Languages |
|---|---|---|---|---|---|
| **North Carolina** | Interact | (919) 828-7740 (domestic violence hotline) (919) 828-3005 (sexual assault hotline) (919) 828-7501 (admin) | 24/7 | * | Spanish |
| **North Dakota** | Mental Health Association of North Dakota | 1-800-472-2911 | 24/7 | * | — |
| **Ohio** | Ohio Domestic Violence Network | (614) 784-0023 1-800-934-9840 www.ohiodvnetwork.org | M-F 8:30-5 (EST) | Referrals | Translators |
| | Open Arms Domestic Violence Shelter | (419) 422-4766 www.uwhancock.org/Open Arms.htm | 24/7 | Referrals | — |
| **Oklahoma** | Oklahoma Coalition Against Domestic Violence and Sexual Assault | (405) 848-1815 ocdvsa-sc@clnk.com | M-F 8-5 (CST) | * | — |
| | Family Crisis and Counseling Center | 1-800-522-7233 (in-state only) (918) 336-1188 | 24/7 | * | Spanish |
| **Oregon** | Oregon Coalition Against Domestic and Sexual Violence | (503) 365-9644 www.ocadsv.com | M-F 8-5 (PST) | Yes | Translators |
| | Oregon Statewide Crisis Line | 1-800-235-5333 | 24/7 | Referrals | Spanish |

| State | Organization | Contact | Hours | Services | Languages |
|---|---|---|---|---|---|
| | Bradley Angle House | (503) 281-2442 www.bradleyangle.org | 24/7 | Groups, sexual minority service coordinator | Spanish, translators |
| | Women Space Crisis Line | (541) 485-6513 | 24/7 hotline, M-F 9-3 drop-in | Groups | Spanish |
| **Pennsylvania** | Pennsylvania Coalition Against Domestic Violence | (717) 545-6400 www.pcadv.org | M-F 8-5 (EST) | Referrals | Spanish |
| | Lutheran Settlement House Bilingual Domestic Violence Project | (215) 739-9999 www.libertynet.org/~luthersh/BDVP.html | 24/7 | Counseling, referrals | Spanish |
| | Women in Transition | (215) 751-1111 www.libertynet.org/~wit | 24/7 | Lesbian services | Translators (Spanish) |
| | Congreso (Latina Domestic Violence Project) | (215) 978-1174 | 24/7 | Counseling, referrals | Spanish |
| **Puerto Rico** | Coordinadora Paz Para La Mujer | (787) 281-7579 www.pazparalamujer.org | M-F 8-5 (EST) | * | Spanish |
| **Rhode Island** | Rhode Island Coalition Against Domestic Violence and Sexual Assault | (401) 467-9940 www.ricadv.org | M-F 9-5 (EST) | Referrals | Translators |
| | Statewide Hotline | 1-800-494-8100 (in-state only) | 24/7 | Referrals | Translators |
| | Women's Resource Center of South County | (401) 782-3990 www.wrcsc.org | 24/7 | Referrals | Translators |
| | Blackstone Shelter | (401) 723-3057 (401) 723-3051 www.the-key.org/transit.htm | 24/7 | Referrals | Spanish |

*(Cont'd.)*

**APPENDIX Table 1   Domestic Violence Resources State-By-State (continued)**

| State | Organization | Contact Information | Hours | Lesbian, Gay, Bisexual, Transgendered, Homosexual Services | Foreign Languages |
|---|---|---|---|---|---|
| **South Carolina** | South Carolina Coalition Against Domestic Violence and Sexual Assault | (803) 256-2900 www.@sccadvasa.org | M-F 8:30-5 (EST) | Referrals, outreach, training | Translators |
| | Statewide Hotline | 1-800-260-9293 | 24/7 | Referrals | Translators |
| | Hispanic Outreach | 1-800-372-3312 | 24/7 | * | Spanish |
| **South Dakota** | South Dakota Coalition Against Domestic Violence and Sexual Assault | (605) 945-0869 www.southdakotacoalition.com | M-F 8-5 (CST) | * | Lakota, translators |
| | Crisis Line | 1-800-430-SAFE (in-state only) | 24/7 | * | — |
| **Tennessee** | Tennessee Task Force Against Domestic Violence and Sexual Assault | (615) 386-9406 www.tcadsv.citysearch.com | M-F 8-5 (CST) | Referrals | Translators |
| | Statewide Hotline | 1-800-356-6767 | 24/7 | * | — |
| | HomeSafe | (615) 452-4315 | 24/7 | * | Spanish |
| **Texas** | Texas Council on Family Violence | 1-800-525-1978 www.tcfv.org | M-F 8-5 (CST) | Referrals, information | Spanish, translators |
| | Family Place in Dallas | (214) 941-1991 www.familyplace.org | 24/7 | * | Spanish |
| **Utah** | Utah Domestic Violence Advisory Council | (801) 538-4635 www.udvac.org | M-F 8-5 (MST) | * | — |
| | Statewide Hotline | 1-800-897-5465 | 24/7 | * | — |

| | Contact | Hours | Services | Languages/TTD |
|---|---|---|---|---|
| **Vermont** Vermont Network Against Domestic Violence and Sexual Assault | (802) 223-1302 vnadvsa@sover.net www.vtnetwork.org | M-F 8:30-5 (EST) | * | — |
| Statewide Hotline | 1-800-228-7395 | 24/7 | * | — |
| Women Helping Battered Women | (802) 658-1996 (crisis line) (802) 658-3131 (office) http://homepages.together.net/~whbw/ | 24/7 | Groups | Translators, Spanish, Vietnamese, Bosnian, TTD |
| **Virginia** Virginia Family Violence and Sexual Assault Hotline | 1-800-838-8238 | 24/7 | Referrals, information | Spanish, TTD, translators |
| **Washington** Washington State Coalition Against Domestic Violence | (360) 407-0756 www.wscadv.org | M-F 9-5 (PST) | Yes | TTD |
| Statewide Hotline | 1-800-562-6025 | 24/7 | * | Translators |
| **West Virginia** West Virginia Coalition Against Domestic Violence | (304) 965-3552 www.wvcadv.org | M-F 9-5 (EST) | LGBT advisory council, information | Translators |
| Statewide Hotline | 1-800-352-6513 | 24/7 | * | — |
| Family Crisis Center | 1-800-794-2335 (304) 428-2333 | 24/7 | * | TTD |
| **Wisconsin** Wisconsin Coalition Against Domestic Violence and Sexual Assault | (608) 255-0539 sjulian@wwwise.org | M-F 9-5 (CST) | Referrals | Translators |
| Unidos | (920) 922-4933 | | * | Spanish |
| **Wyoming** Wyoming Coalition Against Domestic Violence and Sexual Assault | (307) 755-5481 wcadv@vcn.com/~wcadvsa | M-F 9-5 (MST) | Referrals | Translators |
| Statewide Hotline | 1-800-990-3877 | 24/7 | * | — |
| Self-Help Center | (307) 235-2814 | 24/7 | * | Spanish |

## APPENDIX Table 2    Resources for Survivors of Same-Sex Intimate Partner Violence

| State | Organization | Contact Information | Hours | Languages |
|---|---|---|---|---|
| | **National Gay and Lesbian Hotline** (referral service and crisis hotline) | **1-888-THE-GLNH** **1-888-843-4564** | M-F 4pm-Midnight Sa Noon-5pm | Spanish |
| | **Anti-Violence Project** (list of anti-violence projects with domestic violence resources) www.avp.org/index2.html | **(212) 714-1141** | 24/7 | Spanish TTD: (212) 714-1134 |
| **Arkansas** | Women's Project | (501) 372-5113 | 8am-5pm | Spanish |
| **Arizona** | Wingspan Domestic Violence Project | (520) 624-0348 | 24/7 | Spanish |
| **California** | Community United Against Violence | (415) 333-HELP (4357) www.cuav.org | 24/7 | Spanish, Cantonese, Mandarin, Translators |
| | L.A. Gay and Lesbian Center/STOP Partner Abuse/Domestic Violence Program Domesticviolence@laglc.org | (323) 860-5806 www.laglc.org/domesticviolence | Daily, variable times | Spanish |
| | Lesbian and Gay Men's Community Center, San Diego | (619) 260-6380 | M-F 9am-9pm Sa 9am-Noon | Spanish |
| | Shelter for Gay Men and Lesbian Women, San Diego | (619) 692-2077 | 24/7 | Spanish |
| | WOMAN (Women Organized to Make Abuse Non-existent), San Francisco | (415) 864-4722 | 24/7 | Spanish, translators |
| **Colorado** | Anti-Violence Program | Crisis Line: 1-888-557-4441 (303) 852-5094 | 24/7 | Translators |
| **Illinois** | Horizons Antiviolence Gay and Lesbian Crisis Line | (773) 929-2273 | 24/7 | — |
| | Horizons Gay and Lesbian Hotline | (773) 929-HELP (4357) | 6-10pm | — |
| **Louisiana** | YWCA Rape Crisis Center | (504) 483-8885 | 24/7 | — |

*(Cont'd.)*

## APPENDIX Table 2   Resources for Survivors of Same-Sex Intimate Partner Violence (continued)

| State | Organization | Contact Information | Hours | Languages |
|-------|-------------|--------------------|-------|-----------|
| Maryland | Turnaround | Hotline: (410) 828-6390 Office: (410) 837-7000 | Hotline: 24/7 Office: M-F 9-5 | — |
| Massachusetts | The Network/La Red: Ending Abuse in Lesbian, Bisexual Women's, and Transgendered Communities | (617) 423-7233 www.nblbw.org | M-Th 10am-Midnight, F 10am-6pm, Sa and Su 1-6pm | Spanish, TTD |
| Minnesota | Out Front Minnesota | 1-800-800-0127 (612) 822-0127 | 24/7 | — |
| New Jersey | Hotline for Battered Lesbians | 1-800-224-0211 (in-state only) | Evenings and weekends | — |
| New York | New York Gay and Lesbian Anti-Violence Project | (212) 714-1141 www.avp.org | 24/7 | Spanish |
| Ohio | Buckeye Region Anti-Violence Organization (BRAVO) | (614) 268-9622 | M-F 9-5 | Translators |
| | Lesbian and Gay Community Service Center of Greater Cleveland | (216) 651-5428 | M-F Noon-10pm Su 6:30-9pm | — |
| Pennsylvania | Women in Transition Lesbian Services | (215) 751-1111 www.libertynet.org/ ~wit | 24/7 | Translators (Spanish) |
| Texas | Montrose Counseling Center | (713) 529-0037, ext. 316 www.montrosecoun selingcenter.org | M-F 8am-7pm | Spanish |
| Washington | Northwest Network www.nwnetwork.org | (206) 568-7777 | 9am-5pm (PST) | — |

## APPENDIX Table 3   Resources for People with Alcohol or Drug Addictions*

| Alcoholics Anonymous | (212) 870-3400 (general service office) www.alcoholics-anonymous.org |
|----------------------|----------------------------------------------------------------------|
| Narcotics Anonymous | (818) 773-9999 www.na.org/links-toc.htm |

*Local branches of Alcoholics Anonymous and Narcotics Anonymous can be found in the telephone book.

## APPENDIX Table 4    Internet Resources

| Organization | Web Address | Target Audience | | | |
|---|---|---|---|---|---|
| | | Survivors | Legal Profes-sionals | Physicians | Counselors/ Advocates |
| American Bar Association – Commission on Domestic Violence | http://www.abanet.org/ domviol/home.html | | | X | |
| American Judges Association Domestic Violence Booklet | http://aja.ncsc.dni.us/ domviol/booklet.html | | X | | |
| American Medical Association | http://www.ama-assn. org/ama/pub/category/ 4605.html | | | X | |
| Battered Women and Their Children | http://cwolf.uaa.alaska.edu/ ~afrhm1/index.html | | | | X |
| Boston University Community Outreach Health Information System | http://www.bu.edu/cohis/ violence/domesvio.htm | X | | | |
| Center for Disease Control – Family and Intimate Violence Program | http://www.cdc.gov/ncipc/ dvp/fivpt/fivpt.htm | | | X | X |
| Center for Prevention of Domestic Violence | http://www.1079.com/ announce/domviolence/ viorel.html | X | | | |
| Community United Against Violence | http://www.xq.com/cuav/ index.html | X | | | |
| Cybergrrl SafetyNet – Domestic Violence Resources | http://home.cybergrrl.com/ dv/ | X | | | X |

*(Columns continue on facing page.)*

## APPENDIX Table 4    (columns continued)

| Topics | | | | Information | | | | Comments |
|---|---|---|---|---|---|---|---|---|
| Child Abuse | Partner Violence | Same-Sex Partner Violence | Elder Abuse | Domestic Violence* | Legal Issues | Local and/ or National Links/ Contacts | Provider Interventions | |
| X | X | | | | | | | Extremely informative; extensive links |
| X | X | | X | X | X | | | Information for judges and public on the recognition of domestic violence and emotional battery |
| X | X | | | X | X | | X | In-depth discussion of diagnosis, screening, and intervention by providers |
| X | X | | | X | | X | | Offers social services workers PDF-format papers and reports, training materials, questionnaires for screening for abuse, etc. |
| | X | | | X | X | X | | Provides useful information such as state-by-state hotline listings and a step-by-step guide to obtaining legal protection |
| X | X | | | | | | | Describes CDC's tracking of family and intimate partner violence and evaluation of prevention and intervention programs; provides links to relevant research sites |
| | X | | | X | | X | | Offers a "How Do I Know if I'm in a Violent Relationship?" Q&A |
| | | X | | X | | X | | Offers information and resources specifically for survivors of same-sex partner violence |
| | X | | | X | | X | | Offers support for survivors, including resources and survivor stories, as well as educational information for for professionals and annotated list of regional and national resources for survivors and professionals |

*(Cont'd.)*

*For example, clinical presentation, statistics, training materials.

## APPENDIX Table 4    Internet Resources (continued)

| Organization | Web Address | Target Audience | | | |
|---|---|---|---|---|---|
| | | Survivors | Legal Profes- sionals | Physicians | Counselors/ Advocates |
| Domestic Violence Clearinghouse and Legal Hotline | http://www.stoptheviolence.org | X | X | X | X |
| Domestic Violence and Homelessness Fact Sheet | http://nch.ari.net/domestic.html | | | | X |
| Domestic Violence Information Center | http://www.feminist.org/other/ dv/dvfact.html | X | X | | X |
| Family Peace Project | http://www.family.mcw.edu/ FamilyPeaceProject.htm | | | X | X |
| Famvi.com | http://www.famvi.com | X | | | |
| Family Violence Prevention Fund | http://www.fvpf.org | X | X | X | X |
| Guide to Clinical Preventive Services – Screening for Family Violence | http://cpmcnet.columbia.edu/ texts/gcps/gcps0061.html | | | X | X |
| International Society for Traumatic Stress Studies | http://www.istss.org/ | | | X | X |

*(Columns continue on facing page.)*

## APPENDIX Table 4    (columns continued)

| Topics | | | | Information | | | | Comments |
|---|---|---|---|---|---|---|---|---|
| Child Abuse | Partner Violence | Same-Sex Partner Violence | Elder Abuse | Domestic Violence* | Legal Issues | Local and/ or National Links/ Contacts | Provider Inter- ventions | |
|  | X |  |  | X | X |  |  | Provides a description of legal services for survivors and training for students, doctors, counselors, and legal professionals offered through the organization |
|  | X |  |  | X |  | X |  | Details the connection between domestic violence and homelessness; provides statistics and bibliography |
|  | X |  |  | X | X | X |  | Provides extensive Internet resources, hotline information, fact sheets, and news, including a link to the Violence Against Women Act of 1994 |
| X | X |  | X | X |  |  | X | Offers information on abuse and screening for abuse in clinical settings; provides good information on intervening and dealing with abuse |
|  | X |  |  | X |  | X |  | Offers information on domestic violence and links to resources and support for survivors |
| X | X |  |  | X | X |  |  | Extremely informative and comprehensive site detailing information on abuse and the prevention of abuse, legal and policy issues, developing safety plans, etc. |
| X | X |  | X | X | X |  | X | Summary of existing data on screening for abuse, value of early detection, literature on interventions, and recommendations for dealing with abuse in clinical settings |
|  |  |  |  | X |  | X | X | Primarily offers links to a research network for professionals interested in traumatic stress; also offers public education information on PTSD and links to *Journal of Traumatic Stress* (Cont'd.) |

*For example, clinical presentation, statistics, training materials.

## APPENDIX Table 4    Internet Resources (continued)

| Organization | Web Address | Target Audience | | | |
|---|---|---|---|---|---|
| | | Survivors | Legal Profes-sionals | Physicians | Counselors/ Advocates |
| Metro Nashville Police Department – Domestic Violence Division | http://www.police.nashville.org/ bureaus/investigative/ domestic/default.htm | X | X | | X |
| Minnesota Center Against Domestic Violence and Abuse | http://www.mincava.umn.edu | X | X | X | X |
| My Sister's Place | http://www.eurekanet.com/ ~ebfinc/mysis.html | X | | | X |
| National Center for Post-Traumatic Stress Disorder | http://www.ncptsd.org | X | X | X | X |
| National Coalition Against Domestic Violence | http://www.ncadv.org | X | X | | X |
| National Council of Juvenile and Family Court Judges – Family Violence Department | http://www. nationalcouncilfvd.org | | X | | |

*(Columns continue on facing page.)*

## APPENDIX Table 4 (columns continued)

| Topics | | | | Information | | | | Comments |
|---|---|---|---|---|---|---|---|---|
| Child Abuse | Partner Violence | Same-Sex Partner Violence | Elder Abuse | Domestic Violence* | Legal Issues | Local and/ or National Links/ Contacts | Provider Inter- ventions | |
| | X | | X | X | X | X | | Provides women with information on abuse, what to expect when the police are called, and Nashville area counseling and shelter resources; also offers training materials for legal and social services professionals |
| X | X | X | X | | | X | | Offers an impressive number of annotated links to reports, organizations, resources, and sites focusing on research, discussion, and prevention of all forms of domestic violence |
| | X | | | X | X | X | | Regional organization serving three counties in Ohio; provides support for survivors and basic information on identifying battering and how to get help |
| X | | | | X | | | X | Wide variety of information on PTSD and its treatment, types of occurrence, indications, etc.; provides summaries of research on specific PTSD-related topics, links to further information, bibliographies, etc. |
| | X | | | X | X | X | | Provides a wide variety of information, including safety planning, how to get a new Social Security number, starting a shelter, public policy updates, and links to other sites |
| X | X | | | | X | | | Provides information for legal professionals on domestic and family violence, including current policy issues, training publications to download and order, and a "DV Law" search engine |

*(Cont'd.)*

*For example, clinical presentation, statistics, training materials.

## APPENDIX Table 4    Internet Resources (continued)

| Organization | Web Address | Target Audience | | | |
| --- | --- | --- | --- | --- | --- |
| | | Survivors | Legal Professionals | Physicians | Counselors/ Advocates |
| National Domestic Violence Hotline Site | http://www.ndvh.org | X | | | X |
| National Organization for Women – Violence Against Women | http://www.now.org/issues/ violence/ | | X | | X |
| Partnerships Against Violence Network | http://www.pavnet.org | | X | | X |
| Safe Horizon Victim Services | http://www.dvsheltertour.org/ main.html | X | | | X |
| Sidran Traumatic Stress Foundation | http://www.sidran.org | X | | | X |
| Silent Witness Project | http://www.silentwitness.net | | | | X |

*(Columns continue on facing page.)*

## APPENDIX Table 4    (columns continued)

| Topics | | | | Information | | | | Comments |
|---|---|---|---|---|---|---|---|---|
| Child Abuse | Partner Violence | Same-Sex Partner Violence | Elder Abuse | Domestic Violence* | Legal Issues | Local and/ or National Links/ Contacts | Provider Inter- ventions | |
| X | X | | | X | | X | | Offers survivors a description of hotline resources and education on identifying abusive behavior |
| | X | | | | X | | | Geared towards political activists; includes articles on recent issues pertaining to domestic violence, legislative updates, and links to important legislation |
| X | X | | | | | X | | An online "virtual library" of links and resources for violence prevention professionals, including program listings of education, prevention, and treatment programs, and search engines for current research and funding sources |
| | X | | | X | | X | | Offers information for women and communities on domestic violence, the role of a shelter in helping survivors leave, the impact of domestic violence on children, and a listing of U.S. and international resources |
| X | X | | | | | X | | Organization "devoted to education, advocacy and research to benefit people suffering from traumatic stress"; offers list of publications and training courses, information on PTSD, and links to other sites |
| | X | | | | | X | | Organization dedicated to ending domestic murders; offers  suggestions, information, and resources for advocacy and links to violence prevention programs and other sites |

*(Cont'd.)*

*For example, clinical presentation, statistics, training materials.

## APPENDIX Table 4    Internet Resources (continued)

| Organization | Web Address | Target Audience | | | |
|---|---|---|---|---|---|
| | | Survivors | Legal Profes- sionals | Physicians | Counselors/ Advocates |
| The Standard Times | http://www.s-t.com/projects/ DomVio/ | X | | | |
| U.S. Department of Agriculture – Domestic Violence Awareness Handbook | http://www.usda.gov/da/shmd/ aware.htm | X | | | X |
| U.S. Department of Justice – Violence Against Women Office | http://www.ojp.usdoj.gov/vawo/ | | X | | X |
| University of Minnesota/ U.S. Department of Justice – Violence Against Women Online Resources | http://www.vaw.umn.edu/ | | X | | X |
| WATCH | http://www.mtn.org/~watch/ | | X | | X |

## APPENDIX Table 4    (columns continued)

| Topics | | | | Information | | | | Comments |
|---|---|---|---|---|---|---|---|---|
| Child Abuse | Partner Violence | Same-Sex Partner Violence | Elder Abuse | Domestic Violence* | Legal Issues | Local and/ or National Links/ Contacts | Provider Inter-ventions | |
| | X | | | X | | X | | Regional site offering 60 articles on domestic violence issues and links to resources online and in the southeast Massachusetts area |
| | X | | | X | | X | | Provides information on domestic violence and available resources as well as information on how to prevent abuse in the community and workplace |
| X | X | | X | X | X | X | | Offers downloadable training information on working with victims of abuse as well as information on innovative prevention and treatment programs nation-wide; also provides a complete listing of contact information for the State Domestic Violence Coalitions |
| X | X | X | | X | X | X | | Site offers copious information for legal and social service professionals and counselors, including model legislation, how to handle specific types of family violence investigations, and links to innovative prevention and treatment programs |
| X | X | | | | X | X | | WATCH is a nonprofit volunteer-run organization that monitors the handling of domestic and child abuse cases in Hennepin County, MN; Web site provides information on the program and its impact on the area court system |

*For example, indications, statistics, training materials.

# Index

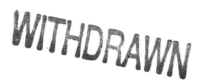